DATE DUE

NOV 2 2 2011			

DEMCO

Patient Encounters

The Experience of Disease

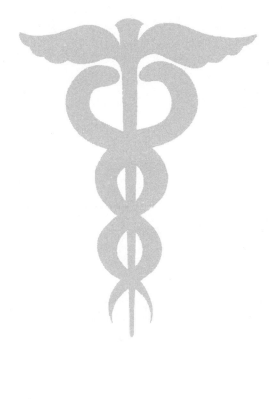

PATIENT

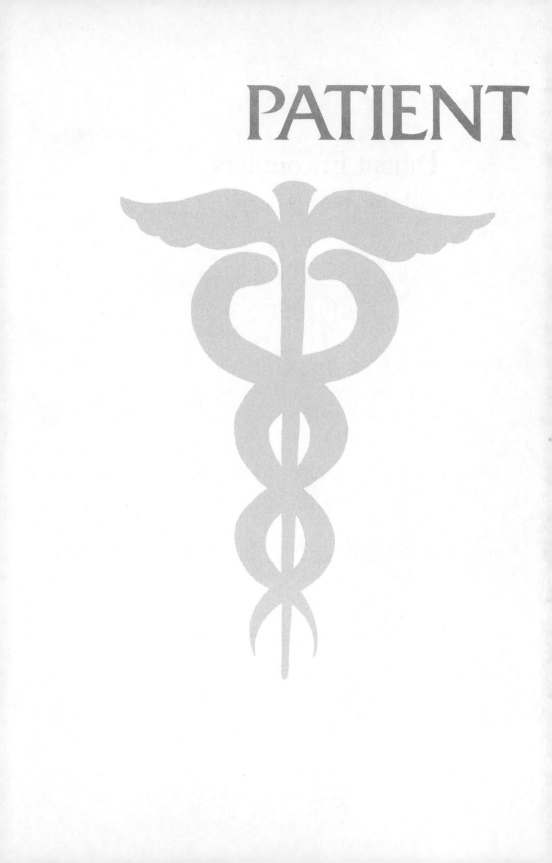

ENCOUNTERS

The Experience of

DISEASE

The status and progress of medicine
ought always to be judged primarily from the
point of view of the suffering patient,
and never from the point of view
of one who has never been ill. Jurgen Thorowald
The Century of the Surgeon

JAMES H. BUCHANAN

University Press of Virginia

Charlottesville

THE UNIVERSITY PRESS OF VIRGINIA
Copyright © 1989 by the Rector and Visitors
of the University of Virginia
First published 1989

LIBRARY OF CONGRESS
Library of Congress Cataloging-in-Publication Data
Buchanan, James H., 1942–
    Patient encounters : the experience of disease / James H.
Buchanan.
        p.   cm.
    Bibliography: p.
    ISBN 0–8139–1184–2
    1. Sick—Psychology. 2. Sick—Biography. 3. Internal medicine—
Case studies. I. Title.
R726.5.B83 1988
616′.09—dc19   88–19803
                                                                              CIP

Printed in the United States of America

For
MARYANNE AND RICHARD
. . . to each in separate measure

Contents

Preface

These *Patient Encounters* are all true stories. Great care has been taken to present the truth and substance of the individual clinical accounts with real and accurate descriptions of the disease processes. Nevertheless, every effort has been made to protect the privacy of the patients by changing names, places, and particulars of their individual stories. It is the moral duty of every writer to respect the privacy of persons and their families, and I have taken this charge very seriously. The characters in twelve of these stories are entirely fictional, and any resemblance to actual persons living or dead is purely coincidental. The only exceptions are those persons whose stories already belonged to the public domain through published biographies, memoirs, or personal accounts; there are four such accounts in this collection. "October" is the story of Thomas Wolfe, the writer, whose death from miliary tuberculosis has been well recounted over the years in many different biographies. "The Face of a Wolf" is the story of Flannery O'Connor, the southern writer, whose death from lupus has been recounted extensively in several biographical sources. "Wilder Had a Sister" recounts Ruth Penfield's battle with a brain tumor and treatment by her world-famous brother the neurosurgeon Wilder Penfield. Dr. Penfield wrote extensively about this case in his autobiography *No Man Alone*, and I have drawn upon his own account for accuracy of detail. Finally, "Cushing's Monsters" is an account of the neurosurgeon Harvey Cushing's work on the pituitary gland. The standard biography of Harvey Cushing by John Fulton along with many individual memoirs by members of his staff provided the source material for this account.

Each of these stories have been read for accuracy—both medical as well as biographical—by a number of different people. There are three persons in particular, however, who bear special mention. The first is Dr. Richard Selzer, Professor of Surgery at Yale University. The second is Dr. Sharon Romm, Associate Professor of Plastic and Reconstructive Surgery at Georgetown University. The third is Dr. Oliver Sacks, Professor of Neurology at the Albert Einstein School of Medicine. I owe these three people a special debt of thanks because they have been more than advisers, they have also become friends. Nonetheless, any inaccuracies in the accounts are entirely my own and not the responsibility of those who have been kind enough to counsel me.

The reader might also inquire about my credentials as the author. My interest in medicine has been an active learning experience for the past twenty years, and during that time I have been exposed to nearly every facet of the medical community. I have taken formal course work in medicine, worked in the Physiological Laboratory at Cambridge University in England, served as consultant for the Ethics Review Boards of several area hospitals, given workshops in medical ethics and medical decision making for clinics, hospitals, and family practice units, and read extensively in clinical medicine as well as neuroanatomy, diagnostics, and neuropathology. I have also published several clinical pieces in medical journals and magazines as well as articles in academic and scholarly journals. In addition to my medical experience, I also hold the Ph.D. in Philosophy with special emphasis in epistemology and the relationship between perception and neurophysiology.

It might be of interest to the reader to learn how each of these stories came to be written and precisely why they were written. In short, what was the process of selection for diseases so diverse and disconnected? In large measure, it was the occasion and circumstance of my own experience that brought me into contact with different people at different times who were suffering from such disorders. Given my interest in medicine and in the people that I met, I would often keep a small diary of notes to record my thoughts, my reactions, and my observations as I grew to know the people better. The accounts in this book are just a part of that journal, of which there is more to come.

Part I treats Diseases of the Soul and contains six stories about different types of neurological illness. The first of these,

"An Island in a Storm," is about the disease amyotrophic lateral sclerosis, in which the patient gradually becomes paralyzed by the death of the motor neurons that control our muscles and voluntary movements. Literally, one becomes an island in a stormy sea, for the cortical neurons are spared and the patient observes all that is happening to him. There have been several prominent persons who have suffered from this disease, and its occurrence seems to be on the increase.

The second chapter—"Whence the Meaning of All This Pain?"—is counterpunctual to the first since it treats of Alzheimer's disease. In Alzheimer's disease the motor neurons are spared, but the cortical neurons die prematurely and in massive numbers. The patient becomes senile and deranged and dies without fully comprehending what is happening. This disease was relatively rare when the German neurologist Alois Alzheimer first diagnosed it at the beginning of this century, but it now has increased in alarming numbers. There is however, some suspicion that our diagnostic instruments simply have improved rather than the number of cases increasing and that today we are diagnosing correctly what used to be placed in the general category of presenile dementia.

The third chapter is "Cushing's Monsters" and treats the spectacular and brilliant life of the neurosurgeon Harvey Cushing. Cushing always had a strong fascination for circus people, magicians, and especially people in the sideshow. Displayed as "freaks," these unfortunates were often ridiculed and tormented because of their disabilities. The story begins with a letter of protest that Cushing wrote to *Time* in 1927 about its story of a woman who was suffering from acromegaly, whom the magazine had referred to as one of the "Uglies." Cushing's defense of the woman and explanation of the disease is the focus of this story.

"October" recounts the death of the writer Thomas Wolfe from miliary tuberculosis of the brain in 1938. Perhaps it was coincidental that Wolfe was operated upon at the Johns Hopkins Hospital by Dr. Walter Dandy, who was one of Harvey Cushing's residents, and that Cushing himself died exactly one year later.

The fifth chapter is titled "Wilder Had a Sister" and is a true

account of the efforts of the Montreal neurosurgeon Wilder
Penfield to save his sister from a brain tumor by performing
the operation himself. Naturally, Penfield wanted only the best
treatment for his own sister, and so, weighing all the facts, he
concluded that he was the best neurosurgeon living and should
do the operation himself. I corresponded with Penfield just
months before his death and knew one of his nieces. At the
time that I wrote this piece, I was also watching a business
associate slowly dying of the same type of tumor as Penfield's
sister's.

The final chapter in this part is "Brother Damian" and is
about a Trappist monk's battle with multiple sclerosis. Brother
Damian is coping with and still suffering from this disease in
the most courageous and spiritual way. I first met him on a
retreat to the Abbey of Gethsemani in Kentucky five years ago.
Since that time I have returned two more times, and during
the last visit I summoned the courage to ask him to tell me his
story. He did so, and I have related the particulars just as he
told them to me. In his younger days he was physically very
strong and did very heavy farm work at Gethsemani's farms.
He knew Thomas Merton quite well and had some very interesting stories to tell about the Christian mystic's encounters
with farm work.

Part II is titled Metabolic Furnaces and treats the two diseases lupus and porphyria. These are both systemic diseases
and produce the most unusual symptoms. They can both be
fatal in one form and merely chronic in another; the difference
depends upon the particular chemistries of each metabolic disturbance. The title Metabolic Furnaces is a very appropriate
term to use in this context because these disorders are the result of metabolic processes that are no longer being kept in
check and balance. Many people know that the southern writer
Flannery O'Connor died of a disease that affected her bones,
but they do not know the particulars or the exact nature of the
disease. "The Face of a Wolf" is an account of her last few
months and of the time that she spent in the hospital. It is so
titled because the name of the disease is taken from the Latin
word *lupus*, which means "wolf." One of the characteristics of
the disease is a rash about the face which resembles the same

markings as those on the face of a wolf. I became interested in Flannery O'Connor when I visited her hometown of Milledgeville, Georgia, in 1982 and talked with several people who had known her. I also went out to her farm, Andalusia, where she spent some of her happiest hours, and I visited her grave as well as the church in which she worshiped.

The porphyrias are metabolic disorders in which physical symptoms often associated with werewolves begin to appear in the patient. These can be very specific and even include heavy hair growth over the entire body, prominently displayed teeth, an adverse reaction to garlic and sunlight, and a need to ingest the heme that is found in blood. There are two forms of the disease, and one is far less severe than the other. I titled the story "The Fear of Light" for the most obvious of reasons.

Part III is titled Diseases of the Heart. The first chapter, "I Grow Old before My Time," is on the developmental disorder progeria. This genetic disease is particularly tragic because babies who appear to be healthy at birth will quickly age to senility within a few years' time. To anyone who has had a child born with a genetic defect—and I have known several—the story will strike a note of harmonic recognition. "Fox-Teeth" treats the disease AIDS, which has become one of the most frightful disorders of the twentieth century. It is preposterous to believe that one's sexual life is either rewarded or punished by the cosmos. Indeed, it is more likely that the universe smiles at love in any form and only despises hate in all of its forms. I have known several people jeopardized by this disease, and this chapter is dedicated to them out of affection for them and understanding of the dangers they endure.

The final chapter in this section is "The Smoker," and it is more real, more intimate, and more personal than any of the other stories. It is about the death of my mother from lung cancer in 1979, and I have excerpted her own diary kept during her illness in order to write this piece. It was, needless to say, perhaps the most difficult story to tell in the entire collection.

Part IV treats of Diseases of Life, and while both stories in this section are true, they are based upon purely fictional characters. "A Cup of Bitterness" is the story of a druggist who committed suicide in a particularly hideous and painful way. "Just

Looking" is about an odd and disconnected relationship between a beautiful woman with flaming red hair and the quiet, shy, retiring jeweler who lusted after her.

Part V deals with Chronic and Acute Illnesses. The first chapter is titled "Faces Frozen in Time" and is about Parkinson's disease. I have found much inspiration and information from Oliver Sacks's outstanding book *Awakenings*, which deals with the history and treatment of parkinsonism. "The Marble Palace" is a story about a young woman dying of Hodgkin's disease and the effect it had upon her family. The final story, "The Vegetative Heart," is my own story. I was nearly eight years old when I became sick with subacute bacterial endocarditis and nearly died of the disease. It was only the good fortune of penicillin that intervened, and until I wrote the story I never realized just how sick I actually was. I have called myself Christopher Campbell in the story, and anyone who knows something about Scottish history and the wars between the clans will understand why I used this name.

These stories are meant to be accurate accounts of the medical and historical facts that surround each disease. In addition, however, each story focuses on the experience of the disease as it is suffered as well as the experience of the disease as it is treated and diagnosed. Patients and physicians, sufferers and healers, victims and survivors come together in this odd, dynamic network of sickness which involves the entire community as well as the patient. Diseases both frighten and fascinate us because while we want to learn about them we also fear the infectiousness of this knowledge. Part of the purpose of these accounts is simply to show that despite all their mystery, every disease has a clinical structure and course which are understandable, natural, and not nearly as frightening or mysterious as they might first appear to be.

An author's greatest pleasure next to writing is to acknowledge the many people who have made that writing possible. If it is true that every writer is the sum total of all the books he has ever read, then so much more is it true that he is the final product of all the people he has known. I am particularly fortunate in knowing several people who counseled and encouraged me along the way and without whom this book could not have been written.

First and foremost is my wife Maryanne who believed in me when I had already stopped believing in myself. To her I owe a debt which can only be acknowledged but never fully repaid. To Richard Selzer, who is my inspiration and my friend, I am indebted for showing me the way, providing me the maps, and then guiding me back again when I wandered off in the wrong direction. To these two dear friends, this book is dedicated.

Sharon Romm gave of her time and of her talents so often in my behalf that mere gratitude seems little recompense. Oliver Sacks always seemed to find time for me even when he could find little time for himself. Without the counsel of these two friends, this book could not have survived its own impoverishments.

Sylvia Juscak typed, edited, advised, and improved upon this manuscript in far too many ways to mention. Suffice it to say that I have come to trust her instincts above my own. I also owe a debt of gratitude to James Childs, Professor of Law at the University of Akron, for his counsel and advice.

I am grateful to *Pennsylvania Medicine* for kind permission to reprint "An Island in a Storm" and "Cushing's Monsters," which previously appeared in the February 1986 and February 1987 issues, respectively, of that magazine. I am also grateful to *Medical Heritage* for kind permission to reprint "October" and "I Grow Old before My Time," which previously appeared in the Nov./Dec. 1985 and Sept./Oct. 1986 issues, respectively, of that magazine.

Finally, grateful appreciation is also due to Father Timothy Kelley, the Abbot of the Abbey of Gethsemani, for permission to publish "Brother Damian."

Patient Encounters

The Experience of Disease

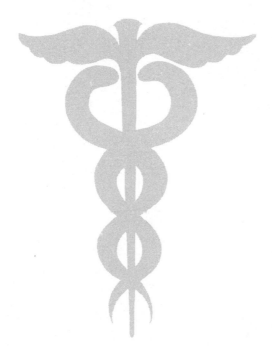

Introduction

Do diseases have a signature? That is, do they sign their names on our bodies while infecting us in those peculiar and curious ways that define the difference between functional and organic disorders, chronic and acute illness, curable and terminal disease? The answer to that question has puzzled anatomists, physiologists, and clinicians for centuries. At one time it was thought that every disease was forced to follow anatomical routes that confined it to the tissue boundaries of the infected organ. However, the discovery of systemic diseases led to the rebuttal of this anatomical thesis and to the promotion of the physiological claim that diseases are defined by the physiological trails and passages they follow within our bodies. Compounding the simplicity of such explanations, however, are phenomenon such as the blood-brain barrier that securely divides the physiology of the brain from the rest of the body and in most cases specifically forbids the infection of the former by the latter.

In spite of all these failures to understand the obvious, it does seem perfectly clear that each disease has a characteristic mark which distinguishes it from each and every other disease. Patients can actually feel, experience, and sense this signature of their disease without being able to give adequate explanations or reasons for possessing such intelligence. One "knows," for example, the aching heart from the fevered brain, and one can sense a serious acute attack upon the system apart from the chronic drudgery of continuous pain. The first is a sharp, violent, and angry pain of steel teeth that devour the flesh in huge, ferocious bites, whereas the second is a weary, continual digestion of the flesh that devours slowly in a methodical, plodding, planned way. Moreover, one knows when one is dying and when one is not, when "it is nothing" and when "it is something" (though we often lie to ourselves about the body's truth), when it will go away and when it won't. How do we know, and

1

why can we not give reasons for our wisdom? Perhaps because such things are known in that savage, primordial way that all animals know about their bodies. Sensing deep within us the presence of some dark, primal source, we can monitor the metabolic fires that may conserve or consume us.

These accounts are an effort to write large the signatures of the diseases discussed. The people involved know that they are sick and in some cases know that they are profoundly sick even to the point of dying. Still, this "savage sense" makes no sense to the doctors, family, and friends who surround the patient, and efforts to explain are a dismal failure. When the patient begins to look at himself as an object and an illness—such as a tumor, a fever, or an infection—his disease becomes as opaque and mysterious to him as it does to the physician who treats him. Norman Cousins in his book *Anatomy of an Illness* focuses his attention on the self-healing properties of the body and on this strange, mysterious "savage sense" that seems to know what is biologically right and wrong about us.

In my own experience, I have known many such people. I knew a woman who could tell if you had cancer by simply looking at the color of your skin. I know another who treats herself with all kinds of strange potions and elixirs of her own construction and at ninety-seven still drives her car to work, takes her three-mile walk every evening, and looks to be in her late sixties. I also knew a woman who was married thirty-five years to the same man and then discovered that he was having an affair. She confronted him with the facts and promised to forgive and forget this indiscretion if he would be faithful in the future; to her surprise, he instead asked for a divorce to marry the other woman. In the course of the court proceedings, she developed cancer of the liver and was given six months to live. Her husband agreed to stay with her to the end and be faithful during that time. In six months' time, she was still alive, and one year later she was diagnosed as free from the disease. Believing that he had discharged his duty, he reinstituted divorce proceedings, and two months later her liver cancer returned. This time, however, he did not agree to stay, and she died before the court issued the final divorce decree. Dr. Bernie Siegel in his book *Love, Medicine, and Miracles* relates many similar cases.

One of my patients, as soon as she was diagnosed as having cancer, went home and donated all her clothes to Goodwill Industries. More clearly than anything she ever said, this act showed her belief that the disease would inevitably kill her, so she might as well give up without a fight. [p. 101]

. . . Jennifer had been entered in a hospice program by her doctor, who expected her to die within six months. But she kept on living. When the hospice staff asked if she looked forward to spring, she said, "Oh, yes, I love to watch the flowers come up." They asked her if she liked summer. "Very much." Fall? "Oh, I just love the leaves changing color." Even winter? "Yes, the snow." Eventually the hospice personnel told her they had to stop coming. They would return when she was ready to die. . . . When winter approached, however, Jennifer told me, "I don't think I'm going to be buying any winter clothes." This indicated that perhaps she was getting ready to die. Then she came to one of our meetings wearing a lovely winter suit. I said, "Aha! I see you decided to buy some winter clothes." "No," she said, "I just brought some down from the attic." To me that said that she'd made a compromise. She was saying, "Let's see how the winter goes, I'm not going to invest in it, but I'll give it a try."

Another cancer patient I know, named Matt, went to his physician one day looking awful and came home looking fine. His family asked, "Gee, what did the doctor do?" Matt said, "Oh, he gave me my allergy shot." That let him know that the doctor expected him to live through the spring, and his body responded. [p. 108]

Is it possible that we have lost touch with our bodies somewhere along the way and in so doing have also lost touch with the property of self-healing?

To observe or treat a disease is not the same as to suffer from it. Jurgen Thorowald in *The Century of the Surgeon* makes this point so very well when he says, "the status and progress of medicine ought always to be judged primarily from the point of view of the suffering patient, and never from the point of view of one who has never been ill" (p. 26). It is certainly true that diseases seem to hide themselves from the searching eye of the investigator but to reveal themselves in shocking exhibitionism to the patient. I remember very well the summer that I was sick with endocarditis, and I still recall vividly the texture, tone, and composition of that illness. And yet, when I researched the textbooks to write an account of my

3

illness from endocarditis, included in this volume as "The Vegetative Heart," it seemed like an entirely different disease. The medical books said that you could die of it, and yet I never once had the sense that I would die. The descriptions were clinical and objective in their discussions of irregular fevers and heart disturbances, but I had an entirely different perspective of these same clinical facts as I suffered and underwent them. The fevers were awful because they were so unpredictable and left me with a desolate sense of isolation, distance, and aloneness. I remember one night waking up and seeing my own body as if projected down the long end of a telescope. I looked and felt bony, starved, and feverish. I seemed to be floating, and when I reached out to touch my face, I bit my fingers instead. When I woke the next morning, my fingers were bruised and bloody as if I had tried to claw my way to freedom. It was this claustrophobia of disease, this utterly intolerable sense of being suffocated by my illness that I felt but could not relate to the objective, intellectual discussion of symptoms and causes. To understand a disease, it is not enough to study it; you must also endure it, suffer it, survive it, perhaps even die of it as well.

These stories are intended to be phenomenological descriptions of disease processes and not merely textbook rehearsals of anonymous symptoms belonging to anonymous patients. One reads, for example, that "a 77 year-old composer had left occipital lobe haemorrhagic infarct giving him a severe reading disturbance with well-preserved writing and without appreciable aphasia" (Judd, Gardner, and Geschwind, "Alexia without Agraphia in a Composer," p. 435). However, what is not made clear by such medical descriptions is how this same composer was able to continue to read and compose music despite these neurological deficits. What, moreover, were his experiences as he suffered, and can these experiences be phenomenologically described? That is, can the feelings, experiences, and inner dynamics of the illness be revealed as clearly as the anatomical, physiological, and visible aspects of the disease? It is in answer to these questions that *Patient Encounters* has been written.

I

Diseases of the Soul

Nature saw fit to enclose the central nervous system in a bony case lined by a tough, protecting membrane, and within this case she concealed a tiny organ which lies enveloped by an additional bony capsule and membrane like the nugget in the innermost of a series of Chinese boxes. No other single structure in the body is so doubly protected, so centrally placed, so well hidden. Her acts being purposeful, she must have had abundant reason for this, and man's prying curiosity impels him to ask what they were.

Harvey Cushing
"Neurohypophysial Mechanisms:
From a Clinical Standpoint"

1

An Island in a Storm

Oh roses for the flush of youth
and laurel for the perfect prime;
But pluck an ivy branch for me
Grown old before my time.

Oh violets for the grave of youth
and bay for those dead in their prime;
Give me the withered leaves I chose
Before in the old time.

Christina Rossetti
"Song"

AMYOTROPHIC LATERAL SCLEROSIS: This is a combined upper and lower motor neuron lesion which may involve either the spinal or bulbar level, or both. It is a chronic progressive disease of unknown etiology associated with fibrillation and atrophy of the somatic musculature. It is predominately a disease of middle life, with onset usually between the ages of 40 and 60 years. Degeneration of the motor cells of the spinal cord and brain stem and, to a lesser extent, of the motor cortex may occur, with secondary degeneration of the lateral and ventral portions of the spinal cord. There may be spastic weakness of the trunk and extremities, with associated hyperactive deep reflexes and extensor plantar responses. If the fibers of the bulbar nuclei become involved, pseudo-bulbar or

7

bulbar paralysis may appear. The initial symptom is often weakness and wasting of the extremities (usually the upper extremities). The course is progressively downhill without remission. The average duration of life from the appearance of the first symptoms is about 3 years.

Krupp and Chatton
Current Medical Diagnosis and Treatment

I

The first symptoms of amyotrophic lateral sclerosis (ALS) are coquettish, even demure, in their malevolent innocence. You will notice a slight weakness, even a gentle lethargy, about your arms and legs. Then, perhaps one morning in the shower, the weaving fasciculations will appear. They are gentle, oceanic ripplings of musculature that pass almost orgasmically across the flat plains and prairies of stomach, chest, thigh, and hip. It is irritating but not unpleasant or painful. But soon the shy and retiring illness will break all bonds of propriety and good manners as it explores and explodes the terrain that it shall shortly claim as its own. If only it could be satisfied with merely local destruction, occasional forays into the enemy zone of healthy tissue, we could forgive its uninvited presence. But no! It insists upon announcing itself globally, even internationally, in the most haughty and arrogant manner. The disease is not sympathetic to this most sympathetic of systems. The motor neurons that control arms and legs and even those that cry and those that caress are all territorialized and so dominated. Only the majestic cortical neurons—with their thoughts, reason, logic—are too powerful for such submission. One becomes an island in a storm.

7:00 A.M. Neurology Clinic
"Gentlemen. This morning's lecture is on motor neuron disease and, in particular, amyotrophic lateral sclerosis. Its etiology is idiopathic—with the possible exception of hereditary factors in certain patients—and is one of the commonest neurological diseases after disseminated sclerosis. Nonetheless, it must be carefully dif-

8

ferentiated from other disorders with which it is sometimes confused. For example, we sometimes see patients in clinic with metabolic disorders such as hypoglycemia or uremia whose symptoms are remarkably similar. Again, lead or triorthocresylphosphate poisoning will frequently present itself in like fashion. My colleague McDuff now has a case of Creutzfeld-Jakob disease which was first given a presumptive diagnosis of ALS. Geographically, there is a motor neuron disease endemic to the Chamorro tribe on Guam. In addition, the Kugelberg-Weylander syndrome has been observed in Sweden wherein the patient undergoes a similar spinal muscular atrophy.

"Are there any questions? Good!"

II

Within two years or so, you will be dead! Most likely you will suffocate and drown in an ocean of your own fluids without the strength even to cough or cry out for help. But first, your body will grow weary—oh, so very weary—day by exhausting day until gradually your arms, legs, feet will be too weak to move. They will be heavy. So heavy that the mere thought of lifting them is too burdensome to contemplate. And always the spreading blanket of paralysis will be with you, nuzzling you and overcoming vital areas of your life. The smile that you took for granted, the frown that so often you used to win your own way will be frozen now into a mechanical mask which shows neither joy nor sorrow. You will not feel the slow atrophy of neurons in the corticospinal tracts and anterior horns, but you will see their presence and feel their effects. Now you will no longer be able to speak even simple words, and if you do, they will be too garbled and incoherent to be understood.

"Gentlemen, to continue. It is known that males are affected twice as often as females and that the disease usually appears between the ages of forty and seventy. Naturally, these are merely statistical ranges, and I have personally seen a patient as young as twenty-three and as old as eighty-six with the disease. The first symptoms are often experienced as a weakness or clumsiness of fine motor control. The patient frequently drops things or evidences dysarthria and various swallowing syndromes. When the hands are affected—and they always are—it will be muscles of the thenar

9

eminences that first announce themselves. Then the forearm muscles—with flexor involvement preceding extensor—will fall prey as well. Usually, if not always, the anterior tibial groupings as well as the peronei are compromised. Any questions? Good!"

Family, lovers, friends will draw near to comprehend the weakened gaspings that you now count for language. But should they brush against you or reach to caress your withered shoulder, you will no longer feel their warm touch within the solitude of your cold prison of atrophied marble. Across your chest, legs, back, and face the muscles will hang in atrophied sheets of ragged immobility. The hurricane of your illness will pass over you and yellow your skin like the broken sails of a drowning ship. Even to touch your face, wet your lips, blow your nose, or clear your throat will seem a task too divine for your humble means.

"Do not fail, gentlemen, to note the invariable presence of fasciculations; if they are not apparent upon first inspection, then passive articulation of the muscle mass will always elicit them. Now we enter the second stage of degeneration in which the bulbar muscles are affected. There will be considerable atrophy of the tongue with concomitant fasciculations. Interestingly enough, the orbicularis oris will degenerate but not the orbicularis oculi. Naturally, speech, eating, and facial expressions all undergo deformation at this juncture. The interesting stage of the disease is reached when degeneration of the upper motor neurons occurs. Deterioration of lower motor neurons depresses reflexes, but deterioration of upper motor neurons heightens and exaggerates them. Here you may expect to find your Babinski reflex in full regalia, gentlemen. In the final stages, of course, the sphincter muscles will collapse, and ocular sympathetic palsy might occur. As subcutaneous fat decreases from muscle atrophy, the patient will appear more and more emaciated. The respirator muscles will finally succumb to the progressive atrophy, and the patient will die of respiratory failure. There is, of course, no treatment and the disease is always fatal. Questions? Good!"

You will find death a gentle, even a considerate friend, who will understand your circumstance and only desire to lead you out of it. You will accept this invitation enthusiastically because slowly, ever so slowly the prison of stone that you have become is closing in, and it is terrifying to behold!

III

Professor Stanley Ackyrod, who looked far older than his forty-four years, seemed unable to insert his office key into the latch. He had tried three times without success and now decided to set his briefcase down and try again. It worked! Thank God. How ridiculous to have to fumble with a simple key, especially in the presence of colleagues who were always on the lookout for your weaknesses. But no one had said a word, and although Anderson had watched the whole show, he had pretended not to notice Ackyrod's clumsiness. But in truth, notice he did indeed, and so had everyone else at the office. In fact, Stanley had become the academic klutz in the department because he was always dropping something.

For instance, last week he tripped over his own briefcase, and the week before he spilled hot coffee all over himself. Actually, his colleagues found the whole matter to be quite amusing. Naturally, they had noticed that he made less and less sense when he talked, but then Ackyrod had never made much sense before either. It was probably just old age—they reasoned and he assumed—and so Stanley's colleagues dismissed the whole matter as rather boring.

But Stanley was alarmed. In fact, he was quite worried. Yesterday morning when he first awoke, his left thumb and index finger were twitching uncontrollably almost as if they were caught in a spasm from which no exit could be found. It was almost noon before they became calm and returned to normal. Also, he had been very embarrassed the other day in committee meeting when his right eyelid began to twitch involuntarily. It appeared to others—or so he thought—that he was winking in a seductive manner to everyone around him, and yet he had no control over the lid's movement. If all of this continued, he would see a doctor. But for the time being, he was certain that a good rest would take care of the matter.

There was no time for such nonsense anyway. This afternoon Professor Descombes would be lecturing in the amphitheater, and this evening there would be a faculty reception in

11

his honor. Then the following day, Stanley himself would be taking the shuttle to the city to deliver a lecture. No, there simply was no time to be bothered with these minor health problems. Perhaps when the term ended and things were less hectic, he might have lunch with his colleague Winthrop from the medical school and ask his advice.

Descombes's lecture was clever, suggestive, and, of course, very subtle. But isn't it always true of the French that they imply more than they actually state? For these reasons, and others, Ackyrod found the argument to be rather thin and insubstantial. He was certain that he could have handled the topic much better. But Descombes had an international reputation whereas Ackyrod did not, and that was the end of the matter, wasn't it? Even in the academic world the great names frequently have mediocre minds.

Still, Maurice Descombes was of some interest as a person, and when he was more relaxed at the faculty reception, Stanley rather liked him. With the French, of course, you never know what they are thinking. You suspect you do, but you can't be sure. Stanley asked him a somewhat delicate question about his theory, and instead of defending or acknowledging the point, Descombes raised that elegant French eyebrow and replied: "Oui." Now, what the hell was that suppose to mean, after all?

Stanley had always been somewhat cynical and intolerant of others, but recently he had become even more so. Everyone this evening seemed so common, so ordinary to him. The faculty wives who always attend such parties appeared to him to be fat, stupid, and dumpy gnomes who were only good for having babies and cooking quiches. They didn't understand their husbands or anything about their work, their ideas, their thoughts. How grateful Stanley felt that he had never married and was therefore free of all such insufferable nonsense. By ten o'clock the reception had transformed itself from a somewhat amusing affair to a quite boring ordeal. Naturally, everyone was drunk by this time, or so it seemed to Stanley, and the witty academic conversation had degenerated to who was sleeping with whom. Such talk did not interest Stanley in the least. Also, he had long ago discovered that when you begin discussing the private lives of others, they in turn will soon begin to discuss your own personal life. Stanley was not at all certain that his privacy could tolerate such close scrutiny. But most important was his own lecture tomorrow morning. Like every senior scholar—and Ackyrod was a senior scholar if not an international one—he needed time this evening for final revisions, editing, and a last superlative polish to each of his ideas. Therefore, he excused himself.

Later that night in bed he found sleep difficult and elusive. To sleep by yourself is not to sleep alone. Frequently, it is to lie in bed with monsters, demons, and malformed creatures of the night. And to cohabit with these devils is a most terrifying and tormenting kind of business. So it was with Stanley Ackyrod tonight. He thought of graduate school so many years ago; he thought also of his lecture so close upon him; he thought of his colleagues; of his lovers past and present; he thought of what he was and indeed of what he might become. Deep within him there grew the seeds of destruction, and within general parameters, he knew them to be there.

Encapsulated by the night and focused by the darkness, Stanley had the opportunity to assemble the disconnected and fragmented prophecies of his disease. The twitching in his fingertips, the grimaces, and the convulsions and tics of muscles that obeyed laws quite different from the ones he sought to impose upon them were all evidence of some malfunction that he could neither identify nor define. In short, the illness was as elusive and ambiguous as the confusion by which it sought to celebrate itself. Confusion, yes, that was the word, confusion! His system was somehow in a state of confusion, disorientation, and even fragmentation. When he sought to move his left leg, he instead frequently moved his right. When he reached for one object, he might pass it by and grasp another instead. It was confusion, chaos, and cacophony. As if the whole geography and landscape of his body had been repolarized so that the geometry of north now pointed south, that circles were squares, and no angle was any longer equal to any other. It made no sense, this new body with its melting polar caps and reorganized magnetic directions; it simply no longer made sense. In short, it was the anarchy of a system which

13

having always been trustworthy in the past now decides to betray us without any explanation. Why? Why indeed! Why do our bodies, having behaved themselves for years, one day suddenly begin to disintegrate for no good reason whatsoever? And why do these former good servants enact their betrayal in such ungrateful and audacious ways? The glands, muscles, bowels, lungs, and various interstices of the body fill themselves with tumors, cysts, fluids, and all sorts of matter of an unimaginable kind and degree. They make spectacles of us and publicly humiliate us in the most private ways. Yes, for whatever reason, Stanley Ackyrod's body was vigorously, even enthusiastically, disobeying his every command and plotting in secret against him. He knew not what was happening to him, but he felt suffocated, enveloped by an evil presence which was, in fact, his very own flesh and blood.

The next morning he awoke to the worst day he had experienced so far. His legs were weak; his arms felt rubbery and unresponsive. He found it impossible to shave because he had virtually no fine motor control in his fingertips or hands. Moreover—and this was the frightening part—he trembled. He trembled all over. He did not shake but rather trembled in minute, microcosmic shudders that spread oceanically over the surface of everything that he did. For instance, he spent twenty minutes tying his tie and another twenty minutes combing his hair. Everything took so long because he had to wait for the shudder to pass, the earthquake to calm before the simplest task could be accomplished.

But then it passed. Well, it subsided. By the time he was comfortably seated on the shuttle to the city and had consumed a double scotch, he felt good again. At least, he felt in control. When he arrived for his lecture at McNerry Hall, he was convinced that all this was behind him and a good rest would put things right again. And perhaps he was right; the next two weeks were quite uneventful. Yes, he felt tired, and yes, he had some trembling. But nothing significant. The whole damned matter was finally behind him!

But Saturday, November 12, at 7:32 in the morning, he was unable to get out of bed. And if he had been able to do so, he would not have gone very far because he had no control over any part of his body. It was unsettling because by 8:30 he was fine again. But it was also the most terrifying and frightful manifestation of his illness thus far. He knew then that he was ill, seriously and profoundly ill, and that he must seek medical attention.

IV

Stanley Ackyrod found himself the following Monday morning outside the offices of Dr. J. J. Sylvester. He was extremely fortunate to be here and probably would not have been without the intervention of his good friend and colleague Edgar Winthrop, who was Professor of Internal Medicine and Associate Dean of the Medical School. He had phoned Edgar Saturday afternoon following his attack and described the last few weeks in detail. Edgar asked no questions and suggested no answers, but rather remained silent for a few moments and then flatly stated, "You must see a neurologist at once, Stanley."

"Do you think it's serious, Edgar?"

Oddly, Edgar had not even responded to the question but instead reaffirmed the importance of seeing a doctor at once.

"Whom do you suggest?"

"Well, young Sylvester is the best man available in motor neuron disease. I would recommend that you see him."

"Is that what I have, Edgar, motor neuron disease?"

Again, there was no response to the question. "I'll be back to you within the hour, Stanley."

"Well, should I call this Dr. Sylvester and make an appointment, or what should I do?" He was frightened and filled with questions. Indeed, he now felt totally dependent upon Edgar Winthrop, a weakness that Stanley had always despised in himself and in others, and this only heightened his increasing sense of vulnerability.

"No, Stanley. Don't call him. You would never get through. Let me arrange things for you."

"Thank you, Edgar."

For the next hour, Stanley Ackyrod ran the gamut of fears, terrors, and frights that affect us fragile human beings. It seemed an endless wait until finally the phone rang.

"Stanley? Edgar here. He will see you Monday afternoon at

15

1:30 at his office. He is leaving for Paris that evening to deliver a paper, so we were lucky to get you in at this late date."

"Thank you, Edgar," and the phone fell silent.

Silent so also did Stanley fall. For the rest of the weekend, he saw no one and waited in terrified expectation for this ominous, most unwelcome interrogation of his body. And now, at 1:23 on a Monday afternoon it was about to begin.

The offices of J. J. Sylvester, M.D., Ph.D. were not at all what one would expect. Usually physicians seek out the most ordinary and pedestrian of structures within which to conceal the instruments of their profession. Squat, ugly buildings of prestressed concrete and glass with tiled floors and rooms divided into perfect cubic feet are the natural habitats of these scholars of disease. But not so with the offices of J. J. Sylvester. In fact, Professor Ackyrod was certain that by 1:23 on this Monday afternoon he had gotten himself completely lost. For here there were no office buildings whatsoever, only elegant brownstones with carved wooden doors and wrought-iron railings. Then, suddenly, he saw it—the bronzed nameplate upon a square of precisely cut black onyx.

J. J. SYLVESTER, M.D., PH.D.
PRACTICE LIMITED TO NEUROLOGY

Stanley approached the front door—quite hesitantly it must be admitted—only to find that it was securely locked. Beneath the nameplate, however, was a door chime, which he rang. Momentarily, the door was opened, not by a nurse in starched white uniform but by a sophisticated young lady in a tailored herringbone suit with an appointment book in hand.

"You are Professor Ackyrod?" she inquired.

"Yes, I am."

"The doctor is expecting you. Do come in."

It seemed much more in the nature of a social call than a professional appointment. He did not sit anxiously in a waiting cubit with five or six invalids but was ushered into an elegant room which was clearly a library rather than a consultation room. At the far end of the room burned a roaring fire in front of which were two large leather wing-back chairs.

Gazing about the room, Stanley encountered a marvelously astounding sight. From floor to ceiling, in each and every available place there were books. Dear God, there were books everywhere! A very conservative estimate would place the sheer quantity of volumes at about 6,000, and they covered the entire range of scholarly literature. Looking at the spines, he noted the complete works of Shakespeare, Milton, and Johnson as well as Pope, Melville, Hawthorne, and the classical and romantic poets as well. In addition, there were the modern novelists of the twentieth century as well as the poets Pound, Eliot, Auden, Stevens, and Williams. However, there were no medical books within the collection—presumably these were reserved for a special room of their own—but there was a very substantial inventory of contemporary scientists including Einstein, Bohr, Prigogine, and other contemporaries working on the unification of physics. Near the French doors, which looked out upon a now bleak winter garden, there stood a massive library table carved of finest woods and obviously dating back to the early nineteenth or late eighteenth century. Upon its leather surface rested the latest literary periodicals including *Vanity Fair, Atlantic Monthly,* and *Harper's,* as well as *Architectural Digest.* It was, indeed, a scholar's haven, and because of this Ackyrod immediately was put at ease. In fact, he was so deeply absorbed in an eighteenth-century edition of Burton's *Anatomy of Melancholy*—to be precise, that wonderful section in volume 1 where Burton speaks of the "miseries of scholars"—that he barely heard the door open and Sylvester enter.

"Professor Ackyrod. It is a great pleasure to meet you. I am J. J. Sylvester."

He was a solidly built man in his late thirties or very early forties. With dark, piercing eyes and darker hair combed straight back with a slight wave, he appeared to be of either Greek or Sicilian descent. A prominent mole upon the left cheek, high up near the cheekbone's sphenoid ridge, gave him a rather malevolent, even a dangerous and brooding look. But it was with the greatest warmth that he clasped Stanley's hand in both of his.

"I have followed your work with the greatest interest over

17

the years, Professor Ackyrod, and in particular your most recent book, *The History of Theoretical Systems.*"

"You have read it?" Stanley was astonished and suspicious at the same time.

"Yes, of course, and each of your other works as well beginning with the very first, *Theoretical Equations and Methodological Models.*"

"I must say that I am both flattered and surprised, Dr. Sylvester."

"I thought you might be," Sylvester replied with a good-natured laugh. "Academic scholars do not expect the medical community to know very much about these sorts of things."

"Oh, . . . but I . . ." Ackyrod was very embarrassed. He had perhaps offended this very intense young doctor, and it was only proper to make amends.

"Nonsense," Sylvester silenced him with a single gesture. "I am not in the least offended. Actually, it is rare to find my interests combined with medicine, but there it is and what can we do about it?"

By now, Stanley was thoroughly enraptured by Sylvester and would have welcomed a good academic discussion on the spot had not Sylvester abruptly redirected the conversation.

"Now, Edgar informs me that you have been having some problems. Tell me all about it."

"Well, I'm sure that he told you the details . . ."

"No! I prefer to hear the whole story from you. Begin at the very beginning and tell me everything without leaving out the slightest details. Take your time, include everything that seems important, and we shall have coffee while we talk."

And so it was that Stanley confessed—for it seemed to be just that—the entire seam and substance of everything that had been happening to him for the past few months. He told Sylvester about the leg spasms, the slurred speech, and, of course, about the fasciculations—those terrible, terrifying quakes and tremblings—and of all that he had suffered, feared, agonized, and undergone. Within an hour, he had told it all and had recalled, also, things that he had been too frightened to admit before. At the end, Sylvester was silent. He had said not a word for the full hour but had listened intently, and now he seemed almost meditative and even grave and troubled in his thoughts.

Then he said gravely, "I will arrange to have you checked into Good Sam hospital by this evening, Professor Ackyrod."

"By this evening? But . . . but . . . that's impossible!"

"On the contrary, Professor, I assure you it is absolutely necessary!"

"But surely there is time; I mean, my classes, my lectures."

"Yes, yes, I understand." Sylvester seemed almost weary and certainly impatient with this whole debate.

"You apparently believe that I have some grave and dangerous illness. You have frightened me."

"Frankly, Professor Ackyrod, I am not certain what to make of the symptoms you bring me today. But on the basis of your history of the past few weeks, I am reasonably certain that they will return and perhaps more aggressively than before."

"Will I die?" He regretted the question even as it was asked. It was, of course, an unanswerable question and far more an inquiry about his present feelings of vulnerability than about his present state of health.

"Let's first determine whether you are sick, shall we? We'll do some tests, give you a complete workup, and observe you in the hospital a few days. Then we'll know more."

It was a most unsatisfactory end to an otherwise pleasant visit.

v

Admission to hospital with a presumptive diagnosis of ALS entails a costly and complex series of tests. There are several other possible disorders from which a differential diagnosis must be extracted. For instance, syringomyelia, syphilitic amyotrophy, or even intramedullary tumor of the spinal cord may imitate—at least for a while—the characteristic symptoms of ALS. Multiple sclerosis or, less frequently, chronic cervical spondylosis are also possible candidates. In the final analysis, it must be admitted that certain diagnosis is possible only upon autopsy. Still, a competent diagnostician, clear X rays, good myelograms, and common sense are the most important tools of the profession. But even then, to disentangle ALS from the several myopathies associated with carcinoma, chronic forms of polymyositis, or even myasthenia gravis is a lengthy and expensive process.

In Stanley Ackyrod's case, the full workup took about a week. By the time his chart was complete, Sylvester had returned from Paris. He spent most of Monday morning reviewing the test results in the hope that something had been overlooked, some nuance forgotten whose inclusion would change the diagnosis entirely. But no, everything was accurate and everything was complete. By 11:30, he was certain of his diagnosis, and nothing now remained but to inform Ackyrod.

"Professor Ackyrod, we know now what has been causing these symptoms."

"Is it cancer?" was the first question Stanley asked. Isn't that always the first question asked, as if only cancer were the most lethal and fatal of diseases?

"No!"

"Thank God!"

In every way imaginable, amyotrophic lateral sclerosis is worse than cancer. But such information cannot be delivered to the patient wholesale and without sufficient preparation. Rather, time and circumstance, as well as the disease process itself, must purchase their retail absoluteness over a proper duration. Between patient and physician, there is always a duet, a dance of complex curtsies and bows. It is a ballet, a dialectic between the weak and the strong, between ignorance and knowledge, between death and life. As one advances, the other in turn withdraws; as one acts, so also does the other react. Finally, the synthesis is complete, and the patient grasps profoundly within what the physician could not bear to speak from without. The exact particulars and precise details of degeneration, vulnerability, degradation, and death can only be hinted at prosaically and never fully confronted poetically. And thus, in this strange dialogue of half-spoken truths, Stanley Ackyrod could only ask in the most inarticulate fashion: "Is it serious?"

And Dr. J. J. Sylvester, M.D., Ph.D.—last year's recipient of the coveted Cushing Award and recently invited keynote speaker to the College de France's Symposium on Cerebellar Astrocytomas—could not halt answering: "Yes."

And Professor Stanley Ackyrod, M.A., Ph.D.—who had lectured at Harvard, Yale, the Sorbonne, and Freiburg universities and who had received international recognition for his work as well as winning the Medal of the Centre de la Recherche Scientifique last fall—could only respond: "How long?"

And the sophisticated, elegant, and wise J. J. Sylvester could but ineloquently reply: "Not long. Perhaps a year. Not more than two."

"Will there be pain?"

"Some. We can manage most of it."

"And the rest?" Ackyrod's bitterness began to assemble itself. "Who will manage the rest?"

"Professor Ackyrod, we know so little about this disease . . ."

"What is the disease," Stanley demanded; "what is its name?"

"Amyotrophic lateral sclerosis."

"Is that like multiple sclerosis?"

"Yes, somewhat, only . . ."

"Only worse?"

"That's right, Professor, only worse."

Even the most intelligent among us is reduced to clichés and hackneyed expressions when confronted with our own mortality. Were the positions reversed, no doubt J. J. Sylvester's questions would be more technical but no less bitter.

Stanley was released from the hospital that very afternoon. After all, why keep him and for what purpose? With such a judgment placed upon him, there was little else to do but return to his apartment. There, dwelling among his books, his ideas, and within his world, he sought to make some sense of this utterly senseless situation.

VI

To die alone is, alas, the lot and destiny of each of us. To withdraw from the sounds, smells, lights, colors of the world into darkness and the void is a demand that nature makes upon both the willing and the reluctant. But to live alone while dying is the most hollow, stale, and bitter of states. It is to suffocate slowly and atrophy deep within yourself. For things are not persons, and they understand so very little the burden of being mortal. See them there: the books, china vases, Buddha statues, and all the paraphernalia of the lonely scholar— how could they even begin to know human suffering? Almost arrogant and insolent in their immortality, they mock and flaunt their privileges of fate. Do not turn to books, papers, and scholarly articles for solace in your misery, Stanley Ackyrod, for they do not care! But rather turn within to your gentle and fragile ideas that cower and hide with fright in the corners of your mind. What will become of them when they no longer can feed upon the oxygenated blood that is their diet and main staple? Will they wither? Will they die? Will they evaporate along with you into the darkness and the void? All your great ideas, all your precious ideas that you have labored and nurtured and fed for so very many years are about to die. The great books, the scholarly articles that you would have written are but empty promises now unfulfilled. The lectures that you would have given, the conversations that you might have had, the thoughts that you might have thought are now but dust and ashes. They are forgotten, Stanley, even before they are remembered. You are a dream about to be awakened. You were these ideas—they were you—and they made you what you are, but now even these are abandoned to themselves and will disintegrate like drops of water upon a red-hot stove. What did it all mean, Stanley, what was the meaning, the purpose of all of this? Why did you labor, study, learn, love, cry, and laugh if in the end it was simply to die? Why did you hope, plan, build, and create if only to be destroyed along with all that you become? In the end, what is the point of this madness that causes us to labor and suffer if in a single curvature of time it all unwinds and reverses itself?

For days, who knows how many, Stanley sat among his books and thoughts. Could it be true? Could it be avoided? Could it be a mistake? After all, he was a scholar, and so he sought to learn all about his disease, but the information was all so theoretical, abstract, and stale. There was nothing here about fear, hopelessness, despair, and the terror of darkness and death. "Amyotrophic lateral sclerosis is a fatal disease (cause unknown) characterized by destruction of motor cells in the anterior grey horns of the spinal cord together with degeneration of the pyramidal tracts bilaterally" (Gatz, *Manter's Essentials of Clinical Neuroanatomy and Neurophysiology,* p. 29).

But what of death and what of pain? What of humiliation and what of paralysis and of eventually drowning in your own wasted and diseased body fluids? Where, within these technical words, was to be found solace for despair, comfort for agony, and hope for the hopeless?

Neither was Sylvester of any help. The great Sylvester, the savior of all who suffered, was impotent and silent upon this disease. Stanley was quite alone and without allies or redemption. There would be no magic potions for him; neither herbs nor minerals nor elixirs of extraordinary power and promise existed that could argue his case with death.

After two weeks, he was surprised to discover that he still felt fine. Not perfect, you understand, but not nearly so bad as he had imagined or feared. In fact, when he went to his office that afternoon it seemed, there among old familiar things, as if nothing had changed. His colleagues did not seem to notice his absence any more than they remarked about his return. In fact, the indifference and anonymity of the department was a reassurance that things couldn't be all that bad if so much remained the same.

One day he decided to call Edgar for lunch in order to touch base with old friends and familiar surroundings. There is a certain belief—call it magical if you like—that we can return to what might have been by returning to what once was. But he had not calculated the exact longitude and latitude of his new situation and thus failed to realize that he had been transformed by his disease. Edgar, of course, was a physician and so knew with the keen eye of a clinician all that Stanley was undergoing. In fact, throughout the meal Stanley felt himself observed, diagnosed, and even evaluated with each morsel of food. Of course, it was Stanley and not Edgar who thought such thoughts, but one could not help wonder, Did my hand shake, is there a slight fasciculation there on my brow? Was Edgar thinking, even now as they ate together, Yes, he's getting worse, or Yes, yes, a typical case of amyotrophic lateral sclerosis; nothing exceptional or extraordinary here.

But Stanley Derek Ackyrod, Ph.D., was an extraordinary and exceptional person now reduced to an ordinary and perfectly predictable disease. You may present to a physician all the good evidence in favor of your health and in rebuttal of your disease and still elicit a customary "Yes, yes, nothing new here; just a slight readjustment of symptoms." At least so felt Stanley in Edgar's presence, and he therefore carefully avoided all further contact with him thereafter. Instead, he sought out the company of people who were ordinary, uninformed, and even quite unsophisticated. Formerly the thought of exchanging pleasantries with a cabdriver or a bellhop would have seemed preposterous, but now it had its charm. They were, after all, innocent, naive, and safe. To them he was simply another normal human being, and thus within their company there was a salvation which he had never sought or desired before: the province of simply being average, common, and ordinary. "Nothing unusual here with this fellow; he's just average, just an ordinary Joe."

The curious word *exceptional* is often applied to children who are extraordinary both in what they have as well as in what they lack. Geniuses and morons, rich and impoverished are all collected within the confines of this curious designation. Stanley had always wanted to be exceptional in the richest and best sense of that curious word and now instead found himself to be exceptional in the worst and most impoverished sense. Thus, he sought anonymity among common people who were neither scholars nor doctors nor even men of learning. Perhaps it was a compensation, perhaps it was a form of withdrawal, but for whatever reason it worked. The unsophisticated accept you for what you are. Life has made no great claims upon them, and so they expect less in return. They do not expect to write the novel of the century or to be offered the Emerson Chair at Harvard. Rather, they live for summer picnics, Monday night football, and a game of poker now and then. Should one among them be eccentric or peculiar, they pay it no mind unless it is excessive or aberrant. Stanley liked these people, and they offered him both the community and the nonjudgmental acceptance he needed. The store clerks, bank tellers, postmen, and shopkeepers of this world became his friends. They were good people with solid lives and clear-cut goals. Their day was not filled with the political intrigues of the Academy but was organized around hard work and getting the job done. They had names like Bud, Joe, Tom, Bob, and Ed, and they told you what they thought straight out and with no apologies. Unlike his colleagues at the university, who gave with one hand and took with another, these fellows were generous, unassuming, and honest with their friends. They were, of course, tough with their enemies, but at least they knew who their enemies were. In the academic world, everyone was your enemy, and most especially those who professed to be your friend.

Stanley had his rounds, so to speak, and he made his visits each day according to the same regular and orderly schedule. Recently, he had come to like routine and coveted the familiar and known rather than the new and unpredictable. In the mornings, he would have breakfast at the Home Cafe; now, unlike before his illness, he knew almost everyone at the counter, and they, in turn, knew him by first name as well. Sitting at the counter, drinking coffee and eating doughnuts, there was no class distinction between laborer and professional but simply men and women who had become friends with one another over the years. Stanley thought—at least he hoped— that he had become their friend as well and a member of this regular, orderly, predictable, and secure community. After breakfast he did his shopping for the day and often stopped to chat with stockboys and checkout clerks. In the past, he never would have paused to talk with any of them, believing they had nothing in common with him. But now, all of that had changed, and he found endless things to chat about, whether it be the price of lettuce or simply a change in the weather. Stanley had come to have great affection for the trivial and ordinary things of life and much less patience with grand ideas or theories that never touch concrete reality. It was not the substance of his life that changed but the style and manner in which that substance

25

was executed and lived. He was still a university professor; he still had amyotrophic lateral sclerosis, and he still was dying of it. None of that would change. What had changed was not the melody but the pitch and timbre of his life. It was because he no longer hoped to transform himself that all of his longitudinal change now became transverse.

But even magic as powerful as this is insufficient against an enemy as deadly as amyotrophic lateral sclerosis. Gradually, the disease began to subdue and domesticate Stanley Ackyrod. Soon, what had only weeks before been a limp now became a gait and then a shuffle, until finally he could not walk without benefit of a cane. Even this inconvenience became an asset, for the cane gave him an air of dignity which he had previously lacked. But even as the disease dignified, so also did it degrade, and gradually his fine tenor voice began to slur and slip over delicate words. At first, it was no more than a slight lisp, but then his jaws weakened, his lips trembled, his tongue grew heavy and old, until finally each word was a total confusion of vowel and consonant held in unsteady articulation. His eyes trembled; his cheeks flinched; and what had been a cheerful wink became instead a grotesque and hideous spasm. In short, he was coming apart at the seams. He knew it, and he had known it for some time. All the tricks, devices, distractions, and changes of life-style that had worked for a while were now revealed as only momentary pauses on a continuous arc. Having now come full circle to his disease, he realized that he had never left it in the first place. Rather, it had only expressed itself in degrees and kinds that appeared to be longitudinal changes whereas in fact they were only transverse. He was right back where he had started. And he was dying. And he was alone. And he was afraid!

VII

Now it was that the disease took hold of him with absolute fury and destructiveness. No longer a mere parasite which nonetheless retained its individuality, it had become a part of him much like an arm or a leg. Where healthy spinal tissue began and diseased tissue ended was now a distinction without difference.

He had become his disease; and it, in turn, him. Thus, the struggle and fight for conquest of the one over the other had been fought and lost. As a mother becomes the fetus that she bears within her, so now Stanley Ackyrod became this embryo of death which blossomed within him.

By mid-November he was unable to walk without his cane, and by the end of December his shuffle had rendered the cane useless as well. By January he was as bound to a wheelchair as any prisoner is to his cell, and by February he could barely hold a pencil in his quivering hands. All within the span of six months—180 days—his body had become the product of its own internal decomposition. Indeed, he was decomposing even as the integration of a solid is resolved by centrifugal force into its several separate elements. Legs, thighs, arms, fingers that had been the orchestration of a corporeal symphony were now but abandoned instruments in a dissolving melody. Nothing worked; nothing obeyed orders, commands, or directives. The brain had lost control over its provinces and now found itself isolated and alone.

Stanley Ackyrod, whose intelligence was frightful in its power and intensity, had always relied upon his mind for survival. In grade school he fought with his brains and not with his fists. When the battlefield was intellectual, he was a dangerous and clever opponent who nearly always won. It was for that reason that he felt safe and comfortable in the academic world where the bullies all try to destroy you with ideas. But if his mind had been his haven of rest, then surely his body had always been his garden of pleasure. Sexuality, especially among intellectuals, often assumes complex and unpredictable forms. No longer restrained by the provincialism of the bourgeoisie, the intellectual prides himself on his willingness to experiment, investigate, and venture forth into new territories. Stanley Ackyrod had ventured more than once into these somewhat forbidden lands, and he found them delightful! But now his body refused the sexuality it had so willingly—and not so very long ago—indulged with such abandon. Erection, orgasm, satiation—all the instruments of pleasure—now failed him. He was imprisoned within a demotorized and somewhat desensitized tomb which rang hollow when struck with instruments that had previously elicited melodies of monumental volume and tones most lovely in their degree.

How strange the mind is! It is like the body, but again so different, so very different, in so very many ways. Herein there are no movable parts, no motorized aspects, but rather the swiftness of an instant thought upon a single contemplation. But here too, despite all of its differences from the body, the mind also grows weary, sluggish, even as exhausted muscles do. For here too there is fatigue, exertion, renewal of strength and loss thereof. In truth, Stanley had always relied upon his intelligence without really ever understanding it. Now that knowledge was forced upon him.

It seemed that as his body weakened, so in turn, the power and strength of his mind increased—as if the energy lost from the one was being transferred to the other. Ideas that had previously been indistinct, even ambiguous, now clarified and resolved themselves with a power, a crispness, a sharpness he had never experienced before. A thought previously interrupted by a demand of the body was now free to expand and enlarge itself unencumbered. Even ordinary notions such as the title of books, the place where a most-needed object was last seen were far more vivid and structured than ever before. Then, too, his concentration increased in width as well as depth. Before, a moment's thought would be shattered unpredictably by some distraction or other. Not so anymore! Now he could maintain a thought for an instant or an hour, and as he measured its length, so also could he calibrate the depth of such new concentrations. Not one thought, not two, but even a dozen held in parallel planes of composition were quite possible for him now. And as his concentration of thoughts lengthened, so did it also deepen. Layers, one upon the other in horizontal plateaus, were exposed with little effort. Thinking became for him an archaeological dig in which not merely the contents but also the structure of his mind were exposed and illuminated. He could easily become lost in this kaleidoscopic world of myriad reflections and lights. And he frequently did! Each individual illumination was a phosphorescence of the whole, and thus he grasped in a single stroke the orbit of thought that surrounds an otherwise solitary idea.

But the renewed energy now pouring into the funnel of his mind was emptying out of his perfectly paralyzed body. Like granite or marble it had become, and with the same cold surface shine that such dead things have. By April he could not move a muscle below his neck, and yet his entire body shook with the quakes and tremors of fasciculations. He was like a rock in an ocean: perfectly still amid unceasing waves and cascades. And in the center of it all there existed the terrible indignity of wasted muscle and nerve. His bowels did not work; his bladder was useless; he could not speak a single intelligible sentence. Neither could he swallow his food nor scratch his cheek nor even rub his eyes. Dear God, not even to be able to rub your eyes! Should an insect land upon his body, he could neither protest nor aggress nor even disagree. He was a stone in a field which could not be moved. When visited by colleagues or friends, he was horrified to discover the horror in their eyes. For to see him now was, in truth, to see a totally transformed effigy of what had once been the proud, somewhat arrogant, brilliant, and dynamic Stanley Ackyrod.

In his wheelchair he slumped, rather than sat, restrained by two thick webbings of strap. His head was unable to support itself and so hung at an angle to his wasted body. Beneath the cotton shirt and pants, one could see how thin his arms and legs had become. Now the bones were as visible as the hull of a broken ship, and his skeleton seemed to almost float to the surface even as his skin receded to the depths. He was an exoskeleton with just a thin wrapping paper of skin and hair for elegant decoration. A colored bow tied upon a gift of doom.

The visitor must now approach slowly, cautiously, and with great care so as not to make a sudden move. "Stanley? . . . Stanley? It's me. How are you today? Yes, yes, I understand. Don't try to speak. I just came to say hello and now I must be going. Goodbye . . . goodbye." That, and nothing more. They are terrified of him, and after all why shouldn't they be? Look at what he has become. He is contaminated; he is poison; he is the residual of what each of them fears they might become.

"Oh, dear God," they think as they leave. "Oh, dear God, what has he become?"

Stanley, of course, was well beyond caring. He no longer felt in any touch at all with that hollow and uncertain world that others inhabited and into which he could not enter, could not move, could not breathe. Without, within, he was the inside of his outside and the inner surface of his awful, frightful outer.

> "Gentlemen, to conclude, as labioglossalaryngeal paralysis established itself, you will find that muscles of the cranial nerves—as well as the corticobulbar tracts—are compromised. Thus, chewing, swallowing, and, of course, talking will become increasingly difficult and finally impossible. Dysphagia greatly complicates prognosis, but you may expect your patient to succumb to his illness within three years at the outside from respiratory failure.
>
> "Any questions? Good!
>
> "Do be certain to read your Ripers and McCall for next time and especially the sections on myasthenia gravis, which will be our topic of discussion. If I may add a personal note, I find this entity—and I think you will as well—almost as fascinating as amyotrophic lateral sclerosis. Note especially pp. 1394–1427 in your text on neurological diseases.
>
> "Dismissed."

Stanley Ackyrod awoke that morning with some disorientation but also with a certain pleasurable giddiness. It was as if he had held his breath too long—as indeed he used to do as a child—and now felt rather dizzy and about to faint. But soon he realized exactly what was happening to him. His breathing was heavy and labored, and the harder he tried to draw more air in, the more air, in turn, he seemed to lose. He was suffocating to death!

Perhaps it was not unexpected, for, after all, he had noticed his own heavy breathing for the past ten days. So had everyone else around him, and they knew—even if Stanley didn't—that the end was near. It sounded like a billows, a fireplace billows, to hear him breathe. Each breath was a labored gasping which grabbed rather than reached for the air available. Even to hear those wheezing grunts was maddening since one could not help but draw more air into his own lungs in sympathetic collaboration. But it did no good, and each day Stanley's lungs grew weaker and more fragile. He was as dizzy as a young schoolgirl about to swoon at her first dance. In fact, he could barely summon the strength to breathe at all, and when he did, it was of such shallow capacity that only one-tenth of what was needed was actually drawn.

Of course, Stanley little knew and little cared about these technicalities. He knew only that his lungs felt on fire as if they were winged chariots. He pushed and pulled; he tugged and coaxed the reluctant muscles, and they seemed ignited, inflated by their residual weakness; and yet amid all of this labor, he felt strangely safe, secure, and even calm within himself as if he were sitting on a sunny hillside one spring day and heard, far off, the labored rise and fall of a distant pump. It had, or so it seemed, altogether everything and altogether nothing to do with him.

But now the slow revolutions of dizziness turned instead to an increased spinning which accelerated even as it deepened. A vortex opened up, and therein a cone emerged into which he seemed to tumble effortlessly. As the walls closed in, so did the apex of the cone expand as if to welcome him. It was not unpleasant; it was neither painful nor even frightening, but rather moist, pliant, and rather delicious—or perhaps delirious—with its smooth, textured slopes. He fell—rather floated to a fall—within this immense pleasure dome of gyrating moisture, gloss, and substance.

Suddenly, just as suddenly as it had started, it stopped. He stopped as well! Suspended in midair like a bird in gliding flight, all motion ceased. And then he fell; he fell straight and with immense speed, in a perfect gravitational drop, to the very bottom of the cone. Whether he reached it or whether he didn't, he could little tell, for all light ceased as he approached the opening. It was at an end; it was finished; he became what he was not!

2

Whence the Meaning of All This Pain?

And she forgot the stars, the moon, and sun,
And she forgot the blue above the trees,
And she forgot the dells where waters run,
And she forgot the chilly autumn breeze;
She had not knowledge when the day was done,
And the new morn she saw not: But in peace
Hung over her sweet basil evermore,
And moisten'd it with tears unto the core.

And, furthermore, her brethren wonder'd much
Why she sat drooping by the basil green
And why it flourish'd, as if by magic touch;
Greatly they wonder'd what the thing might mean:
They could not surely give belief, that such
A very nothing would have the power to wean
Her from her own fair youth, and pleasures gay,
And even remembrance of her love's delay.

John Keats
"Isabella"

ALZHEIMER DISEASE: Alzheimer disease is characterized by atrophy of the cerebral cortex that is usually diffuse, although it may be more severe in the frontal and temporal lobes. The degree of atrophy is variable. Brains of affected individuals weigh between 850g and 1250g at autopsy. On microscopic examination, there is loss of both neurons and neuropil in the cortex and, sometimes, secondary demyelination in subcortical white matter. With qualitative morphometry, it has been shown that the greatest loss is that of large cortical neurons. The most characteristic findings are the argentophilic senile plaque and neurofibrillary tangles. The senile plaque is found throughout the cerebral cortex and hippocampus, and the number of plaques per microscopic field has been correlated with the degree of intellectual loss. The senile plaque is composed of enlarged, degenerating axonal endings surrounding a core composed mainly of extracellular amyload. The degenerating axonal boutons contain lysosomes, degenerating mitochondria and paired helical filaments. These paired helical filaments, which are about 20nm wide with a twist every 80nm along their length, constitute the chief element found in the Alzheimer neurofibrillary tangle. These tangles consist of accumulation of these filaments within the body of the swollen neuron. Neurofibrillary tangles first occur in the hippocampus, particularly in region CA1 and subiculum; later, neurofibrillary tangles may be found throughout the ce rebral cortex. Other less prominent but still common features of Alzheimer disease include granulanacualar degeneration of pyramidal cells of the hippocampus and congophilic angiopathy. The Hirano body, a rod-like body containing paracrystaline material, first described in the Guam, parkinsonism, dementia complex, is also found in Alzheimer disease.

H. Houston Merritt
Textbook of Neurology

I

Is it out of malice or is it out of mercy that we are condemned to watch our own death? No other animal is so cursed—or so blessed—as to observe with horrified detachment its own disappearance into the thin envelope of nothingness. For them, death comes silently and quickly from nowhere; the knife blade is sharp, clean and cuts rapidly. But for us it is different. We must watch—even meditate—over what we shall become, and knowing this we study the illnesses that inhabit us with the calm seriousness of one who is unaffected. How very strange!

There are diseases that take their time with you. Leukemia, lymphoma, myeloma, and melanoma—poetic in their deathliness—and permit you to watch as the great systems of your being unravel: gut, gizzard, lung, bone, and brain. Others cannot afford this leisure; they attack brutally and with savage intensity and so demand immediate recompense. While yet a few—but only a very few—are far more merciful in their malice, for they destroy not what is seen but the act of seeing itself. As the brain becomes mortally wounded by the gradual blinding of its intelligence, the falling victim gropes for some sense, some meaning, even some purpose to all this pain, agony, and decomposition. But herein the body raises questions that the brain cannot answer but instead must endure uncomprehendingly. In 1907—just eight years before his death at the age of fifty-one—Alois Alzheimer placed himself in medical history by naming one such disease.

There had been a change in Murray. The children hadn't noticed it, of course, but then they were all grown up and out on their own. Danny was in his second year of law school, Linda had just become engaged, and David was working for a firm in California. How would they know if things were different at home? But things were different, and Murray had definitely changed. Beatrice might not have even noticed the change herself were it not for the bridge club. Yesterday afternoon, her friend Margery had confronted her with the fact that she had declined every invitation to play cards with the girls for the past six months, and frankly wanted to know why. Why? Why indeed! Beatrice did not know herself except to say that something had come up every month which made it impossible. But what? Well, last month—it was April—she had the taxes to do, and the month before she had worked with the accountant to get their investments in order, and the month before . . . oh yes . . . the month before she had settled that insurance claim for Murray's accident. So there, that was the reason she had been unable to play bridge because of all these unexpected things which kept coming up. Maybe next month she could. But then—almost as a afterthought, and it struck her like a thunderbolt—Margery asked: "But doesn't Murray do all of that?"

"Well, no, he doesn't. He used to, but he doesn't any more."

"Why not?" Margery persisted.

And the very best that Beatrice could answer was simply: "I don't know; I really don't know. He used to."

Now having thought about the matter, Beatrice realized that Murray didn't do any of the things these days that he used to do. She did the taxes for the first time three years ago because when April 15 arrived Murray had not even assembled the receipts and seemed so forgetful about the whole thing that she had to file a late extension and do them herself. She had been doing the taxes ever since. When Murray had his accident last month, she had taken care of the insurance because she knew, she absolutely knew, that he would forget to do so. And when the bills came due, it was she who paid them because Murray would postpone and postpone and then forget what needed to be paid until it was simply easier to do it herself. Yes, that was why she had no time for bridge, or for anything else such as getting her nails done or visiting Mother or even writing to David, because she was doing all of Murray's work. And she had been doing it for almost three years! Why— quickly now her mind raced to assemble the disconnected fragments and aspects of obligations, responsibilities, and commitments that she had assumed instead of Murray—had she been doing her jobs and his as well? Quite simply because otherwise they would not get done. Murray would be sorry, of course; he would promise to do them the next time and wouldn't; he would make lists out and then lose the lists. Even the accident last month had happened only because Murray got confused in rush-hour traffic and hit the car in front of him. But that wasn't like Murray, was it? He had always been responsible, even meticulous, about finances and details around the house. Why was he now so . . . so damned lazy?

And there was one other thing as well; it even embarrassed her to admit it, but they had not made love for almost three months. She had tried—even putting on that naughty night-gown from France—but Murray just didn't seem very inter-ested. That was all right. At their age, she reasoned, it didn't matter all that much whether they made love or not. But still that was just not like Murray because he had always been the one chasing her around the bedroom. Maybe they should talk to someone. But who? A counselor or maybe Father Black? Maybe they should see a doctor? Maybe he should see a doctor!

Actually, Murray felt pretty good. Not perfect you under-stand; he didn't feel like a teenager or anything like that. Just pretty good. But that was all right for a man in his mid-fifties, well, fifty-seven to be exact, a fellow doesn't expect to feel like a kid anymore. Sure, he forgot things once in a while, but didn't everybody else? He looked at himself in the bedroom mirror and was happy with what he saw. He wasn't fat and his stomach was nice and trim; he had good arms and a strong chest. Yes, he looked fine for a man of fifty-eight or fifty-seven. Which was it? It was fifty-seven! So there couldn't be very much wrong with a fellow who looked that good, could there?

But he was tired. Sometimes he just didn't seem to have any energy at all. This business with lovemaking was fine, and he knew that Beatrice felt he wasn't interested, but that wasn't true. He was interested, but then when the time came it just seemed to be too much effort. Lots of things were like that now: just too much effort, too much of a burden. He had no energy left for anything except his job, and even there prob-lems were constantly occurring. Last month his boss was mad as hell about that interim report that Murray had forgotten to file on time, and the other week he completely lost his train of thought in the middle of a routine presentation and had to start all over again. It was kind of embarrassing. Maybe he just needed to rest or to take his vacation a little early this year. That was probably all there was to it. Certainly, no need to waste money on a doctor when the problem was just a question of nerves. Actually, the only thing that really worried him at all was this thing of getting lost. It had happened twice in the last week, and although he did not tell Beatrice this, that was really how the accident had occurred in the first place. He had decided to go down Chester Boulevard—just in order to avoid the rush-hour traffic—and then got so turned around that he was lost and in his confusion hit the car in front of him. He could not tell Beatrice the part about getting lost; it was too embarrassing.

In private practice, a doctor sees a hodgepodge of different kinds of diseases but nothing too much out of the ordinary after the first five years or so. By that time, you basically have seen the same kinds of illnesses that you will be treating for the next forty years. Occasionally, something interesting comes along, but not too often. Herbert Medcalf, M.D., was not very disappointed that his cases were routine. These days—with insurance premiums, angry patients, and malpractice suits—he was content to treat the basic stuff with no great challenges to get in the way.

Murray and Beatrice Wasserman had been his patients for the past twenty-two years. Medcalf had delivered each of their three children, had removed Murray's appendix sixteen years ago, and had biopsied a benign lipoma in Beatrice's left breast last April. They were an average, hardworking middle-class family who always paid their bills on time—but not before exhausting all insurance options—and seemed to be in good health for a couple in their middle fifties. Medcalf was not surprised to see the Wassermans scheduled for a three o'clock appointment the following afternoon. It was no doubt another routine complaint, and after all, it was a good idea to have these little aches and pains checked out as one gets on in years. Actually, come to think of it now, he had noticed Murray at the gas station yesterday, but Murray had not seemed to recognize him.

Medcalf was shocked when he saw Murray Wasserman close up. True, it had been well over a year since his last visit, but a man doesn't age that much in a year, does he? Murray looked far more like a man of sixty-five than one of fifty-seven. The skin along his cheeks and eyes had lost its tautness; his face was puffy and bloated; and he walked with the slouch of an old man, of a very old man. Perhaps his wife had failed to notice the profound changes that had occurred only because she had not achieved sufficient distance. But to an observer, it

37

was perfectly clear that dramatic changes had occurred and of an irreversible kind.

Sometimes, a physician can learn as much about a patient by simply watching—instead of closely examining—him. Medcalf watched very closely this Thursday afternoon, and what he saw was as much diagnostic proof of advanced Alzheimer's as any cortical plaque or neurofibrillary tangle. The patient's personal appearance was slovenly, if not entirely neglected. He walked and even talked with a weariness that was deep and most profound. Moreover, both what he did and how he did it were characterized by a slippage, an asynchronous rupture which interrupted every movement that should otherwise be smooth and rounded. One had the impression that his gestures were mechanical rather than organic. But the most striking thing about Murray was the shroud that surrounded him. It seemed as if he was sequestered within the darkest of cerebral cloaks, which prevented him from either comprehending or being comprehended. More than a distance, far more than an abyss, there was a curtain which circumscribed his actions and so isolated them from their meaning. Thus, nothing occurred spontaneously or easily, but rather every thought, every idea or concept was dredged up with weariness from a solitary cell where it had rested within itself while remaining in isolation from all other ideas that might provide depth, width, and proportion. This was not a measurable or quantifiable ingredient of the patient's makeup but a qualifiable loss or deficit which could be noticed only when it was missing. Medcalf had learned some time ago to take gross and large measurements first before attending to minute details. Thus, he was struck immediately by the disintegration, the discontinuity of Murray Wasserman's behavior.

"What happens when you forget or can't remember?"

"Well, Doctor, it's like the ideas are there, but I can't touch them. You know how things look through the wrong end of a telescope: they're distant and small, and if you could bring them close it would be all right. But your arms don't reach that far. Does that make any sense?"

"Yes, I think it does. You mean your mind isn't quite in touch with itself?"

"That's right! That's what I feel. As if there is a gully or a ditch that divides everything from everything else."

"Are you ever confused or disoriented?"

The hesitation in answering was itself an answer. "Sometimes. Just sometimes." Murray looked with embarrassment toward his wife. Surely, there is nothing more infirm and vulnerable about a man than when he is not in control. "Sometimes, I guess I am sometimes," he repeated.

II

Are the laws that govern the development of intelligence also those which govern its disintegration and destruction? As a concept or idea is formed, does it so also deform in the same manner and by the very same principles acting in reversal? Or is the destruction of a mind—literally its de-structuration—a chaotic and disorderly process in which random events collide with one another, thereby producing an internal holocaust having neither structure nor configuration? Certainly there is much about birth and much about death that is brotherly and familiar. Indeed, there seems to be a strange adagio between these two forces of our beginning and our end in which each bows and curtsies to the other. For some of us, our ferocious will to survive is counterbalanced by an equal weight of self-destructiveness, a will to consume ourselves and become nothingness. For some of us, the impotence of old age is merely a revisitation of birth's innocence and vulnerability. For some of us, death is far easier than birth: far kinder, far gentler, far richer than we ever imagined life could be. For some of us, life is simply overrated when compared with its brother death. Yes, there is much about the end of life that is so much like its beginning that the two seem but a continuous arc with only moments of relief between them.

Accordingly, Alzheimer's disease—this writhing, coiling convulsion of axonal fibers baptized by a man's name—was neither cruel nor savage in its quest for Murray Wasserman. Rather, strange to say, it was much like a lover courting the beloved. It did not deform, devour, or degrade as other illnesses often do. Instead it was gentle, even patient, as the beloved was slowly wooed, seduced, and charmed into sleepfulness. And since he could not feel the buildup of argento-philic plaque upon his cortical tissues, since he could not discern the neurofibrillary tangles 20 nm wide but with a twist every 80 nm, since he had no certain knowledge of the slow degradation of axonal boutons filling now with the dirt of wasted mitochondria, since his gentle brain could feel so much but could not feel itself, Murray was little aware of this dance of death in which the lover courts the beloved. In fact, he felt quite at ease and even calmer and calmer as the sea about him became more dangerous and desperate. Is it mercy or is it malice when death seduces rather than rapes us?

The second stage of Alzheimer's disease is more subversive, but also more anesthetizing, than the first. The memory losses, the confusion and disorientation are alarming and worrisome documentaries to the patient of his gradual disintegration. But now the disease disarms him by increasing the degree of its destructiveness while minimizing the warning signs of pain and discomfort. It is a dialectic of reversals and oppositions in which the deepest wounds ache with exquisite pleasure while the least of these is too painful to behold. Now laughter and tears freely associate with one another at inappropriate times and places. Restless, discontent, and haunted by an anxiety which can be neither registered nor understood, he is driven by blind forces that seem both merciful and kind in their terrible, aching malevolence. And so it was with Murray Wasserman as he gradually became less what he was and more what he would become.

Ideally, a husband—at least for most wives—is either an equal or a superior, but never an inferior. Should the latter become the case, or be the case, then a profound reorganization of powers and priorities will most usually ensue. She will not, after all, assume responsibility for everything while also forfeiting control and leadership. No! Beatrice now rightly decided that if Murray could be entrusted with nothing, then neither could he be empowered with anything. This recalibration of their roles and responsibilities exercised itself with amazing swiftness, and Murray found himself a child once again while Beatrice rediscovered maternalism.

"Murray," she reminded him, "eat your peas; they're good for you."

"No, Murray, don't touch that; I'll do it myself."

"Murray? Did you remember to take your medicine?"

In his more lucid moments—and they became fewer and fewer—Murray knew that he was a fallen angel, a wounded animal which could not survive except as a scavenger feeding from its host. Such dependency both comforted and terrified him at the same time. On the one hand, he needed her, but on the other hand she—increasingly now—no longer needed him. The transfer of power at first had been subtle and tentative, but all that changed after diagnosis, after what was really troubling Murray Wasserman had been given a name: Alois Alzheimer's disease. Now, Beatrice seized command with force and determination and so reduced Murray to a child who received but could not give direction whether to his own life or to anyone else's.

What is a man? What constitutes his gristle, muscle, gut, and testicle? In short, what makes a man a "real man"? Does a man, in order to be a "real man," need to dominate, tyrannize, and subjugate everyone around him? Does he always have to be the smartest, the strongest, and the best, or can he rather be a man who is gentle, kind, caring, loving, and even sensitive? Is not such a man still every bit a "real man"? Certainly, there are some who believe that men only become "real men" when they succeed in elevating themselves by degrading and demeaning others. But a man, in the best and most perfect sense of that word, does not strive to master others but instead strives to master himself by taming and domesticating all of the lusts, fears, doubts, weaknesses, and agonies of his daily life. Such a man is in control; and yet, not of others is he master but only of himself. He has learned through sheer force of will to control all that is bizarre, weak, wicked, woeful, destructive, and petty about himself. He is not free of fear or immune to terror, tragedy, and tears but has learned to bridle these hostile forces within himself for greater reasons and higher goals. This simple and elementary fact about the nature of "real men" has been misunderstood repeatedly by those who could not claim

41

it for their own. To focus energy while maintaining it, to be courageous while feeling fear, to be assertive while admitting doubts, to be secure while trembling within, to be strong in love while being gentle as well, to stand independent while leaning upon those you love, to reach out when everything within you wants to withdraw, to stand tall while feeling small are the simple equations by which men become "real men."

The greatest challenge for anyone—man or woman—is to achieve control of themselves while focusing their energy into socially acceptable and profitable manners and forms. But some men have misunderstood this challenge and failed utterly in their efforts to achieve it. Such men have become the bullies, the thugs, the beaters, and the breakers of all that is gentle in order to prove their power and strength, first to themselves and then to others. In the end, such men have nearly always destroyed themselves while destroying everyone around them as well.

In many ways men have always been the more fragile and delicate members of the human race. They die sooner, suffer more, and agonize constantly over each weakness, infirmity, and defect within themselves. In so many ways a man is soft flesh within protective gristle, fear within terrible anger, vulnerability within presumed strength, and dependency within need for independence. Without his protective covering, he is all soft underbelly waiting to be gutted and fearing every enemy that comes along.

For Murray Wasserman, the real threat to his existence was not the loss of cortical tissue but the exfoliation of all that was vulnerable, fragile, and delicate within him. He was a fallen angel beating his wings violently in order to gain elevation and yet finding himself falling only the more heavily and all the more certainly into despair.

"No, Murray," she yelled from the kitchen, "I'll do that!"

"But Beatrice, I can do it; . . . I can do it."

"No, Murray, I said leave it be and I will do it later."

"Yes, dear."

For Murray, the most excruciating pain was not in what his illness did to him but what other people did to him. He was treated as a child, an invalid, and a guest in his own home. It was all the big things and the little ones as well. Beatrice allowed him to pay no bills, write no checks, and have no spending money; neither could he drive the automobile, cut the grass, fix the roof, or even be alone with himself for more than five minutes; nor was he permitted to answer the phone, greet people at the door, talk to salesmen when they visited, or even go next door to see the neighbors. Everything about him now was suspect and suspicious. His least and every move was watched intently by someone not in order to see what was right about it but only to wait for him to do something wrong. With the naming of his illness, his life had suddenly become a negative reversal in which only the shaded areas were observed, with all the positive images disregarded as exceptions to the darkness of his impending situation. They knew—his family, friends, and associates—that he was losing control of himself, and so they assumed that he had already lost it. They believed—for each of them had run to some dictionary or other and read about his illness—that he would not be able to remember things, and so they assumed that he had already forgotten them; that he could not be counted on to do the appropriate thing, and so it was taken for granted that he would do what was inappropriate. They knew—perhaps they knew too well—that Murray would die old before his time, humiliated by incontinence, confusion, and incompetence. And so, they believed him to already be so. In short, he had lost more than his manhood; he had also lost his freedom. Thus, being neither man nor person, he became instead an obstacle which simply got in the way but was quite forgotten when it remembered its place, much like a dog or a cat which the family merely tolerates only when its behavior is perfect but seems to loathe and despise at the slightest provocation. Yes, that was it exactly: having lost his manhood—and then his personhood as well—Murray had become a pet whose charming incompetence got in the way of more serious business.

Lying that night in bed, Murray reached with gentle, searching fingers to find Beatrice. Sensations had become important, even exquisite to him, and it was sensual just to feel the satin and silk on her nightgown. But when satin finally became flesh, it had turned rigid and taut with the expectation of his arrival. He felt the race of her pulse, especially in her loins, and sensed the tight muscles forming a protective shield about her. Beatrice was afraid! And she was afraid of him! He knew that without even asking, but nonetheless did ask.

"Would you like to make love?"

"Oh no, Murray, not tonight."

The embarrassment in her voice was heavy but not sufficient to mask the greater fear assembling now behind it. He blurted out the very question that he most feared to have answered:

"Are you afraid you'll catch it, Beatrice, is that what worries you?"

"No, Murray, of course not. It's just that I . . . well, I just feel tired tonight."

He never asked again. He knew; he could see it in her eyes and when she kissed him on the cheek instead of the lips and when she never used his bathroom and when she washed his dishes twice and when she did a dozen little things to avoid becoming what he already was. And he hated her for it. She had not only reduced him to a child; she had degraded him to a disease. He was no longer her husband, her lover, her provider and protector but simply Alzheimer's disease. And he was disgusted with her for all of that because finally he was becoming disgusted with himself.

Stage II of Alzheimer's disease creates a hurricane of unpredictable and unexpected emotional storms. One day the sky is clear and brilliant, and then suddenly the air is broken with a profound sadness almost too grave to bear. But then, instantly, as if a ray of intense sunlight should illuminate this interminable rain, the clouds part in joyful exuberance. You know how it is on a summer's day when the rain parts to permit sunlight and light bends to permit the rain. A rainbow forms of sun and storm which forecasts danger while promising good fortune. That's how it was within this most humid and self-contained vessel of Murray's emotional life. He knew not when everything would change from joy to sadness or back again. He felt no control, no inner diaphragm of regulation over these productions of his cortical chemistry. Nor could he have ever hoped to grasp the equations, the physiology and physics of those neurofibrillary tangles and senile plaques. Rather, he was their victim, their puppet who danced or cried most wildly to their slightest command or directive.

By mid-November, Murray's speech had become so distorted, so twisted upon its own axis that when he spoke it was no longer language that he uttered but only degraded signs and gestures. Oh, they knew what he wanted well enough, but not because of what he said but rather what he did. He pointed, looked, gestured, and tried to speak, but it was simply a rambling confusion. Oddly enough, in the midst of all this disconnected, mispronounced, and dislocated word-salad, Murray made perfect sense to himself. Why were they too stupid to understand? He knew clearly and precisely what he wanted to say, and yet the family looked at him in bewilderment and confusion. But the words did not seem the wrong words to him; the grammar, the vocabulary, the context, and the content all seemed properly integrated to him. What was wrong with them? Why couldn't they understand? Why were they becoming so distant and disconnected as if they were being miniaturized in direct proportion to the greater distance they had established from him?

Of course, it was Murray's own microcosm that had so expanded that now it incorporated everything else. As he became more self-contained, everything else was forced to move to the very periphery his most intense center had created. Accordingly, there was no longer room for anything within this walled-off confinement but Murray himself. His needs, his point of view, his perspective had become the central law and gravitational force of this new universe he now inhabited. Giving space for no one but himself, everything else grew distant in polarized opposition to his own greater distance.

III

The third stage of Alzheimer's is surely the most benevolent, the most understanding and merciful, of death's trimesters. All the confusion, embarrassment, and agony of self-observation are forfeited in favor of grateful amnesia. Family and friends become as strangers while the familiar and the foreign lose the elasticity of their boundaries and become as one. Relieved of recognition and responsibility, Murray is free to enter a sanctuary in which any behavior is permitted and every law, rule, or sanction can be disregarded as one pleases. One is a child again.

The original development of a self—of a geometric center to one's life—is achieved through a series of topographical measurements and calculations. First, the immediate environment—breast, bassinet, blanket—are negated and so disentangled from the living, organic center that will become the self. Gradually, even incrementally, these measurements increase in their complexity until everything that is different from, other than, and dissimilar to self has been inventoried. With such notations in place, it now becomes possible to circumscribe a limit or domain within which self is contained and everything else is excluded. It appears that one must first have a world, a universe, before one can have a self.

But, in turn, the closing down of a world in order to open up a self will also obey the same principles and laws in reverse. As the universe constricts, so also does the self dilate and expand. It is, in fact, a sort of aging in reverse, a kind of rejuvenation which develops inward instead of outward. All that Murray had become now unraveled and disentangled itself in order to simplify his life. He was an air balloon in search of elevation and so threw overboard all that was unnecessary sand in order to gain greater height by maintaining lesser weight. What, after all, did he need of those thousand memories, thoughts, lists, and memorabilia with which we burden ourselves for daily life? What difference did it make whether the conversion factors for weights and measurements were stored away or whether the exact number of inches in a foot or the correct telephone numbers of everyone he had ever known were properly remembered? What difference did it make? Such information is useful only to those who commerce in such worlds. Be gone with it all, be gone with so much sand and irrelevancies!

For survival, only simple tools are needed: air, food, water. Life at its most basic and most elementary level has no need for anything unnecessary or burdensome. Murray simplified all that he had become for the purpose of concentrating what little he had on that which remained. Indeed, he was a child again. His bowels and bladder were liberated from social customs; he slept when he wished and ate when he wanted. Rules and regulation, which formerly had corseted and structured his behavior into predictable and orderly formats, were now abandoned in favor of more immediate concerns. He had become a child again.

Of course, his family and friends saw none of this. Rather, they saw an old, emaciated man who now wore diapers and wept to himself alone, and sometimes cried in grateful acceptance of the slightest things. For them, his behavior was quite simply inappropriate. They pitied him because his life was now only one of survival and nothing complex or compound remained of him. He had become a child again, but an old and aging child who was not precious but hideous. No one wanted to hold or rock Murray to sleep; no one looked at him in sleep and dreams with a sense of endearment in their hearts. He was disgusting and grotesque to behold. For if Murray had become a child, he had also become a monster.

What of Murray throughout all of this? Did he feel deformed and misshapen? Was he disgusted or frightened for himself? Or did he enjoy becoming a child again? One wonders what it must be like to surrender every obligation and responsibility of the world—even the appropriate time and place of moving one's bowels and bladder—and regain independence again. Is there a giddy sense of release and freedom in knowing that one is no longer bound by any social convenience or custom or rule? To do or think or be whatever you want to be, to lie or sleep as long as you want to, to laugh or cry or even sing without regard to the Chorus's demand for conformity.

Lest it seem that the terribleness of Murray's condition can be somehow idealized, it must be admitted at once that dark and dangerous things were occurring within his gentle brain. Within the hippocampus—that hippopotamus of memory— there resides a latticework of the most delicate and integrated of circuitries. At one end of the hippocampus lies the amygdaloid nucleus and at the other rests the ventromedial aspect of the temporal lobe. Fanning out in every direction are connections to the cingulate gyrus, other aspects of the limbic system,

47

and, of course, the hypothalamus itself. It is thought that the affective markers of sensory information reside herein and these associations are transmitted to the hypothalamus to play their decisive role in learning, remembering, forgetting, rewarding, punishing, and everything else that makes sense of our behavior. But it is just here—specifically at CA1 of the hippocampus—where the neurofibrillary tangles first enunciate themselves. Spreading then throughout the cortical complex, they invade pyramidal cells and gradually all other areas of the cortex.

Strange to say, however, as important as the cortex appears to be, it remains a covering, a convoluted surface protecting deeper and more important ingredients of the brain. One must therefore wait for the neurofibrillary tangles, plaques, and cell death to reach the centers of respiration, heart regulation, and metabolism. Which they, of course, eventually do.

When Murray awoke that day, it was to the odors and sounds of breakfast being made. He liked breakfast, always had, in fact, and thought with some anticipation of the good things that this meal always brought with it. But then his thoughts changed to other matters entirely. A deep crimson hue surrounded by a luster of cobalt blue; it was very beautiful. A sound of high-pitched intensity with modulations and modifications of scale, pitch, and harmony. The sensation of a cool breeze across starched sheets and new-mown grass from morning dew. These most elegant sensations were as precise and well defined to him as any concept or idea had ever been. In fact, more so now that the machinery of cognition no longer gobbled up and robbed emotion of everything that was new. Thoughts are, after all, greedy and voracious in their desire to consume everything and make it their own. It is rare that a feeling or a sensation is free to float unmolested in these treacherous waters where thoughts are always in pursuit of feelings. But purified and rid of such ideational carnivores, Murray was free to luxuriate in more tranquil and less hostile waters. Here a sudden ocher yellow would flood his vision and turn with deeper hue into the cobalt blue from whence it came or the violet lavender it sought to become. Sounds—especially the integrated and musical ones—appeared to diagram and structure themselves in ways never before possible. For example, a melody would rise or fall in geometric arcs, peaks, and valleys of its increase and decrease. It was a new world, a new universe, composed of sensations, feelings, and perceptions rather than the brute hardness of idea, thought, concept, as if the disintegration of the cortical surfaces—with all their heavy six layers of tissue—had sensitized and enriched the trio of delicate hippocampal tissues beneath. Surely, this was a world of organic and visceral boundaries rather than the cognitive walls that closely guarded one idea from another. Here things flowed and melted together; here identity and difference were the same and indistinguishable rather than isolated and hostile to one another. Here things were . . . well, they were . . . familiar, common, not antagonistic but sychronistic. It is hard to explain, hard to conceive these diameters of light and sound and scent. Perhaps one had to be there in order to really understand.

Beatrice—close by his bedside this sunny morning in springtime—watched it all without understanding any of it. But then how could she? For her, later this spring afternoon, there would be the light chatter of gossip, with tall cool drinks in frosted glasses and sweet perfume upon a balmy evening. That night she would stretch lazily upon cool, crisp sheets and drift off to sleep with neither pain nor a particular care in the world. She, after all, was well and in good health. But Murray was engaged in a desperate struggle for his life, for his existence, for some shred of solidity against the possibilities of death and nothingness. There were no springtimes for him, no lazy afternoons in which he rested or serene evenings of languid, catlike comfort. Instead, every minute, every hour, every day was a desperate struggle to remain something against forces that sought to make him nothing. How could she understand any of this? She was well, and he was desperately, deathly ill. She talked about diseases whereas he suffered them; she spoke of "poor Murray" while remaining enriched; she sat by his bedside dressed in cool linen while he sweated, twisted, and turned in soiled and diseased sheets all the while his disease devoured him. She said she suffered to watch him, while Murray did in fact suffer. It broke her poor heart to see him so—so she said—while his poor heart did actually break. She basked; he broke. She commiserated; he suffered. She

49

worried herself to death; he suffered himself to death. No, she could never understand what he underwent as there she sat in a linen dress, with cool brow, and in perfect health.

In the end, all death comes from anoxia. The heart may stop; the brain may die; the lungs may quit. The circumstances do not really matter, for these are but the several occasions by which anoxia comes to us. But when it does—and by whatever means it does—we are sequestered unto ourselves and thus deprived of this most elemental and primal force of air that sustains us. To suffocate—to feel the lungs grow weary and distended with incompetence—must be the most claustrophobic of experiences. To taste and feel the thick ropy mucus as it clogs the bronchi and alveoli is certainly a most maddening, a most terrifying ordeal. The lungs grow dense and heavy with their watery weight, and still one tries to draw in the precious air. The nostrils dilate and burn with the desperation of their effort, the throat cracks and breaks and bleeds from its failed efforts, the chest aches and heaves with exasperation, and still it is not enough. With all of this, the air won't come, and what little finally does bubbles through a slime of infected snot which mocks its desperation with further choking coughs. One tries not to breathe, to end it all quickly, but the body is too desperate to obey such intellectual suicide. It wants to live even if the brain desires to die. And so like a heaving, straining animal, the frightened lungs continue again and again their futile efforts until coma and unconsciousness discontinue this malice of self-observation and self-torture.

Murray died in such a way; he died wrapped about himself—actually holding on to himself for dear life—in a fetuslike position. Were it not for the gray hair, the wasted six-foot body, the wrinkled and puffy face, one might have thought him a child who had died of crib death, for so he seemed to be as he held himself in tortured silence. But Murray Wasserman was not a child but rather an old—a very old—man who died before his time and looked far more ancient than his sixty years could ever foretell. Is there some recompense, some justification to this cruelty of nature, that he suffered much and understood little? Where, after all, are meaning, purpose, and sense to be found if they cannot be understood?

3

Cushing's Monsters

Briton Hadden, Esq.   May 3, 1927
      25 West 45th Street
      New York City

Dear Mr. Hadden:

"Time" is an excellent journal which I read with interest and often with entertainment. I am quite sure that you would not wish to be entertaining at the risk of being cruel.

May I accordingly tell you something of the woman whose picture you published on page 17 of your issue of May 2nd under the caption of "Uglies"?

This unfortunate woman who sits in the sideshow of Ringling Brothers "between fat lady and Armless Wonder" and "affects white lace hats, woolen mittens and high laced shoes" has a story which is far from mirth-provoking. Could it have been written for you by O. Henry, it would have provoked tears rather than laughter. The facts are as follows:

She is, as you say, a peasant of Kent and four times a mother. The father of these four children, a truck gardener, died some years ago and left her their sole support. She, previously, a vigorous and good-looking young woman, has become the victim of a disease known as acromegaly. This cruel and

deforming malady not only completely transforms
the outward appearance of those whom it afflicts
but is attended with great suffering and often with
loss of vision.

   One of Mr. Ringling's agents prevailed upon
her to travel with the circus and to pose as the ug-
liest woman in the world as a means of livelihood.
Mr. Ringling is kind to his people and she is well
cared for. But she suffers from intolerable head-
aches, has become nearly blind, and permits herself
to be laughed at and heckled by an unfeeling people
in order to provide the wherewithal to educate her
four children. Beauty is but skin deep. Being a
physician, I do not like to think that "Time" can
be frivolous over the tragedies of disease.

Very sincerely yours,
Harvey Cushing, M.D.
Selected Papers on Neurosurgery

ACROMEGALY: The chromophil adenoma leads to the endocrine symptoms of hyperpituitarism, especially in the sphere of the growth hormone. When the tumour arises before growth has ceased, gigantism occurs. When, as more frequently happens, the tumour begins during adult life, acromegaly is the result. This is characterized by slow changes in the skin and subcutaneous tissue, bones, viscera, general metabolism, and sexual activity. The skin and subcutaneous tissues, especially of the fingers, lips, ears, and tongue, exhibit a fibrous hyperplasia. Overgrowth of the bones is most evident in the skull, face, mandible, and at the periphery of the extremities. The calvarium is thickened, the malar bones en-larged, and as the result of overgrowth of the mandible the lower jaw becomes prognathous and separation of the teeth occurs. The hands become broad and spade-like, and hyperostoses may develop on the terminal phalanges ('tufting'). Similar changes occur in the feet, and the patient frequently notices that he requires a larger size in gloves and boots. Kyphosis in the upper thoracic spine is common and enlargement of many of the viscera has been described. Carbohydrate metabolism is often disturbed, leading to hyperglycaemia and glycosuria. The metabolic rate is usually increased. Impairment of sexual function occurs in both gigantism and acromegaly.

Roger Bannister
Brain's Clinical Neurology

I

One Sunday afternoon Harvey Cushing sat back in his book-lined study to ask himself whether he had entered the right profession. It occurred to him that one should not trust nature. Do not ask of it aesthetic questions requiring the beautiful to be distinguished from the grotesque. For it knows no such differences and rather believes that all is beautiful, all is sublime and precious that is its own. Instead, it is we humans who speak of goddesses and monsters, of misformed and well-formed, of beauty and ugliness. Nature knows nothing of this. Wherein consists the difference between the sculptured brow of an Adonis and the prominent supraorbital ridge of fronto-metaphyseal dysplasia? Is it not merely one of degree, of curvature and kind? What is the proper dimension and proportion of the cranial vault? Should it be ten or twenty or thirty or forty inches in circumference? Are microcephalics more beautiful, more perfect, more delicate in their symmetry than macrocephalics? And what of eyes and spines and bones and brains? Should they be large or small, hidden or revealed, of this color or that? Nature accepts them all and believes that anything it creates is therefore beautiful and good.

These endless experiments of nature—for which life serves as the display room within which to place its products—are conducted without regard to beauty and ugliness. Blind natural forces palpitate by touch alone the rightness or wrongness of their creation and seem pleased with life at any level, at any cost, of any structure, shape, or degree. So there are no monsters but only the experimental entanglements of repeated architectural designs, different motifs, varying shapes and sizes in a constant quest for adaptation and survival. We have devised our own categories of perfection that nature quite ignores. For us, it is the average, the multiple imprints of the same design, the copies upon copies with nothing remarkable about them that are most ideal. For therein are safety, solace, and security in repetition.

But nature's ennui—its weariness with itself—causes it to tire easily and in its discontent to devise distractions, amusements, and differences of an extraordinary kind. It prefers the unusual within the usual; and while the average, the ordinary and common multiplicity will be tolerated, there must also exist extraordinary kinds and degrees of creatures. Not limited by a few overused templates, these are the latest and most recent inspirations of a restless nature which constantly becomes bored with itself.

It is only our vision, which constantly seeks similarity rather than difference, that reduces the something which is special, unique, and powerful about these specialties to the monstrous and malformed. One wonders with what vision monsters see themselves, whether they feel their monstrosity or rather their special uniqueness: are they frightened of themselves; disgusted with themselves; do they see themselves as glorious testimonials to the extraordinary—and therefore privileged—or as failed productions of the ordinary and usual?

On Sunday afternoon, April 11, 1909, Harvey Cushing sat down to write his father a letter. Despite endless interruptions from his own son about stamp collecting, it was quite a long letter, filled with all the usual things a son writes about to a father until near the end when he mentioned an acromegaly patient sent to him by Charles Mayo from Rochester, Minnesota.

J. H. was a farmer from South Dakota who was relatively healthy until the age of twenty-seven when he began to have intolerable headaches. These continued, increasing in severity, over the next eight years while several other alarming symptoms also appeared. His hands and feet grew not only in size but also in thickness and density; his fingers and toes elongated in a fibrous and spadelike fashion. His lips became thick and rubbery, and the skin upon his face became more leathery, more hidelike as subcutaneous tissues underwent fibrous hyperplasia. Most alarming of all, however, was the growth of his tongue, which was soon a cumbersome protrusion too dense to perform the subtle measures required of it. Finally within the last two years, the disturbance of his carbohydrate metabolism left him hyperglycemic, lethargic, and fatigued. His impotence and lack of energy were particularly troublesome to him, and at the age of thirty-five he sought medical counsel at the Mayo Clinic.

The only successful pituitary operation had been performed three years earlier by the German surgeon Schloffer in 1907. Cushing decided to attempt pituitary removal on March 25, 1909, just eighteen days before writing to his father. Access was achieved through the frontal sinuses, the route recommended by Schloffer, and invasion of the sella turcica disclosed a greatly enlarged anterior lobe of the pituitary. About one-third of this was removed—a technique often used with the thyroid in exophthalmic goiter—and the patient was up and about within six days. His photophobia and headaches were immediately relieved, and within weeks the thickening of hands, feet, tongue, and face was greatly reduced. It was—as Cushing himself remarked—a brilliant success!

Harvey Cushing at this time was within two weeks of his fortieth birthday and was already an established neurosurgeon; however, his work on acromegaly would soon earn him an international reputation. In fact, he reported on this case at the International Medical Congress held in Budapest during August 1909. By the time his monograph on *The Pituitary Body and Its Disorders* appeared in 1911 (the preface being dated September 11, 1911), Cushing had had forty-five patients with pituitary dysfunction, most of whom had undergone operations.

In addition to Cushing's professional interest, however, he had a fascination for anything that was extraordinary or unusual. For years, he wrote back and forth to the magician Karl

Germain, who was incidentally from Cushing's boyhood town of Cleveland, Ohio, and he liked nothing better than to visit the circus. He maintained a correspondence over the years with a large number of circus personalities, including giants and midgets, and visited them frequently. It was during one of these visits that Cushing came to know the English woman whose picture *Time* published under the caption "Uglies," and to whose defense Cushing rushed in his letter to the editor of May 2, 1927.

What then of Cushing and monsters? Mrs. Albert Bigelow, the Cushings' next-door neighbor in Brookline when they lived at 305 Walnut Street, remembered when Cushing first visited his acromegalic patient at the circus. We shall call the patient Edith for convenience' sake. We know certain facts about her from Cushing's judgmental letter to *Time* magazine on her behalf. She had four children whose support and education she provided through her work at the circus. This work consisted of becoming a spectacle, a monster of ugliness to the gawking ridicule of the paying visitors who stared at her night after night. The year was 1909, and such entertainment was regarded as proper for the whole family and in the spirit of good clean fun. One need only recall John Merrick, whose neurofibromatosis baptized him the "Elephant Man" at London's Bartholomew Fair just a few years before, to appreciate the climate of those times. Edith had been on display for some years at the Ringling Brothers Circus where her life had adjusted to a familiar routine among the midgets, giants, and other freaks. Originally from Kent, England, she was left with four children and no means of income when her husband died. An entrepreneur suggested that she profit, rather than merely suffer, from her illness, and she accepted the proposal.

To Cushing's biographer, John Fulton, Mrs. Bigelow recounted Cushing's first visit to Edith's living quarters in a circus railroad car.

> In one corner at the end of the car Harvey made his call on his strangely pathetic patient. She had arranged her children's photographs on the walls and had a few little knick-knacks about and had courageously made a semblance of a room of her own. She intro-

duced him to her friends, Half-a-Lady and the giants and dwarfs
before he left, and he said it was all such a strange combination of
something slightly comic and yet really so exceedingly tragic that
he felt torn between smiles and tears in telling about it. [p. 304]

Cushing's interest in acromegaly would continue for the
rest of his professional life. There is the charming story that his
curiosity about a giant's skeleton on display at the Hunterian
Museum was powerful enough to gain him access to the skull
so that he could measure the sella turcica. Yes, indeed, it was
enlarged.

On June 13, 1927, Cushing gave one of his last public
addresses on acromegaly to the Medical Society of London,
"Acromegaly from a Surgical Standpoint." His surgical work
continued, and on April 15, 1931, Cushing performed his
2,000th verified brain tumor operation; it was, of course, for
the removal of a pituitary tumor.

II

Edith Kennelworth-Hughes was—considering all that fate had
done to her—a kind and generous woman who forgave far
more readily than she forgot. She never forgot that she was
different and therefore quickly seemed to forgive those who
ridiculed her. In fact, the more she suffered at the hands of
others, the more accepting and gentler she became. Why this
was so, no one can truly say. Perhaps it was simply her nature
to be so, perhaps some deep psychological compensation so
compelled her, perhaps the Divine had blessed her with this
special gift of forgiveness. Who can say, and does it matter?
Sufficient to note that she was a good and decent woman who
was grateful for all that she had despite the fact that she deserved far more. She was grateful for her children, Stephen,
Robert, Elizabeth, and Stephanie, and grateful as well that
they were all healthy and had not inherited the curse that she
so bravely bore. It had occurred to her now and then that she
might be cursed, but if so, she just as quickly concluded, only
because she deserved it. What a strange person, she who
blamed herself more readily than others, but there seemed
within her nature to be some quality of acceptance that si-

lenced outrage, anger, and bitterness within her. She was not happy with life, of course not, but she was content and far more grateful for what she had than bitter over what she didn't.

What did she think of those long and no doubt boring hours spent in display upon the Freak's Rack at Ringling Brothers Circus? Well, frequently of her children, of course, and how they were doing at school. Robert and Stephanie were still in school in England, where they lived with relatives; Robert would soon go on to the university on scholarship. The children knew nothing of their mother's profession, and she had always insisted that it remain that way. So she thought often of them, worried about their grades and their friends, and longed to see them. But also there were her friends at the circus, and she spent much time attending to their needs. These were special friends, for in their company she was ordinary, common, and absolutely unremarkable; it was all the more for these reasons that she worried about their safety, their health, and their well-being. After all, they were more than merely friends; they were her community, her support group, and her confidants. She knew who among them suffered from desperate illnesses, and who slept with whom, and who plotted, revenged, and tried to destroy whom. She knew it all because the circus community was a close family in which nothing could be kept secret.

Did she sometimes long for a lover? Yes, indeed, what woman would not, and she just as often thought of her beloved husband Richard and of how beautiful she once had been. But survivors—and make no mistake, Edith Kennelworth-Hughes was alive today only because she was a survivor—quickly learn not to yearn and quest for that which is strictly forbidden to them. They—how best to say this?—learn to bend in the storms of misfortune rather than break, and that is precisely why they do survive. So, yes, indeed, a man who was loving and kind would have been very welcome on some of those more desperate and darker nights. But she adjusted. She survived. She endured.

Need it be noted, however, that the world is generally not kind or forgiving to the unfortunate, the deformed, and the misbegotten? It is a cruelty born out of the outrage and bitterness that such persons should impose themselves upon the rest of us. John Merrick certainly felt this prejudice, as did Richard Severo's Lisa H., whose neurofibromatosis often elicited similar comments. One day when she rode the school bus with the other children to grade school, the driver "looked at her now and smiled and cupped both his hands around her face, tenderly, as though he were her own father. Then he leaned over, put his face close to hers and said to her softly: 'My God, you are the ugliest thing I have ever seen in my life'" (p. 68).

So, yes, every monster knows that he or she is a monster, for we of the normal world insist upon so reminding them. But why is that so? What mixture of hatred and pity could inspire such loathing, and why are we so monstrous to monsters? Do we fear becoming one of them and thus inoculate ourselves against infection through a defensive aggression? Or is it rather that monsters do in fact litter the beautiful with their deformities and need to be reminded of their capacity to contaminate? Whatever the reason, it is certain that Edith was repeatedly reminded of the disgust she inspired.

"Oh, my God, look at that! Look at that. What is it?"

"Is it a man or a woman? Or a what!"

"Bertie, Bertie, over here, look over here. By God, did you ever see anything like it?"

"Oh, God, I can't look; I can't look at it."

"God, are you ugly!"

No doubt Edith had heard them all before and could even predict on any given night the hideous words her hideous self would inspire. Perhaps it no longer even hurt to hear, having now heard them all already. Perhaps, during such times, she thought of her children, of her husband Richard, of how beautiful she once had been, of how her friends were, of what she had had for dinner or a dozen other commonplace topics of immediate interest. The public had become—in their savagery—strangely predictable and therefore harmless. After all, the true cutting edge to the violent and the vicious lies precisely in being unexpected. When they lose that edge, they are no longer dangerous but only a nuisance. Yes, at best, they were an annoyance, a bother whose sting had departed from their barb through overuse and continual repetition. She forgave them. She forgave them everything and anything both because they were harmless and because they were boring. In the meantime, she thought of other things and simply tolerated their anonymous, annoying presence.

Although, it must be admitted, there were days when she regarded them and herself as well in quite different terms entirely. For, you see, there was a sense in which she had been baptized royalty by reason of her infirmities. After all, they came to see her; they paid to see her and even paraded in courtly fashion before her throne. In being singular and unique—while they were multiple and many—she enjoyed a specialness which they could only dream about. They were her public, her fans, her congregation, and she could do with them as she liked: withhold herself, flaunt herself, and in every possible way so glorify herself. There was an immense and sinister power in being feared and mocked by so many. It made her almost giddy, certainly prideful to realize that she occupied such an indispensable place in their lives. For once having seen her, they could not forget her; she held their memory captive and subject to her will through the most powerful emotions of revulsion and disgust. Yes, in her own domain and by her own rules, she was a queen without successor, having a following of subjects who were bound and captive by their very own fear and disgust.

And yet, there were the headaches. Those terrible, sinister, flesh-provoking headaches which seemed to tear her brain apart and then reassemble it the following morning. Dear God, the pain was incredible in its intensity and was often more than she could bear.

III

The pituitary gland celebrates its importance through the sella turcica that guards and protects it. No other gland, no other structure can make such boastful claims on its own behalf. And yet it has a right to boast, for herein lies the metabolic factory for somatotropin, corticotrophin (ACTH), thyrotrophin, and half a dozen other factors responsible for growth, lactation, thyroid function, sexuality, and metabolic equilibrium. Moreover, it resides in the company of other great systems. Not far away is the hypothalamus whose regulatory factors harmonize the metabolic tunes emitted from the ever active pituitary. Just above lies the great optic chiasm with its decussating fibers fanning about the sella turcica. All in all, perhaps we can forgive the arrogance of an organ which lives in such a neighborhood and controls so much around it.

And yet, it sometimes misbehaves. Perhaps not out of mischief but rather from the influence of either chromophil or acidophilic adenomas, but misbehave it nonetheless does and thereby creates tremendous havoc and confusion within the delicate chemistry of its own metabolism. Strange that these epithelioblastomata should choose this closely guarded sanctuary for their proliferation, but perhaps it is just the secretiveness of such environs that so attracts them. The effects of such mischief are not readily discerned by the heavy, gross measures of our daily behavior. Indeed, it never shows its subtlety or discernment in such delicate matters until the very last moment, although occasional and intermittent forages known as "fugitive acromegaly" do occur. But eventually all this haphazard and erratic chemistry makes its point, and the increase in glove or shoe size, the prognathism of jaws, the hyperostoses of the fingers inscribe an unmistakable configuration that refuses to be ignored. Should the eosinophilic aspect of the pituitary begin its hypersecretion of GH before epiphyseal closure is achieved, pituitary gigantism will result; but if the same events occur after epiphyseal closure, then periosteal and cortical thickening will increase the acral parts, and acromegaly results. It is all very strange this series of contradictory consequences from identical causes; it appears that if growth cannot be promoted at a gross level, it will be promoted at a discrete one. Thus, heart, kidneys, and other internal organs also increase in size, as well as fingers, jaws, hands, and feet. As intracranial pressure increases, headaches become frequent and finally constant in bitemporal distribution. At the same time, the optic chiasm begins to choke upon the ever expanding sella turcica, and compression produces optic atrophy. The bitemporal hemianopsia, headaches, and endocrine dysfunctions produce an internal caldron of agony which marches in symmetrical step to the external evidences of the disease process.

There are so many afflictions of bone and tissue that can twist the plasticity of the developing face into the strangest designs and diameters. The dysplasias—such as craniometaphyseal or frontometaphyseal—have the power to bend and boss bone into outrageous formations, while hyperostoses of bone—such as craniotubular or endosteal—will distort by overgrowth and entrapment what would have otherwise been a pleasing mandible or brow. These are, as it were, the cost-overruns of a metabolic chemistry which has totally lost its sense of proportion and priority. Here chemical equations and formulas transcend their invisibility to enunciate bone and tissue into patterns and avatars of their own structure.

This then is a monster: a metabolic furnace which consumes itself in a desperate search for balance and equilibrium. Its agony causes it to experiment constantly with overproductions and underproductions of chemical combinations as it strives to discover the proper integration that will finally restore harmony. But ultimately exhausted and disoriented by internal chaos, it will employ radical measures to correct minor miscalculations and thereby only intensify the fuels that consume it. What is hideous, ugly, and repulsive to behold about such creatures is precisely all this inner chaos, disorder, and confusion which merely madden and inflame the source with its own failures.

IV

About twelve years before his death, and within five years of his retirement from Harvard, Cushing was invited to give the annual oration before the Medical Society of London in June 1927. The paper he delivered, "Acromegaly from a Surgical Standpoint," was so long that it had to be published in two sections in the *British Medical Journal*.

After reviewing some experimental evidence on acromegaly with animal studies, Cushing proceeded to recount some of his own surgical cases. These are interesting as much for what they tell us about Cushing, who inherited Sir William Osler's charm of personalizing everything he observed, as for what they reveal about the early treatment of acromegaly. Despite Cushing's own confession "that in the report of these few cases I have put my best foot forward so far as it concerns the influencing by operation of the secondary effects on hyperpituitarism," it must be admitted that his results are impressive. Two cases in particular should be mentioned as well as the details of his 2,000th verified brain tumor operation on April 15, 1931.

(Surg. No. 26204): A Russian tailoress, 23 years of age, unmarried, was admitted to hospital on April 22, 1926, with the usual complaint of severe headaches. She had been known to have acromegaly for a number of years, and on the advice of her physician she had been given a series of deep x-ray treatments, which had failed to alleviate her discomforts. Meanwhile her catamenia, which had set in at the age of 14 years, continued without interruption, though she had become somewhat masculinized and, for her sex, extremely hirsute.

She had the typical enlarged extremities, hypertrophic nose, lips, and tongue of a fairly advanced case of acromegaly, and the spine showed well-marked kyphosis. Her height was 171 cm., and her weight 84.6kg. The sella turcica was not greatly enlarged and there were no local pressure signs. The basal metabolic rate was +24 per cent, though the thyroid was not palpable.

On May 10, 1926, by the customary transphenoidal route a fairly radical removal of the glandular contents of the sella was accomplished by pituitary rongeurs and sucker. The tissue showed a typical acidophilia adenoma. Within a week after the operation there had taken place a marked diminution in the puffiness of the hands, the skin having become thinner, softer, and more pliant. [*Selected Papers on Neurosurgery*, p. 387]

There are several interesting points to be noted about Cushing's working methods. First is his compulsion for detail and precision. He was known to be an avid doodler and a very accomplished sketcher, and thus one usually finds quite detailed drawings accompanying his surgical notes. But this same precision also demanded absolute quiet within the operating amphitheater unless the conversation was on the business at hand. Cushing's need to control every aspect of the situation made him a great surgeon, but it also made him a fair number of enemies. It is said that he and Walter Dandy, who once had been his resident, would only acknowledge one another's presence with a curt nod. One day during neurological rounds Cushing had asked another one of his residents to examine a patient's eye carefully. The resident described the eye as perfectly normal with no signs of pathology whatsoever. At this point Cushing produced a ballpoint pen and snapped it against the glass eye that the resident had declared to be perfectly normal. However, to his patients—and especially to children—he was kind almost to a fault. When necessary, he could remove a cerebellar tumor from a youngster using only local anesthesia and charm. Cushing was a remarkable man, and part of what made him a great surgeon was not simply his willingness to go where no man had ever gone before—after all, Horsley had done that with humiliating failure—but rather the strict attention to detail that personalized everything he did. It was this characteristic which led him to develop the transphenoidal access route to the pituitary rather than the more direct but far more disfiguring method through the frontal sinuses used by Schloffer. In fact, as with the case above, he always insisted upon using this method with women, who were especially sensitive about their appearance.

Cushing's diagnostic and surgical skills are clearly illustrated in the next case, a twenty-two-year-old female whose headaches began after her first pregnancy and delivery. Her features increased in size and density, along with a weight increase to 213 pounds and considerable hirsuteness.

> (Surg. No. 25410): She had an enlarged and palpable thyroid and a basal metabolic rate of +25 per cent. There was also a slight glycosuria. She was looked upon as a possible case of acromegaly, but there was some uncertainty about this, and as her sella turcica was not definitely enlarged she was given some general directions and referred to the ambulatory clinic.
>
> She was kept under observation for a month of ineffectual study. She might well enough have been regarded as having polyglandular syndrome of some sort, not necessarily hypophyseal in origin, though, as a matter of fact, all hypophyseal disorders are polyglandular. On the basis of her enlarged metabolism and enlarged thyroid, Lugal's solution was given a prolonged trial, but this failed to lower her basal metabolic rate in the slightest. It was finally decided that primary hyperpituitarism could alone account

64

for her symptoms, and in spite of the small sella, it was proposed to operate, with the double purpose of checking her subjective discomforts, if possible, and at the same time combating the constitutional effects of the disorder.

Accordingly, on September 20, 1926, by the customary transsphenoidal route a fairly radical extirpation of the sellar contents was made. The tissue proved histologically to be a typical chromophil adenoma.

She made an excellent operative recovery with immediate cessation of the headaches. Her glycosuria, which had been constantly present during the preoperative period of study, had disappeared on the following day, and the urine remained sugar-free for the next month while she was kept under observation. There was a coincidental drop in blood sugar to below 0.1 per cent. Successive 48-hour metabolism determinations showed a progressive fall from +25 per cent on the morning of the operation to +3 per cent on Sept. 30, 10 days afterward, at which level it remained. There was a definite diminution in the measured size of her hands, the previously wet and puffy skin became normally dry and supple. At the time of her discharge, on Oct. 20, without dietary restrictions, she had lost 3kg in weight. [Ibid., p. 389]

Both of these cases were patients with few radical secondary characteristics of hyperpituitarism. Moreover, in both instances, improvement of symptoms was immediate and dramatic, probably because there was very little bone malformation; bone is not, of course, reabsorbed as is soft tissue. Cushing did, as he himself admitted, present his most encouraging cases, but they were not all such splendid successes. By May 1, 1927, he had performed 291 operations for suspected adenoma with 264 of these being verified. Of the 253 operations performed by the transphenoidal route, there was a 6.7 percent mortality rate (17 patients); and of the 38 performed by the transfrontal route, there was a 5 percent fatality rate (2 patients). He gave no figures for postoperative recovery, nor was he certain whether "the fragments of adenomatous tissue almost inevitably left behind may not revive and produce further hyperpituitary symptoms" (ibid., pp. 389–90).

Cushing's 2,000th verified tumor operation was quite an affair. He was sixty-two years old, soon to retire within months.

His entire staff assembled for the occasion on Wednesday afternoon, April 15, 1931, and Louise Eisenhardt took care to provide tumor statistics that demonstrated a steadily lowered mortality rate over the past ten years. The operation was photographed by both aerial camera and conventional cameras. Afterwards, there was a tea party which rivaled—so John Fulton tells us—only that of the party held for his sixtieth birthday. Cushing's postoperative notes detail the procedure:

> This woman has a mild grade of acromegaly associated with bad headaches and a moderately enlarged sella. The fields of vision have not been particularly definite and I consequently was somewhat uneasy in regard to what we would find, fearing that there might be a prefixed chiasm between the legs of which I would be unable to accomplish very much in the way of removing the adenoma. As a matter of fact, the chiasm was found widely expanded and I am sure that the bitemporal hemianopias must have been much more definite than was supposed. The operation was relayed with Dr. Horrax. It happened to be our 2000th verified tumor which led to a display of cameras and searchlights somewhat inhibiting one's customary surgical reflexes which are at their best when a surgeon is unconscious of his surroundings and the fact that anyone is looking on. [Fulton, *Harvey Cushing*, p. 604]

Of all that Harvey Cushing did for medicine—and he did so very much—it would be difficult to find a single disease process which more fully consumed the length and breadth of his professional life than the surgical treatment of hyperpituitarism. The only near rival would, of course, be his monumental monograph on *Meningiomas* published in 1938 but started in 1915 immediately after completion of his 1912 monograph on *The Pituitary Body*. Thus, not planned but evolved, there is a natural integrity to Cushing's life, which appropriately began and ended with disorders of the pituitary body. Even satellite and suburban interests—such as circuses, magicians, monsters, freaks, and the curious in general—find their centrality in this consuming interest.

v

The world is very unforgiving. It will forgive evil, injustice, and cruelty far more readily than it will forgive ugliness. Perhaps

66

the crimes of the latter are more hideous precisely because they are the more irresponsible. Horatio was right in saying that "we can forgive men for what they do in the name of evil, but God help us for what they do in the name of good!" In the name of good, the monsters of the world have been persecuted by decent folk. In the name of good, the ordinary, mediocre, and unexceptional have been glorified precisely for what they lack rather than what they have. In the name of good, monsters have been jailed, sequestered, and institutionalized in order to contain the seeds of their infectious deformity. In the name of good, we isolate ourselves from all that endangers our averageness. In the name of good, persecution becomes pardonable, fear becomes righteous hatred; and in the name of good we draw the standard that distinguishes the beautiful from the grotesque.

But precisely what is it that we find so hateful about monsters? Do we fear infection or contamination? Is it perhaps natural to despise the unnatural, and how does one distinguish the biologically acceptable from the biologically repugnant? There appears to be a security, even a salvation, in isolating ourselves from the disorder of differences. Blacks with blacks, whites with whites, men with men, and women with women, normals with normals, and the beautiful in careful contradistinction from the ugly. It is a form of prejudice this business of identifying the monsters of the world and then exiling them to their own domain of sideshows, circuses, and institutions. One is safe in knowing that one is not one of them. And safe also in realizing that the immense chasm between the privileged and the damned cannot be traversed by a single leap or bound.

We shall therefore glorify ourselves through their damnation. We shall ennoble, enrich, and empower ourselves precisely through their impoverishment. And all that is wrong, disabled, and depraved about them shall be right, good, and proper about us. For we are the chosen privileged of the earth; it is the certainty of our genetic fitness that provides for our continuance in just the same way that their imperfections demand extinction and discontinuance of all that they are and have become. They are weak, whereas we are strong. They are damaged, whereas we are perfect. They are turned, twisted

67

upon their very chromosomal axis, and therefore wrought asunder, whereas, we are straight, to the mark, and correctly formed. Moreover, we know who we are precisely because we know who they are. As such, they are the yardstick and measuring device by which we calculate the dimensions of our own health. How grateful we are for monsters, for without them there could not be gods and goddesses!

4

October

Something has spoken to me in the night, burning the tapers of the waning year, something has spoken in the night, and told me I shall die, I know not where.

Saying: To lose the earth you know, for greater knowing; to lose the life you have, for greater life; to leave the friends you loved, for greater loving; to find a land more kind than home, more large than earth—

Whereon the pillars of this earth are founded, toward which the conscience of the world is tending—a wind is rising, and the rivers flow.

Thomas Wolfe
Of Time and the River

MILIARY TUBERCULOSIS: When metastic foci are located near blood vessel lumina, development of hypersensitivity and its attendant necrosis may result in secondary reseeding of the bloodstream, causing early postprimary tuberculous septicemia (hyperacute miliary TB). High fever and general toxicity are usually present. Tuberculous meningitis is a common complication, particularly in young children. Early in the course, the X-ray may be negative because inflammatory foci are small; the tuberculin test may also be negative. Chorodial tubercles are usually present and are important in diagnosis. Cultures of sputum or gastric contents are often positive; urine cultures are occasionally positive even without demonstrable GI involvement. Examination and culture of the bone marrow or liver may provide the only evidence of tuberculous infection; fiberoptic transbronchial lung biopsy is more often productive than either bone marrow or liver biopsy.

Late hematogenous dissemination or chronic hematogenous TB follows breakdown of a longstanding, previously quiescent and undetected, usually extrapulmonary focus of TB. Multiple, widely spaced episodes of bacteremic seeding may occur from these foci. This may produce a serious febrile illness much like that occurring soon after initial infection, but may produce a less acute process with low grade of absent fever, anemia, and wasting. In some, the usual cellular components of the inflammatory process may be lacking, a process termed nonreactive TB, in which myriads of tubercle bacilli exist in the tissues with only a sparse nonspecific cellular response. The clinical manifestations may be extremely subtle, consisting simply of loss of appetite and weight, and failure to thrive. Fever may be absent. Marrow involvement occasionally produces syndromes resembling primary hematologic disease such as refractory anemia, thrombocytopenia and leukemoid reaction.

Robert Berkow
The Merck Manual

I

Later, the day would break clean and brilliant across the Johns Hopkins University Hospital. But now it was still dark and rather cool for September 15, 1938. High up, against the darkness, there was at least one room illuminated by the vigil of family members waiting for a loved one to die. For the past three days, their brother, their son, their friend had lain in a coma from exploratory brain surgery. At first he rallied, but then yesterday—or was it the day before?—the old and subtle enemies of pneumonia and pulmonary infection had sought him out and found him without defenses. Now it was almost 6:30 A.M. on a Thursday morning, and within minutes Thomas Wolfe would be dead. Had he lived but another eighteen days, he would still have only been thirty-eight years old. How strange that death should find him there, in that place which also had claimed his father.

When the details of his death became known, some would claim that all of his genius, all of his power and eloquence were simply the insanity of a diseased brain seeking to free itself from its misery. Cruel? Yes, of course, certainly cruel. But far more strange than cruel. How strange to reduce a human spirit to the agony it endured. How strange to denounce in a single judgment all that was rich, poetic, glorious, and supremely human to the erratic cell division of a pathological process. Such denouncements, in effect, deny that the artist has seen beauty and claim instead that he has simply suffered madness.

Others, however, would hear of his death and feel the earth shudder for just a moment. They mourned for him, but far more for themselves and for the lost words, the beautiful phrases, and the powerful insights that had now disappeared from history. And still others cared little about his death or his life because he meant nothing to them, and they felt no change in the climate or condition of the earth.

What shall we make of an artist's death? After all, is there anything to be made of it at all? He is not special or different from other men who have lived and suffered in similar ways. Does the artist enjoy any special privileges that should make him immune to destruction? Why then should we be surprised or even disturbed by his death? Is the world any better for having entertained briefly Chaucer, Shakespeare, Michelangelo, Dante, Eliot, and Wolfe? Their words, their works were beautiful to behold, but what of that? They often agonized more and certainly spoke more about their agony and in finer words, but what of that? They thought about their lives and often about their deaths, but we have also seen what they have seen and has it made us any better? So what of all this?

Perhaps it is true that these artists are howling madmen who overexaggerate their suffering and break vows of silence that the rest of us choose to keep sacred. Perhaps too much can be made of an artist's death in September. He wrote fine words, yes, and saw great things, yes, but what of all that for us who have seen the same and remained silent?

Tuberculosis has always been a disease of artists. One cannot think of Keats, of Chopin and fail to associate the suffering of their lives with the suffering of their art. Pale, wan, and emaciated from the power of their remarkable gifts, those who create seem ultimately to be destroyed by internal engines too powerful to be contained within the slender frame of the poet. It is a most romantic notion, but appropriately so when used to describe artists such as Keats, Chopin, and Wolfe.

However, tuberculosis is not simply of the lungs or of the bone or of the brain, but rather of each and all of these. It is especially fond of seeking residence in the great dynamic centers of our lives: where we think or where we breathe or even in the skeletal cement that holds us together. For herein it can do what it does best: consume. Tuberculosis is a disease which devours, consumes, and finally digests its victim, and in this regard it is a disease much like cancer. But the latter is a madness gone wild which consumes without reason and without plan; whereas, tuberculosis is a madness in perfect control of itself. So true is this that the disease may wait patiently in remissive tissue for years until some sudden spark of inspiration causes it to roam in search of new histological territories. Certainly this was true of Thomas Wolfe that ill-begotten summer of 1938.

Wolfe was invited to speak at Purdue University on May 19, 1938. It was the usual academic affair with professors from each department waiting to meet him and get his autograph. After his talk at Purdue, he traveled to Chicago, and then a few days later he boarded a sleek and powerful train—the Burlington Zephyr—and left for Denver with the claim that both coach bars on board would be dry before he arrived. From Denver, he went to Portland and from Portland to Seattle. His arrival and eventual return to Seattle were interrupted by a two-week hiatus in which he traveled with two other companions to eleven parks in the western states. Back in Seattle, he departed once again for Vancouver on the steamer *Princess Kathleen*. But in transit he caught a very bad cold and shortly thereafter returned to Seattle. Within days, Wolfe's cold had turned into pneumonia, and at the urging of friends he entered a private hospital for treatment. Despite three days of high fever and alarming symptoms, Wolfe considered himself to be out of danger by July 15. In fact, however, the danger was just beginning, and in his euphoria at being cured of the pneumonia he failed to recognize an even more insidious enemy at work.

There are diseases whose power and fury overwhelm the victim with a savage intensity. They neither court nor seduce nor beckon with sly and retiring ways but instead rape, pillage, and plunder what few reserves remain. But tuberculosis is not one of these. Rather, it toys, experiments, and tantalizes in the most unpredictable ways. There are days when you seem almost symptom free and days as well when your very bones and tissues are rent asunder by pain of indescribable proportions. It is a strange illness which seems either to sleep or to roam with restless energy as it did with Thomas Wolfe that summer of 1938. For within him, the lesions of a past tubercular scarring began to blossom once again very much as a rose in springtime responds to warmth and soil and moisture by bursting forth. Breaking all bounds of propriety and limitation, the tubercular seeding freed itself from the confines of the lungs, sought out the large bronchial blood vessels, and migrated in dozens of different directions.

There exists an invisible but extremely powerful blood-brain barrier which captures most illnesses within its entanglements before they can invade that closed casket of thoughts, ideas, and feelings. Even the great viral infections are usually stopped by this overseer which carefully inquires into the precise credentials of each traveler. But tuberculosis can be so very charming, so innocent and pure of malevolent intentions that even this most powerful governor is often deceived and thereby allows to pass a Trojan horse of insidious design which masquerades as another. Climbing slowly from lungs to brain, the metastatic foci are in search of fertile ground in which to raise their violent young. They pass by the smooth, pink cardiac tissue and mount even beyond the airy, wispy stretch of alveoli, reaching higher, ever higher. Quickly traveling beyond the most inviting carotid arteries—tempted but not seduced by their loveliness—even beyond the fierce, powerful sternocleidomastoid muscles and still yet beyond the white, barren

73

starkness of mastoid and maxillary bone, the tubercles pursue their mission of metaplasia. They wish to transform, to claim healthy tissue into the geography of their own domain. Finally, finally, there is a landmark seen in the distance. There, wrapped and coiled about itself like an endless snake, entwine the cerebral twists of puffy gray cortex.

The tubercles are excited—even erotically aroused—by the moist, delicious fields of gray flesh that await them much as an outstretched lover invites penetration. They kiss—but ever so lightly—the delicate pink folds, and even as they do so also does the flesh, in turn, seem to sigh its sweet consent. Stroking now with eager fingertips, the tubercles—swollen with the fluid serum of their mycobacteria—caress gently, ever so gently, the spirals, twists, and flanges of flesh. Perhaps it would be all right for just a moment to lie serene within those welcome convoluted folds of moist, mauve tissue. Could it, after all, be so very wrong to rest content in such safe havens? Deep within are thoughts, ideas, and perhaps even feelings, lusts, and erotic longings. How delightful it would be to pierce those coils and convolutions in order to diffuse oneself within. Their desire is innocent and pure; it is to penetrate, even as a lover does, the depths of this fragrant moisture, to find warmth and pulse within, to implant the fragile seeds of mycobacteria and death just as a lover conceives the beloved. Can that be so wrong? After all, they are not the aggressive and angry disease rapists such as carcinoma, sarcoma, or myeloma. No, these gentle tubercles rather seduce and woo their beloved with whispered sighs and ruby pouted lips. They penetrate the beloved not by persecution but by persuasion. And yet, penetrate they do indeed.

Just as the lover caresses the beloved, so do they now caress the gentle, tender brain beneath them. It is so moist, so warm that to devour its flesh with full lips would be divine. Deep now, so very deep, they stretch the invitation of their longing only to find the tissues willingly part in welcome—if nonetheless coquettish—acceptance. Intimacy is the attainment of unity between polarities otherwise held in opposition. And within this opposition of health and disease, of life and death, there is the constant beckoning of one to become the other.

The lovers vibrate in rhythmical union of a duality now become one, and so also does the tubercle quiver as it becomes the brain that it invades and the brain becomes it as well. Union is achieved, conception is assured, the promise of birth is portended by the gentle shudder of the brain as its moist and fragrant coils twist in orgasmic acceptance of all that has happened to it and all that it shall become.

But if tuberculosis is like a lover, so also is it like a child. It does not wish death, destruction, or pain but rather life. Its ultimate desire is not to hate but to love and so bring about a rebirth, a reproduction of itself. Can something so completely natural, so innocent as the desire to live be therefore so very wrong? Now the seeds just planted in mutual desire will grow and multiply as the metastatic foci proliferate and exfoliate themselves in dozens, then hundreds, then thousands, and finally millions of tubercles foaming and forming over the delicate brain surface.

II

Dear God, the headaches were terrible in their awful intensity! Starting now at the temple points and then expanding outward like a Chinese fan, they curled and coiled and cantilevered across the brow, down the neck and seemed to vibrate all the cranial nerves from trigeminal to glossopharyngeal. But more than the pain, far more than simply the agony of it all was the terrific and terrible pressure that seemed to verge on the explosion or implosion of the gentle tissues so compressed. And with each and every pulsation of his heart, there emanated a wave of such profound pain and nausea that he thought he could barely stand the passing moments. Every diastole and every corresponding systole produced a contrapuntal expansion and contraction of the nauseating, pressurized pain. It was intolerable; it was unendurable! Dear God, if only it would stop for just a few moments. But neither sleep nor drugs distracted its intensity.

On August 12 the headaches began in earnest, and they did not depart until Wolfe died thirty-four days later. The agony of those thirty-four days was unceasing. On the afternoon of the same day, Wolfe wrote to his former friend and editor at Scribner's, Maxwell Perkins (*Editor to Author*, p. 141):

> Dear Max:
>
> I'm sneaking this against orders—but "I've got a hunch"—and I wanted to write these words to you.
>
> I've made a long voyage and been to a strange country, and I've seen the dark man very close; and I don't think I was too much afraid of him, but so much mortality still clings to me—I wanted desperately to live and still do and I thought about all of you 1000 times, and wanted to see you all again, and there was the impossible anguish and regret of all the work I had not done, of all the work I had to do—and I know now I'm just a grain of dust, and I feel as if a great window has been opened on life I did not know about before—and if I come through this, I hope to God I am a better man, and in some strange way I can't explain, I know I am a deeper and a wiser one. If I get on my feet and out of here, it will be months before I head back, but if I get on my feet, I'll come back.
>
> Whatever happens—I had this "hunch" and wanted to write you and tell you, no matter what happens or has happened, I shall always think of you and feel about you the way it was that 4th of July 3 yrs. ago when you met me at the boat, and we went out on the cafe on the river and had a drink and later went on top of the tall building and all the strangeness and glory and the power of life and of the city were below.
>
> Yours always,
> Tom

Perkins trembled when he read the letter, for it was a certain death knell rung by the one whose passing it would announce.

X rays taken throughout the month of August showed the lesion on his right lung to be contracting in size. By the seventeenth, a large tubercular patch had miniaturized to the size of an egg, and by the twenty-sixth it had been further reduced to about the size of a quarter. The headaches continued, but all tests indicated that he was improving and even recovering. In truth, however, the tubercular assault had simply moved its line of frontal attack from lung to brain and passed the blood-brain barrier in a flash of fever which everyone assumed marked the end of a crisis, whereas, in fact, it merely marked a beginning.

By September 13 Wolfe's new doctor—his brother Fred had dismissed Dr. Ruge and replaced him with Dr. Watts—checked Wolfe's optic disks with an ophthalmoscope. What he saw that fateful day was a severe swelling, or papilledema, of the disk with very prominent veins and small congested hemorrhages emanating out in a fanlike shape. Since the brain is a closed vessel of bony climate and condition, it cannot announce its inner distress except through pressure, and then only at elected sites and in highly restricted ways. One of these ways is by pressurizing the optic nerve and so causing the retinal disk to bulge or choke. These agonizing pleas and cries of anguish from the brain cannot be taken lightly and certainly can never be ignored.

The brain is such a strange organ! It is the first to sense danger elsewhere but the very last to recognize such trauma within itself. The eyes, the ears, and all the cavities of the brain are the sentinels that monitor disorder and chaos everywhere else but are blinded to such confusion within themselves. The eye sees but cannot see itself seeing. The ear hears but cannot discern the subtle tones of its own hearing. The brain feels the body feeling but is anesthetized to feeling itself. Why? Why does it chose to operate according to such contradictory directives? Would it overwhelm itself with feeling if it also felt? Would the eye blind itself with seeing, or the ear become deaf to hearing, if just this additional ingredient of self-consciousness were added to an already overburdened set of responsibilities? Held captive by a bony cranium which permits neither retreat nor advance, the brain is riveted in place. It cannot expand, neither can it contract, but remains a fruit whose outer seed prohibits internal blossoms. Consequently, every swelling, every shift, every movement is experienced not as pain but as pressure. And as the pressure increases, so does it intimidate and pester everything that has the vanity of feeling: eyes, muscles, meninges, and nerves of every length and caliber.

With the headaches, as so often is the case, came confusion and disorientation. By now, Wolfe's family was convinced of his certain and most desperate illness. His sister Mabel contacted a neurologist recommended by Harper's, Wolfe's publisher, and Dr. Swift arrived that very evening to examine Wolfe. He confirmed the observation of choked disks and agreed that Wolfe should be sent to Walter Dandy at the Johns Hopkins School of Medicine. Wolfe and his sister Mabel boarded the Olympian Express at 10:30 the evening of September 6 for Baltimore, Maryland. Within ten days, Thomas Wolfe's agony would be over, for he would die early the morning of September 15 of radically disseminated miliary tuberculosis.

III

Walter Dandy had been one of Harvey Cushing's most loyal and brilliant residents at Johns Hopkins. Unfortunately, the very intellectual energy that made him brilliant also made him independent and often arrogant. Since Cushing himself was both blessed and cursed by the same qualities, the chemistry of the two neurosurgeons was explosive and dangerous in such close combination. For example, Cushing believed that some of his own ideas in the 1917 monograph *Tumors of the Nervus Acusticus and the Syndrome of the Cerebellopontine Angle* appeared five years later in Dandy's surgical note "An Operation for the Total Extirpation of Tumors in the Cerebellopontine Angle" which was published in the 1922 *Bulletin of the Johns Hopkins Hospital* (33:344–45). Cushing immediately sat down and sent a handwritten note to Dandy in which he accused his former resident of "bad taste, bad manners" and suggested the need to acquire "a high plane of professional ethics" (Fulton, *Harvey Cushing*, p. 490). Needless to say, it was overkill on Cushing's part, and Dandy never forgave the insult. It was also quite unfair because Dandy's surgical method represented an advance over the standard procedure introduced by Cushing in 1917. Cushing had argued for a partial and incomplete removal of tumors occurring in this very delicate area of the cerebellopontine angle, whereas Dandy had been successful in completely removing an entire tumor in a patient, who had a full recovery. Dandy's approach to the tumor was different from Cushing's as well, and it was this novel aspect of his procedure that made total extirpation of tumors possible by a suboccipital exposure of the cerebellum. Actually, the tension between the two men extended back nearly eleven years when Dandy had been selected as Cushing's research assistant in the Hunterian Laboratory for the 1910–11 academic year.

All of this is most regrettable, for at the time of Thomas Wolfe's illness neurosurgery was in great need of cooperation rather than competition. It was a very new and very risky specialty with few men of courage choosing to enter these most troubled waters and dangerous undertides. Cushing had retired from active practice just five years before and would himself die the following year on October 7, 1939, just four days past Thomas Wolfe's birthday. (Interestingly enough, Cushing's own autopsy showed tubercular scarring of both lungs.) With Cushing in retirement, neurosurgery was left to his successors, of whom Dandy—along with Wilder Penfield—was probably the shining star. After all, Dandy's radical approach to neurosurgery—in marked contrast to Cushing's more conservative approach—had credited him with the introduction of several innovative measures including ventriculography.

If Walter Dandy was the best surgeon available for Wolfe, then Johns Hopkins was the best hospital. Cushing had once been on the staff, Sir William Osler had planned the curriculum for the medical school, and William Halsted had operated there. Wolfe was suspicious of all hospitals, but especially of Hopkins because it was here that his father had been brought for repeated radiation treatments of his prostate cancer. In his mind, Hopkins could either kill you or cure you depending upon its whim.

Dandy probably deduced the hopelessness of Wolfe's condition immediately. Examination of his choked disks would have shown swelling and perhaps hyperemia of the optic nerve head—caused often by tortuosity of the retinal veins—and the elevation of the disks could be measured in diopters of swelling. Most often it is a brain tumor—but occasionally a hematoma, an abscess, or meningitis—that produces such extreme intracranial pressure. In any case there is always trauma of a holocaustic sort responsible for such optic agony. Frequently, a glioblastoma or astrocytoma will produce such symptoms, but Dandy would have known that such tumors are so invasive that any hope of their removal must be based on faith rather than knowledge or skill. Miliary tuberculosis was equally fatal at the time, and so were the half dozen other conditions that could produce such pressure. In fact, only a perfectly benign tumor or an abscess could be treated, and then only if, first, it was located in just the right place and, second, it was completely encapsulated. Dandy did not give the family very much hope, and he was perfectly correct in so doing.

Nonetheless, Dandy did perform a decompression procedure on Wolfe on Friday afternoon, September 9. A suboccipital decompression of the posterior fossa is accessed by occipital craniectomy and exposure of the dura layers. It is neither a treatment nor a diagnostic procedure in the strictest sense but rather a palliative measure intended to relieve pressure from an intracranial mechanism. This technique is quite ancient—originally referred to as trephining—and consists of introducing a small borehole into the cranial vault in order to relieve the pressure. The pressure in Wolfe's cranium was so intense that cerebrospinal fluid shot several feet into the air. The procedure almost always has the desired result of reducing pressure—and therefore pain—but only for a brief period of time. In Wolfe's case, it had precisely these immediate results, and he was so happy to be rid of his headaches that he thought himself cured. But the relief was only momentary, and the original problem was not solved but only postponed.

On Monday morning, September 12, Wolfe again was taken to the operating amphitheater where Dandy stood ready with his surgical team. Dandy's fourteen-year-old son, who would later follow in his father's professional footsteps and himself become a surgeon, was permitted to watch the operation. It is most likely that operation was conducted under the standard procaine-ether anesthesia with transoccipital osteoplastic flap reflection. The dura and arachnoid layers were exposed to permit access to the cortical hemispheres, and it was then that Dandy discovered hundreds of small tubercular lesions covering their surface. He closely examined the lesions, laid his scalpel down, and instructed his assistant to close up. Elizabeth Nowell, Wolfe's agent and early biographer, recounted the events that followed.

Annie Laurie Crawford [a friend of the Wolfe family and originally from Asheville] had been replaced by Dandy's specially trained surgical nurses, but at the Wolfe family's insistence, she had stayed on with them as a friend. Dandy had given her permission to watch the operation, and the family, still distrustful of doctors and of surgery, had persuaded her to do it so that she could tell them everything that happened. Now suddenly, she came running down the corridor to the little waiting room. Her face was as white as her operating gown, and she was weeping. "He didn't operate," she said. "They opened up Tom's skull, and Dr. Dandy took one look and laid his scalpel down."

Dandy himself came right behind her, still in the white suit and skullcap of the operating room. "The case is hopeless," he said grimly. "He has miliary tuberculosis of the brain. His brain is simply covered with tubercles—there must be millions of them there." Later, after the family's first outburst of shock and grief he explained the case more fully. At some time in his youth, Wolfe had tuberculosis of the lung, but it had cured itself, and the lesion had healed over, sealing up the tubercles inside. Then when he had contracted pneumonia in Seattle in July, the lesion had reopened, the tubercles had gone into his blood stream and finally had been carried to his brain. "He may live for six weeks more," said Dandy, "and we can keep him fairly comfortable. But it is absolutely hopeless. If he can die now, without recovering from the operation—as he may within the next three days—it will be much better." [*Thomas Wolfe*, p. 438]

Wolfe was a dying man at that time in history and under those conditions. In fact, he was a dying man the very moment the tubercles passed the blood-brain barrier.

Today, Thomas Wolfe would still have had a very rocky road to recovery and certainly some irreversible brain damage had he recovered, but he might well have lived. Diagnosed early enough, he would have been immediately placed on a regimen of 10 mg/kg/day of isoniazid, 600 mg/day of rifampin, and 15 mg/kg/day of ethambutol. Surgery would still be completely useless, but a daily regimen of a single oral dose of this chemotherapy would have been effective. The treatment would need to be continued for at least eighteen months and most likely for two years. At first, an intramuscular injection of streptomycin would be given each day for two weeks and then continued twice a week for the next two or three months. At present, with the instituted regimen prescribed and early diagnosis the recovery rate from miliary tuberculosis is close to 90 percent. Isoniazid, the hydrazide of isonicotinic acid, is a white crystalline powder which is water soluble and very effective against actively growing tubercle bacilli. Rifampin is an antibiotic which interacts with the RNA polymerase of bacteria. It is never used alone, however, but always in combination with either ethambutol or isoniazid. Ethambutol hydrochloride is a chemotherapeutic agent effective against the mycobacteria that produce the characteristic symptoms of tuberculosis. It is marketed by Lederle Laboratories in tablet form under the trade name Myambutol.

Thomas Wolfe died at 6:30 A.M. Thursday morning nearly four days after the operation. For most of this time, he was in a coma with delirium and some convulsions. When he did die, it was not of tuberculosis but of pneumonia. The great diseases—cancer, heart dysfunction, tuberculosis—are rarely the cause of our death, although they are certainly the cause of our suffering. Rather, it is the nosocomial infections caused by *Klebsiella*, *Proteus*, *Candida*, or *Enterobacter* that wait in silent expectation of our weakened condition. With a genius and a planning all their own, these opportunistic infections reside within the safe confines of hospitals and sickrooms where the visitor seeking an angel of death obediently comes to them. Their mission is not to degrade, degenerate, or decompose living tissues—this heavy work is left for the catastrophic diseases such as lymphatic leukemia, hypogammaglobulinemia, myeloma, or macroglobulinemia—but rather to whisper the solace and sanctuary of death to the tortured and the damned. Their mission, to that end, is noble, kind, and aristocratic, and even their beautiful names suggest such an elevated office: *Norcardia*, *Aspergillus*, *Cryptococcus*, and *Histoplasma*. Let us therefore honor and respect these merciful diseases of the night which reach out in the most divine hours of our lives to touch us with forgiveness and charity. With death now so near, they are truly the only friends remaining who know our suffering and will relieve us of it. For years, they have prepared themselves for this exalted moment in our lives. Generations upon generations of pneumococcal, staphylococcal, or pneumocystic pneumonias have strengthened and armored themselves against all antibacterial treatments. Millions have been sacrificed in order to insure this most powerful resistance to any known treatment, and now they are prepared to whisper sweet words of reassurance and comfort to this most lonely one sequestered by his immense suffering. We shall sing to them praises of thanksgiving and adoration, for they remember us when others have forgotten; they know our deep misery and carefully administer the proper antidote; they open the only door through which our feeble bodies may now walk. Searching, ever searching, the corridors and alleyways of the sterile environment for their brothers and sisters, they found Thomas Wolfe that desperate day in September. He was afraid, huddled against himself with terrible tubercular storms raging within, and they were gentler, kinder, yes, even more merciful than anyone had ever been before. With extraordinary skill, they begin to fill his pleural cavities with fluids and exudates of their peculiar composition.

One simply drowns! It is not unpleasant; it is not painful or even frightening if one will simply allow these merciful angels to do what they do best. Higher and higher the bacteremic fluids rise within the pleural cavities, and one feels dizzy, perhaps even a bit giddy, as the tide of suffocation encapsulates from within rather than without. The heart begins to triphammer its octaval concordance, and the mucosal tissues blush blue and cyanotic with consent. The skin sweats profusely in a futile effort to empty these immense fluids, while cacophonous disharmonies of rales and asymphonic breaths protest the inevitability of their eventual silence. The body becomes a metabolic oven of blast-furnace temperatures rising now from 100° to 102° to 105° and beyond. The thermostat melts and can no longer monitor itself as cardiac arrhythmia establishes its delirious cadence. But then, suddenly, there is silence, cessation, and an end to it all. Having risen to the crest of a metabolic high, one simply falls through the center of gravity to a hollow vortex and beyond. It was good, it was merciful and even kind that Thomas Wolfe's immense suffering for the past two months should so end in the peace and grace of nothingness.

IV

Is there a poetry, or even a prose, to death? Surely those who watched Wolfe's death saw a great engine slowly come to a halt. They saw—or thought they saw—the cessation of a dynamo which had become too large for life and finally in its rage and frenzy devoured itself. Certainly, it is the very nature of tuberculosis to feed upon itself, devouring its own flesh while seeking at the same time to replenish and renew itself. And yet is this not to describe Wolfe's death in terms of his life, and so falsify everything that was distinctive about each? Moreover, is it not to describe his death rather in his own words and thereby to seek to make poetry out of what is at most prose and at least utterly meaningless?

All death, finally, is the result of anoxia. All death, finally, issues in the deprivation of oxygen without which the fragile, delicate brain suffocates. Whether cancer or heart disease or lung tumor or liver dysfunction was the catalytic factor that resulted in anoxia is irrelevant. In the end, life reduces to these most elementary biological terms: a grave dependency upon the vital but invisible oxygen molecules to which the brain is so addicted that even gradual withdrawal is at once fatal. Physiology, sober and serious physiology, defines pulmonary insufficiency as that exact point at which the gaseous composition of arterial blood fails to be maintained within a certain absolute range of oxygen $[O_2]$ and carbon dioxide $[CO_2]$ pressures. Most precisely that point is defined when the Pa_{O_2} is less than 60 mm Hg and the Pa_{CO_2} is greater than 50 mm Hg. But what does this mean to the withered and wasted lungs gasping for precious air, to the famished brain driven mad by forces incomprehensible to it, to the very substance of life so chemically and mechanically dependent upon powers beyond it that deprivation spells death and disaster? Moreover, this absolute dependency between oxygen and brain cannot be broken—either by slow degrees or by other substitutions—for each is mortally wed to the other. In every case, the result is the same: instant and immediate death. Of course, the predisposing cause is always another factor such as a tumor, bacteria, virus, or functional disorder. But these are never the truth of the matter. No, the truth of life is that only air—simple, elementary, invisible air—stands between life and death.

There is neither poetry nor prose to these facts. In its simplest terms, it means that a veil of the most delicate gossamer separates us from an envelope of darkness and nonbeing. It means that every great thought, every cruel art and practice, every wicked motivation, and every sublime inspiration, as well as every small lust and every great triumph of man, rests upon this slender axis of simply breathing air. It means that every beautiful face, every soft and seductive body in the night, every great genius that ever lived and every monster of history, every fool, every dunce, every sorrowful and every joyful life did so only because of air. It means that air, simple, invisible air, is the tie that binds every great and every small man, every lover and every hater, every master and every slave of history into a brotherhood that can be broken only by death. How strange! How strange that air should have this power.

Death is decompression; it is the evaporation and liquefaction of all that unifies, integrates, and solidifies us. Therefore, all that is noble, good, sacred, monstrous, and marvelous about us stands continually upon the verge of evaporation; and since this decompression occurs instantaneously, it will dissolve without warning all that you thought was proud, noble, and secure about yourself.

So in the end—or so it seems—there is no actual end. That is, there is no transition or gradual habituation of life to death. No, one does not really suffer or waste away. Rather, one evaporates into the thinnest air from whence one came and leaves merely a husk of some degree or dimension behind. Where, after all, is the poetry or prose, the sense or meaning, the nobility or tragedy of it?

Thomas Wolfe's head had been shaved to permit brain surgery, and he had lost over fifty pounds throughout his illness. This, along with the pale and waxen quality by which death always announces its domination, transformed him into a preposterous caricature of his former self. Of course, what is truly absurd is not that he was so transformed from life into death but rather the human efforts made to transform him back again. Why do we cling with such ferocious pride to the effigies we make of ourselves?

The Wolfe family returned to Asheville, North Carolina, with his body, and he was buried in Riverside Cemetery beside his father. Should one visit the grave today and seek to find beneath the clover and grass some energy yet remaining of that intense dynamo of life, there is none. Should one look carefully, even searchingly, at the trees, the ground, the flowers for some evidence that here rests a poet and not a mere man, there is none. Should one look for a sign, a symbol, or an apparition of what was unique about him, there is none. This could well be the grave of a tired old lady, of a young child, of a farmer, butcher, doctor, or potter. It could contain the remains of a violent or lustful or gentle or maddened soul. The earth is inscrutable and most mysterious about the secrets it contains. Of course, it is poetic, most romantic to believe that herein will be found something special or unique that marked and qualified his death just as it enunciated his life. But no, there is nothing of the sort here among these flowers and clover and grass. Rather, there are only the endless rows of gravestone upon gravestone with each much like the other and only this peculiar combination of vowels and consonants—Thomas Wolfe—which separates the one from the other. And yet even that is an illusion. The truth is that there is no diameter which distinguishes the dead from one another. Life enunciates, individuates by contours, faces, and body surfaces that differentiate the living from one another. But death knows no such differences since to die is precisely to lose all such individuality and separation. Death is the evaporation of uniqueness and separateness into universality, collectivity, and anonymity.

The poet, the artist, the writer seeks exactly to distinguish himself or herself through the style and personality of his or her craft. In no other profession is the glorification of self so approved and applauded. And yet nature despises such celebrations and abuses the one who insists upon these triumphs. Thus, he suffers not because he must but rather because he counts individuality higher than happiness and contentment. In so disrupting the center-gravity of unity and integration, nature revenges this hubris by a decompression which brings about its very opposite.

5

Wilder Had a Sister

*We had heard, meantime, about a magician
named Wilder Penfield in Montreal. Half a dozen
folk had suggested that we get in touch with this
renowned surgeon who, like Putnam, has international rank and who, like most great brain surgeons, is a poet. Traeger tracked him down, and he
agreed to come to New York to have a look at
Johnny. It was interesting to notice how impressed
Neurological was with Penfield. The manner of the
whole sixth floor abruptly changed. Previously
Johnny had been a hopeless case; now he was a
phenomenon of considerable interest. Putnam interrupted his holiday, and he, Penfield, Traeger,
and another doctor spent the morning in consultation. We had told Johnny casually how eminent
Penfield was, and his greeting to him was quite
characteristic. He measured Putnam and Penfield
together, and then asked, "Where's Cushing?"*

*Penfield spent an hour on the slides; always, in
a thing of this hideous kind, the possibility exists
of mistaken diagnosis, and the tumor might have
changed for the better or worse. We waited, and
then with everybody listening, Penfield cut through
all the euphemisms and said directly, "Your child
has a malignant glioma, and it will kill him."*

John Gunther
Death Be Not Proud

87

Oligodendrogliomas: The Oligodendroglioma is usually found in the cerebral hemisphere of middle-aged adults. It comprises about 5 percent of all the gliomas and appears as a firm, pinkish tumor which is not demarcated from the surrounding brain and which is often calcified in its peripheral parts. Such calcification, however, does not necessarily imply that the lesion is wholly benign. Its cells are large and rounded, with a well-formed membrane and relatively clear cytoplasm. Mitoses are rare. Seeding sometimes occurs along the cerebrospinal pathways. Although these tumors are usually benign, their size, deep situation, and invasive characteristics make total removal impossible in most instances. Partial removal sometimes results in an extension of useful survival for several years, but in other cases, surgical intervention seems to accelerate the growth, and this factor has to be taken into account in deciding whether surgery is indicated or not.

Frank Eliott
Clinical Neurology

I

There is something special, something profoundly unique, which binds a sister to a brother. Flesh of flesh, blood of blood, they are a unity held within an opposition of differences. This mystery about them cannot be found between brothers or parents or cousins or in any other blood relationship. For a brother, a sister often becomes the measure and model by which all future women shall be judged. Be they cold or be they warm, be they silly or be they serious, be they strong or be they weak, all women will be judged according to these standards. Likewise, a brother is a male in microcosm, for herein a sister can study all the aggressions, doubts, bravado boastings, and humiliations that haunt the male. And yet, since their relationship is neither erotic nor parental, neither brother nor sister is dominated by extraneous demands that confuse the relationship beneath. They are invested but not incarcerated by their sibling bond.

Ruth Penfield was seven years older than her brother Wilder and was protective of him in many ways. Herbert was the first born, in 1881, then three years later came Ruth in 1884, and finally the last born was Wilder on January 26, 1891. She found herself in both a competitive and a cooperative position between the two brothers and must have felt some relief in marrying her high-school teacher in 1905 and leaving the household. Five years before, Ruth had entered into her diary a most insightful observation about her brother Wilder: "It would be a terrible responsibility to bring Wilder up because he is such a firefly and is so willful—and yet he is very affectionate and easily led" (Lewis, *Something Hidden*, p. 17).

When a brother loves a sister, especially one seven years his senior, there must be a certain involution of maternalism which entwines itself within their relationship. After all, when Wilder was four, she was eleven and already partly a mother to him. When he was thirteen, Ruth was a young woman of twenty and soon to plan her own family the following year. In so many ways she was his rock, his support and anchor during the difficult years after their father had deserted the family. In a child as sensitive as Wilder, such devotion no doubt transformed itself into a fierce family loyalty which demanded allegiance and fidelity above all else. One can still discern the heat of this family loyalty in a letter that Penfield wrote at the age of eighty-four to his grandson Jefferson Lewis about his marriage: "In our 58 years of married life the most wonderful source of security and strength and happiness came to us from the awareness of companionship. At 84, soon to be 85, bodily attraction burns low and love continues. It is a thing of the spirit, as companionship is" (ibid., p. xi).

Penfield was a family man. Today he would be regarded by many as antiquated, old-fashioned, certainly out of step with the times, and no doubt a chauvinistic sexist. Indeed, it is likely that he was in fact all of these things and much more besides. And yet, it must be reaffirmed that the secret to Wilder Penfield's emotional and spiritual life was his sense of familial loyalty. It was this sense of loyalty that no doubt sustained his often stormy and troubled marriage; it was this sense of loyalty that drove him to complete his mother's romantic novel *The Story of Sarai;* and it was this sense of loyalty that motivated his decision to operate upon his own sister for a brain tumor in 1928. To fail to understand this dimension of Penfield is to miss the man completely.

Why, after all, should we be loyal to another? In this divisive, treacherous, and altogether brutal world, why should we not be loyal to ourselves alone? One forms allegiances, bonds, intimacies, but are these not in the end mutual contracts to be honored or dissolved insofar as one's original obligation to oneself is fulfilled? All love is conditional and therefore dependent upon a sufficient return for an adequate investment. When this economic principle reverses itself and one receives less in return for what one gives, then such partnerships should be voided. In today's world, the laws of economic recovery apply as much to solid relationships as they do to good business. If one should see another whose turn of ankle, curvature of breast, or length of thigh is provocative, is it not discretionary to invest part of one's funds there also? The laws of diversification are intended to purchase security through multiplicity, for where there is a singular and individual devotion, there also will the risk of emotional bankruptcy increase geometrically. One has no obligations, no enduring commitments, no fidelity except to honor oneself with continual satisfaction. Such is today's world.

But Wilder's world was of a yesterday. Perhaps even he was obliged to first serve himself, but he sought to do so as the circumference of a circle protects and preserves its center. Expanding and ever widening the circle of his commitments, Penfield protected as a family all those who relied upon him. We can see this devotion repeated time and again in all that he did, and even his grandson Jefferson Lewis was somewhat surprised to learn "how much he had cared—in those last months when he knew he hadn't long to live—about the impending marriage of one among his fifteen grandchildren, about the things he knew were true, and, most of all, about telling them" (ibid., p. xii). Even at the Montreal Neurological Institute, Penfield quickly began referring to the surgeons, the staff, and the personnel as "my" people and the institution as "our" place, in an effort to personalize it and so transform it from a place to a family. Penfield stated his priorities in his autobiography, *No Man Alone:* "As far as my own personal philosophy of life was concerned, I had adopted a scale of ultimate priorities: first to be considered was a responsibility to wife and family; second, allegiance to my work in the world and to the teamwork that developed; and third, the friendship and happiness to be found in normal living" (p. 40).

In order to understand the pivotal forces that energized Penfield, then, one must first and foremost understand his fierce sense of loyalty and devotion to those around him. Under no other conditions could his most unprecedented, most remarkable, and most unprofessional decision to operate upon his own sister be understood.

II

Near the end of November 1928 Wilder's mother wired him from California that Ruth was seriously ill and they were on their way to Montreal so that he could examine her. It was a most inopportune time. His wife Helen was sick in bed with the mumps; they had just moved into a new house at 200 Côte Saint Antoine Road, and inadvertently some brain tumor specimens had been hauled to the Rosemount Dump where Wilder spent a cold afternoon searching among grapefruits and rotted junk for their whereabouts. Naturally, he cabled back at once to delay the trip, only to receive in response the following reply from Ruth's husband, Jack Inglis: "Too late to cancel . . . Ruth's condition seems urgent" (ibid., p. 207).

They arrived on Thursday morning at Windsor station where Wilder was waiting to meet them. At once he could see how serious Ruth's condition was by the dazed and lethargic expression on her face, and out of hearing range his mother admitted that she had prayed the whole trip that Ruth would not have another seizure on the way up. As soon as he had them both settled, with Ruth in the upstairs bedroom, he went up to her room with his ophthalmoscope. What he saw upon examination was so disturbing that for a moment he thought he might faint. "The swelling of the head of the optic nerve— dreadful swelling, and there were little red hemorrhages, each bordered by a white margin, that extended out menacingly over the surface of the surrounding retina" (ibid., p. 208).

Wilder knew that he had to act quickly before secondary

optic atrophy destroyed her vision completely. Papilledema is produced by a swelling of the optic disks and is usually caused by intracranial pressure, and so he suspected—especially with the other symptoms he knew about—that she probably had either a tumor or an abscess which had become critical. In fact, his mother had already detailed the events of the last several months for him, and now he began to recall incidents from thirty years ago. It was possible, it was even very likely, that this mass had been slowly growing in her brain all that time.

As if fitting together the disconnected pieces of an elaborate jigsaw puzzle, Penfield began to assemble the events of the past thirty years. There was the incident, for example, when Ruth was nineteen and he still an impressionable twelve, in which he was awakened from his sleep by her agonized cries like the sound of an animal in deep distress. At the time he could not fathom what it meant. And soon thereafter, when the doctor came, Wilder had seen through the thin envelope of the open doorway his sister lying unconscious upon the bed. She must have had, he now reasoned from the distance of time and acquired medical skills, a grand mal seizure. And yes, hadn't it been but five years earlier, when she was fourteen and he was seven, that her headaches began? All of it started to integrate and collate together now, but before he had not seen it, could not have discerned a pattern to such disconnected events. Moreover, there had been deception on this matter for years. His mother had hidden much of this from her youngest child, and the doctor himself had diagnosed the condition as hysteria or girlish nerves. Throughout the years, as the symptoms accentuated, adjusted, and finally enunciated themselves, his mother had denied their reality both to herself and to her children. In fact, it was over just this matter in particular that mother and son had had their first major argument. For example, she had kept quiet the fact that within the last two years Ruth had started to have numerous seizures and, in an effort to cure her daughter, their mother had become a Christian Scientist. Wilder later minimized the whole affair with the following brush-off: "Mother had become a Christian Scientist. Ruth had gone along with her and taken that treatment. Mother's letters had become rather noncommittal then in regard to

Ruth. Perhaps she felt that she and I no longer spoke the same language" (ibid., p. 208).

But Jefferson Lewis informs us that it was much more than simply a question of speaking different languages.

> Three of four years earlier when the attacks grew more frequent, Jean [their mother] had gone with Ruth to a Christian Science healer. Jean was having trouble with her legs, but the real reason for her visit to the healer was her desperation at Ruth's condition. Mother and daughter had both converted on the spot, and Jean had sent Wilder pamphlets and written enthusiastically about the miraculous change Christian Science had wrought. Wilder was not amused, and his dismissal of Christian Science as hocus-pocus had caused the first real strain in their relationship. In a rare letter from Ruth in 1926, wishing him happy birthday, she concluded an enthusiastic account of the improvement in her own and Jean's health with an apology "for this long discourse. I had no intention of dwelling upon this, or preaching any kind of a sermon . . . but it just came out. I'm like mother. She said one day, 'I have tried to be very careful and not talk Science to Wilder, but in every letter he gives me some kind of dig. So I'm not going to be careful anymore, but just be natural, and say what I feel like saying. If he persists in fishing in this pool, I shall rise to his bait.'" [*Something Hidden*, pp. 119–20]

Need it be said that this was exactly the wrong kind of letter to send Wilder? But his grandson is probably right in suggesting that Jean's secretiveness about Ruth's condition had much to do with the fragile and delicate history of Wilder's past reactions. So, it appears that there was a family secret—or even a series of family secrets—when it came to the matter of Ruth's health, and this was partly the result of Wilder's firm opinions about alternatives to standard medical procedure. One can understand why Wilder was out of touch about Ruth's illness as well as his initial shock and surprise to discover just how serious it actually was.

In addition, however, it is standard procedure—both then and now—not to treat one's own family. By and large, Penfield truly respected this injunction; he had first asked his friend Carl Rand, a neurosurgeon in Los Angeles, to look at Ruth, and to Rand she eventually returned after her operation in Montreal. So, in addition to the family deception there was also the ingredient of Wilder's medical ignorance when it came to members of his own family. But finally, there exists the obvious fact that only very recently had Penfield acquired the medical skills to make sense of such symptoms. After all, he was only thirty-seven years old and just beginning his own specialty of neurosurgery; he openly admitted that he had only performed one other operation of the magnitude required for treating his sister, and therefore he had never possessed the medical wherewithal to integrate Ruth's several symptoms into a diagnostic pattern. One can certainly understand his sudden confusion and surprise upon first seeing her and recognizing the importance of her symptoms.

Penfield immediately hid his own fears and misgivings behind a facade of cheerfulness. He seems to have been quite skilled at doing so all of his life, for colleagues around him often were surprised to learn that he had any self-doubts at all. It is a rather admirable quality requiring both self-discipline and considerable courage. He was, his grandson tells us, "a man more ambivalent, self-critical, musing, and troubled than any of us around him would ever have guessed" (ibid., p. xii). And yet he restrained these fears and self-doubts around Ruth and immediately called a conference of his colleagues. They took X-ray films, examined her countless times, and performed all of the necessary workups. Finally it came time to make a decision, and they assembled in Wilder's front parlor at the new home on Côte Saint Antoine Road.

The consultation consisted of Colin Russell, Bill Cone, Edward Archibald, and Penfield. Penfield presented the case to others in the most objective manner and suggested two possibilities: one was to take Ruth to Harvey Cushing in Boston and the other was to find someone else equally qualified. There seemed no doubt that she needed an operation and as soon as possible. Edward Brooks, chief radiologist at the Royal Victoria Hospital, had seen clearly defined calcium granules in the right frontal lobe, and this suggested a very well established tumor of some years' standing. The only doubt was whether it was benign or malignant, and if the latter, of what cell type. If it was a rapidly growing glioblastoma or an astrocytoma, then the case was probably hopeless. But if the tumor was benign or a more slowly growing cell type such as the rare oligodendroglioma, then the picture was much more hopeful. Part of the problem, as Penfield saw it, was that Harvey Cushing was too damned conservative. It is true that his mortality rates were in the 5 to 6 percent range, which was excellent, but this partly due to Cushing's hesitancy to perform radical excision, and it would appear from the films that radical excision of this large tumor was just what was needed. The other problem was that next to Cushing there was no one else with the skill to undertake such a removal except . . . well, as he himself admitted . . . except Penfield. For next to Cushing—and maybe even before Cushing—Penfield was then the best neurosurgeon in the world. Still, he left the matter up to his colleagues to deliberate in the parlor while he went upstairs to visit with his wife, still recovering from her bout with the mumps.

After what seemed like an eternity to Penfield, they called him down to the parlor.

> As I entered the room Archibald asked me this: "If you were to do this operation, could you do it as if she were not your sister?"
>
> I hesitated. At last, I said yes.
>
> He smiled. "I think then that you should go ahead. You'd better admit her to the Royal Victoria the first thing tomorrow morning."
>
> I looked at Colin Russell. "Yes," he said, "Bill tells us you can do it. I think you should. And your sister told me that, if any operating is to be done, she wants her brother to do it." [*No Man Alone*, p. 210]

And so it was decided! Wilder no doubt felt tremendous misgivings and extreme anxiety at the prospect of failure. And yet there is no evidence—as, of course, there would not be—in his account of the next few days. Wanting the very best for his sister, he immediately phoned his old anesthetist Anne Penland from Presbyterian Hospital in New York; she agreed to come at once and arrived in Montreal that evening. It is no small credit to Penfield that he could command such allegiance and loyalty from associates. In addition, Wilder attended to a dozen other details of the procedure. He reviewed the entire operation with Kathleen Zwicker, the instrument nurse, and rehearsed a modification of his own design of Otfrid Foerster's protective screen. Penfield had only weeks before returned from six months of study in Germany during which he had met Foerster and watched him operate. Foerster had devised a screen between himself and the patient by suturing one end of a sterile sheet to the patient's scalp and attaching the other to a metal frame above the operating table. Penfield's modification was to extend the screen another twenty inches and thereby create a shelf; this permitted the instrument nurse to stand at the surgeon's side rather than behind as in Foerster's design. Also, Wilder went over the entire procedure very carefully with Ruth, telling her exactly what would happen at each point:

> "There will be no pain except for the initial needle prick or two. Once the scalp incision is made, you should feel nothing, since the skull and the brain have no capacity for sensation in themselves. You will hear sounds of course. But you can talk to Miss Penland about them. She will be close to you. And Dr. Russel, whom you know and like, says he wants to sit beside you, too. I shall talk to you when I need your help. You may speak to me anytime. I will explain and I'll tell you if there is anything for you to do." [Ibid., p. 214]

And so it was all arranged, most efficiently but also with great brotherly concern for his ailing sister. Wilder's account of the next few days is a strange combination of the professional surgeon speaking most objectively and the concerned family member unable to remove himself from the highly subjective climate of his condition.

III

The operation was conducted the following morning under standard novocaine anesthesia and with the customary osteo-plastic flat reflection. Ruth talked incessantly to her brother during the procedure by relating stories of her children, tidbits of family gossip, and the usual sorts of things that a sister says to a brother. Obviously she felt quite comfortable in his presence, even under these conditions, but then well she might because Wilder had so planned it this way. But finally the distraction was too much, and "I begged her to postpone her talking, since I must begin to concentrate on something else" (ibid., p. 214).

The tumor was located in the right frontal lobe, and although Penfield had already done extensive topographical mapping of these regions, it was altogether uncertain what radical excision of this lobe might mean. But radical excision would indeed be necessary, for now it was apparent that the mass had entwined itself about the entire frontal lobe as wide as the motor gyrus and as deep as the floor of the skull. It was, as Penfield remarked "a gray, firm, malignant looking tissue"; "enormous veins came up through the tissue" (ibid., p. 215). Penfield's reaction to this massive and ominous growth within his sister's brain was that of a brother rather than a surgeon. He does not tell us in *No Man Alone*, but his grandson does later, that for fifteen minutes he was unable to continue and Bill Cone had to take over.

This was certainly to be the largest brain removal that he had ever undertaken, and his inclination was to stop the operation at once and close up. But then he remembered Cushing and why he had insisted on doing the procedure himself; anyone else would have stopped short and withdrawn at this point. Was it not Penfield himself who had confessed just yesterday to his colleagues: "But if I were in her place, I would ask for a radical attempt to remove the whole growth, however dangerous it might be to my life. But I would not want to be paralyzed. I'd rather die. If it can't be removed completely, then I would ask the surgeon to be as radical as he can be, short of paralysis. I would hope then for a year or two of useful life before the beginning of the end" (ibid., p. 210).

Well, that settled it, didn't it? He would go for broke, proceed as aggressively and carefully as possible, but nonetheless go for broke. Is that not after all the mark of a good surgeon? It has been said of Owen Wangensteen of Minnesota that when you operated with him you were well advised to wear a pair of sup-hose and attach a "pilot's friend" because he would not stop until he had gotten everything that needed removal. Perhaps this is good advice. Perhaps it is not. A resident once observed of such surgery that the true marvel is not that some patients die but rather that any of them live! In any case, Penfield had never been conservative in the Harvey Cushing sense and certainly did not intend to be timid today.

But then had not everything so far prepared him for this moment? He had just returned from Germany where he had studied Foerster's techniques and modified some of his methods. Moreover, he had recently operated on young William Hamilton to relieve epileptic seizures. During that operation, in which Anne Penland had also been present as anesthetist, Penfield had found the epileptogenic focus to involve the entire right frontal lobe. The lobectomy that resulted was thought to be the largest thus far attempted by anyone. All the details, all the coincidents were there to suggest that fate was somehow at work here. It is ironic, is it not, that Penfield should choose neurosurgery as a specialty, should have a sister with a brain tumor which has patiently waited these thirty years for attention until her brother was prepared to give it? It is ironic, also, that the tumor should be in the right frontal lobe and that Penfield should have rehearsed precisely the same procedure just recently and also returned only weeks before from studying such procedures in Germany. Penfield believed very strongly in destiny. One need only to recall an early incident from his life to establish that point. As he was returning from Oxford and his study with Sir Charles Sherrington to a surgical internship with Harvey Cushing in the Peter Bent Brigham Hospital, Penfield's boat was sunk by a German torpedo which exploded directly under the forward deck upon which he stood. Thrown high into the air and headed for the dark sea with a badly broken and torn left leg, Penfield at first thought that he was going to die. In just an instant, however, his keen sense of destiny reasserted itself, and he decided instead: "This cannot be the end. My work in the world has only just begun. This cannot be the end" (ibid., p. 37).

Of course, it was not the end and Penfield landed safely on the deck. Can one therefore doubt that Wilder did not summon his sense of destiny and fate to assist him at this moment?

Along with his sense of loyalty, of family obligation, as well as his love for Ruth, it was certain that Penfield would proceed with a radical excision despite advice to the contrary from Bill Cone.

Gently, he passed a silk thread (Halsted had taught them all—Cushing, Dandy, Penfield, and a dozen other young surgeons—the miracles of silk) around the tumor mass and gently elevated its heavy weight. So far, no bleeding. Miss Penland quietly held up for view the blood pressure readings, and everyone began to speak in soft whispers. Perhaps they did not need to do so, for Ruth had fallen asleep, but the moment was truly momentous. Below the tumor resided the venous sinuses whose veritable lake of blood might erupt volcanically at any moment. But so far they were quiet, quite undisturbed, and so Wilder proceeded carefully, very carefully, as if cradled within his hands was something very, very precious. As indeed there was! Already one can perhaps feel, even sense as one's own, the eroticism of fear and jubilation he must have felt. Everything rested on the next few seconds, those moments of intensity as the silk thread gently captured its prey with either success or failure as final reward. So far everything was fine, just fine, and the silk became a smaller and smaller loop while heaving, hefting its malevolent prey toward the surface.

Miss Penland assured the patient's brother that everything was going well, and he was much relieved. The surgeon therefore re-established his grasp upon the delicate silken thread, and slowly "I tightened the knot of my thread, little by little by little, cutting the mass of the tumor gradually free from the dura at the base" (ibid., p. 215). And then, almost without warning, it happened!

Bill Cone had warned Wilder precisely about this possibility, and Edward Kahn certainly would have predicted it also. Kahn was a surgical assistant at Penfield's first frontal lobectomy, performed on William Hamilton. Years later, when Penfield was in his eighties and working on his autobiography, Kahn wrote to say that to his knowledge this was still the largest lobectomy ever performed. Now Wilder found himself in the midst of an even larger lobectomy than the one Kahn knew about, struggling desperately to correct a monumental error in

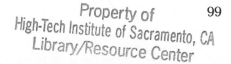

judgment which might well prove fatal to his sister in the next few seconds. Twenty-seven years later, in 1955, Kahn included a section on oligodendrogliomas in his book *Correlative Neurosurgery*. Kahn's observations are most interesting, for the microscopic sections show this to be the very type of tumor that Penfield was now operating on.

> The oligodendrogliomas constitute about 5 percent of all gliomas. In our opinion, they have an unjustifiable reputation as benign tumors with a long life expectancy. In Bailey and Cushing's monograph on the gliomas there were but nine of these tumors. One patient lived for 21 years after his first symptom so that this gave an over-optimistic picture of the average life expectancy in the oligodendrogliomas. Patients do harbor this tumor for years carrying on a fairly normal existence, but that has proven to be more the exception than the rule with our own cases.
>
> Further experience with the oligodendrogliomas has led us to believe that this tumor is usually an infiltrating one which in many cases involves both cerebral hemispheres by way of the corpus callosum. Even when the tumor is limited to one hemisphere it can seldom be totally removed as it is apt to infiltrate deeply.
>
> We have, perhaps, presented too pessimistic a picture of the oligodendrogliomas. Occasionally they may be well circumscribed, as when they involve one parieto-occipital lobe, and can be removed grossly "in toto". In the frontal region, however, where they appear most frequently, a tumor, which at operation seems well localized, may continue to infiltrate into the corpus callosum in the direction of the diencephalon. This is always a disheartening experience for the surgeon and may account for our pessimism with the oligodendrogliomas. [pp. 75–77]

Unfortunately, as Wilder soon discovered, Kahn's observations were neither too pessimistic nor inaccurate. For the moment, however, there was a more immediate and urgent problem than the long-term recovery of the patient, for the surgeon had initiated a crisis in the brother's efforts to save his own sister's life. Just as the two ends of the silken loop met, there "came a rush of blood swirling up from the base of the skull and hiding everything in a rapidly deepening pool of blood" (*No Man Alone*, p. 216). He had cut through the tumor's blood supply line while attempting to extricate the remaining mass. Quickly now, Wilder dislodged the residual tumor parts and then packed the cavity with sterile cotton wadding while Bill Cone systematically suctioned off the pools of new blood forming. The bleeding was finally stopped with a tissue pad fashioned out of temporal muscle, and Ruth was given the first of three transfusions. But the crisis had brought about serious physiological compromises by weakening her pulse and blood pressure rates. When finally she was stabilized and Wilder could reestablish a clear visual field, he saw it.

The tumor had crept silently but maliciously underneath the floor of the midline and up into the left hemisphere's base. As if with a mind of its own, the insidious oligodendroglioma had breached both hemispheres exactly as Edgar Kahn said that it might. It was now that Wilder knew he had failed both his sister and himself. Later in the locker room, he would rhetorically ask C. B. Keenan, an old-timer in general surgery, why anyone would chose to operate on brain tumors since one always fails? Now, at the moment of crisis and discovery, Wilder's strength deserted him, and although he doesn't admit the fact in *No Man Alone*, two days later he would write to Ruth's husband, Jack Inglis, that the discovery "filled me with a sort of frenzy, and I fear I was rather reckless" (Lewis, *Something Hidden*, p. 123).

It had eluded him! With its sly and uncanny knowledge of the brain's interior geography, the tumor had gone where Wilder could not follow. How ironic that this cartographer, this Lewis and Clark of the brain's external routes and highways should pursue the clever oligodendroglioma so expertly only to find it disappear into an uncharted escape route. Could it have known that it would be pursued by an international authority on brain exploration, by a surgeon who had mapped every convolution of the cortical geography and could discern in an instant the thoughtful and thoughtless areas one from another? This brilliant neurosurgeon who had spent years studying the geography of the brain in order to rescue his patients from the jaws of death had been defeated by a swirling mass of crazed, malignant tissues which ran like a forest fire across the delicate brain of his sweet, beloved sister.

"I did not dare to follow it farther," and so they filled the enormous cavity with warm saline solution and packed muscle. But now two problems had arisen like a Hydra's head in place of the original one. First, what were the short-term effects of such a massive excision and would Ruth still be a whole and integrated person afterwards? The second problem was more long-term but also more deadly: how long would it take the ovum of oligodendroglioma to blossom into another child of its own? Already, sinister "daughter cells" had sprung forth to embrace their malicious mother, and the following day "when I saw that some of the cells seen under the microscope were, I thought, giving birth to daughter cells too actively, I had doubts about the future" (*No Man Alone*, pp. 216, 219).

So, Ruth was sent home, and surgeon became brother once again. He worried about her; he fussed and fretted to Helen and seemed in constant contact with her husband Jack. On some days, he felt triumphant, such as the afternoon he received a letter from Ruth telling him: "On the first Monday after arriving, Jack took me to a dinner and dance for Rotary Ladies' Night. It was such fun. Everyone seemed so surprised that I could dance and seem as well as ever. Perhaps they felt I should be in a wheel chair. I wore a tight blue hat I had last summer with my blue dress" (ibid., p. 219).

Her brother was much relieved to receive this letter; she was going to be all right! And yet . . . and yet . . . on the same day, February 24, 1929, dear Ruth had also written and mailed this other letter:

> My dear Dr. and Mrs. Penfield:
> I must add a word of appreciation to Dr. Penfield for setting my brains in order. I must say I have not missed what he took out, not even have I felt light-headed, and if he has the little fungus pickled as a memento of my visit he is very welcome to it. I hope all future patients pay better than I.
> R. P. Inglis

The surgeon felt a shudder run up his back and penciled upon the note: "After Operation. Is this a joke?" (Lewis, *Something Hidden*, p. 124). He then quickly hid both note and commentary away in his file cabinet where the brother could not see.

IV

What, after all, is the effect of removing almost half a brain, especially when that half involves the most important frontal lobes? Penfield could not say; Wilder sought not to guess. The former had seen the effect of frontal lobectomy as a compromise of the ability to plan, organize, and initiate projects; the latter would observe these effects several months later in helping a tearful and confused sister prepare dinner for her guests. But who can actually say?

A. R. Luria argues that the frontal lobes "constitute an apparatus with the function of forming stable plans and intentions capable of controlling the subject's subsequent conscious behavior" (*The Working Brain*, p. 198). Karl Pribram agrees with Luria and adds this interesting observation that "frontal lobe damage impairs those brain processes in which coding of perturbations of states is an essential element. These processes occur in the operations of short-term memory that involve context-sensitive decisions, rather than in well established context-free operations, and are reflected in both problem solving and in emotional behavior. Viewed prospectively, the defect shows in problem solving; the organism is not able to regulate his behavior on the basis of the perturbing events that signal changes in context" (*Languages of the Brain*, pp. 349–50). Certainly, Penfield later admitted the substance of such observations but also added the puzzling note that "removal of very large areas, indeed, of practically the whole frontal lobe on one side anterior to the precentral gyrus, results in an amazing lack of obvious defect" (Penfield and Rasmussen, *The Cerebral Cortex of Man*, p. 192). Is this the brother or the surgeon talking? Whoever it is, he has a collaborator and supporter in Norman Geschwind:

> I have, for example, seen a patient who had what Donald Matson (personal communication) described as the largest glioma he had ever seen and in whom a large left hemisphere resection was carried out. The child was left with a permanent right hemiplegia and was very severely aphasic after the operation. He was still severely aphasic a month later; by two months he had a considerable amount of speech; by three months he was speaking normally. It is inconceivable that the right hemisphere of the child is capable of

relearning English to that degree of complexity within three months. Furthermore, at the time of recovery he was fully capable of discussing his past life. It would be difficult to accept that during a three month stay within the hospital he had somehow reacquired all his previous vocabulary. One must advance a different kind of explanation, i.e., that this was not relearning by the right hemisphere, but that, in fact, the right hemisphere must have been learning language all along. [*Selected Papers on Language and the Brain*, p. 474]

What sense then can be made of these confusing and often contradictory observations about the frontal lobes? Do they, in fact, play a role in our behavior, or do they play none at all? It seems clear that frontal lobectomy does compromise behavior, but it is difficult to determine exactly the degree and kind of this compromise. Part of the difficulty has to do with the complexity of the brain itself and the simplicity of our knowledge about its workings. But another part of the problem is the mind's amazing ability to mask and hide its mistakes and defects. By an elaborate shunting system, an impoverishment in one area is enriched by the power of another area. Thus, the loss of the left hemisphere triggers a compensatory mechanism by which the right hemisphere assumes the burden of the left. The removal of the right frontal lobe signals an elaborate support system in which the left reprograms itself in order to share a double burden of responsibility. Still, the masquerade is not a full-dress affair, for occasionally, even if inconspicuously, the deformed face behind the mask shows itself. Always subtle and always clever about the full degree of its damage, the brain still cannot elude the truth about itself or the awareness that it is not as it was before. Ruth would complain, for example, that "I have trouble getting organized," for the brain that can lie to another cannot often lie to itself. So, too, the surgeon can be fooled by his own optimism, but the brother is a prisoner to the truth: "Outwardly I rejoiced with Ruth and all the others at her recovery . . . but . . . I had doubts about the future. This was a fear, a misgiving, that I kept to myself" (*No Man Alone*, p. 219).

Penfield was an expert at hiding his surgical doubts, often

even from himself, and part of the ability to do so no doubt originated from his certain knowledge that we really have no certain knowledge about the brain. One of his last books, written while he was dying of cancer, was precisely titled *The Mystery of the Mind* and sought to explore that "thrilling undiscovered country" (p. ix). At some deeper level both the surgeon and the brother met, and therein each understood that both were wrong and both were right about Ruth's future. She survived far better than anyone anticipated, but she also died more suddenly, more certainly, and more unscientifically than even Wilder could have imagined and in so doing took that "thrilling undiscovered country" with her.

v

Ruth died on July 14, 1931, at one o'clock in the afternoon. It was a sunny Tuesday in Van Nuys, California, and Jack Inglis telegraphed the news to his brother-in-law in Montreal immediately. Wilder's first response was to call his wife, who had been his solace throughout all this torment that overwhelmed the brother and puzzled the surgeon, and then he wrote to Ruth's family. What a strange and yet ordinary man was this Wilder Penfield! On the one hand, he was a mass of contradictions while on the other he was as predictable and consistent as a sunny day in July.

When a sister dies, does she take only herself or also part of her brother with her into death? "I did want to change the writing on the wall," the sister's brother wrote to the widowed husband (Lewis, *Something Hidden*, p. 125). But why? Why did he want to change fate, control destiny, snatch his sister from the portals of death? After all, he was a surgeon and so he knew that patients die and that neurosurgical patients are especially fragile, even brittle, in the vicinity of death. Well, is not the answer simply that Wilder was also a brother and therefore desperately wanted his only sister to live? And yet this simple answer is too simple, for within the confusion of brother and surgeon there dwells a contradiction of a very personal proportion and dimension.

In one sense, he had failed. Ruth had not been saved by the skill and measure of his training; however many patients

Wilder might save in the future, it could never be forgotten that he failed to save his own sister. He knew this, and despite their reassurances to the contrary, his family knew it as well. In a man like Wilder Penfield, the bitterness of such weakness, of such impotence must have been intolerable. No one could count on him again; he could not count on himself again to perform miracles. Neither the surgeon—however great he might become—nor his family could ever feel safe and invulnerable to disease. For Wilder's failure had cost his family not only a sister but also the privilege of being special, strong, and immortal in the company of death. They would all die, and Wilder would be of no help to any of them in their salvation.

On the other hand, he had not failed but succeeded admirably. For had he not, in fact, given Ruth life, and had she not herself thanked him for this life? She survived another three years after her operation; could this have ever been possible without her brother's intervention? So Wilder could not defeat death, but he could postpone it; he could not conquer disease, but he could negotiate with it. His mother thought well of him, and for Wilder that was very important "for no man should blush to admit that his mother speaks well of him. He should blush if she does not, for he must then know that he has indeed fallen from grace" (*No Man Alone*, pp. 220–21).

And yet, for whatever reasons and whether rightfully so or not, the essence of the matter is precisely that Wilder Penfield had fallen from grace. Moreover, his damnation had not been secured by lusts or sins of his own or by evil manipulations of another, but by a tumor. He had been befallen, undone by an unthinking, unfeeling mass of frenzied cells that had controlled him precisely through the absolute disorder and lack of control that made them what they were. Had he not, after all, traveled to Madrid in 1924 exactly to study oligodendroglia under the great Ramón y Cajal? And had he not published one of his first and most important scholarly papers on just this subject, "Oligodendroglia and Its Relation to Classical Neuroglia," in 1924? Everything that he had done and everything that he had studied or even thought up to this moment should have prepared him for this singular great test which destiny had especially prepared for him. It could not have been more perfect. The moment was right; the tumor was properly located; the cell type was ideal; the patient was precious. How could he fail to succeed? But now, having failed, could he ever succeed again? Indeed, something of the brother had died with the sister, and neither held the hope of resurrection.

There are inconsistencies, ambiguities that puzzle us when we think of Penfield's precision. For example, he is unclear about the date of his sister's death. He claims in his autobiography, *No Man Alone*, that she died in September 1931 "almost three years after my operation" (p. 362). But in fact, she actually died earlier, in July 1931. Why the difference of two months in such an important date? Was it urgent for Wilder to round off the numbers in order that the duration of her salvation might be ever so slightly extended in his own behalf?

Again, his ambivalence is clear when he asked C. B. Keenan, right after Ruth's operation, why anyone would want to be a neurosurgeon. (Keenan's only response was to look down at Penfield and grunt!) Or when he reviewed how much he knew about oligodendroglia except "what causes them to grow or how to stop the growing." Or finally when he simply admitted the "resentment I felt because of my inability to save my sister" (ibid., p. 221). What then shall we make of Wilder Graves Penfield, half surgeon and half brother, self-confident to arrogance and self-doubting to tears?

In so very many important ways it must be said that in spite of all his inner turmoil—and just as often because of it—Penfield was a survivor. He had an uncanny ability to feast upon his own weaknesses and so devour them to the enrichment and eventual strengthening of himself. Admirable, most admirable when it can be done! For example, with all the ambivalence, resentment, and self-doubts about Ruth's surgery, Penfield decided just seven years later to publish the case, along with two other frontal lobectomies, in the March 1935 issue of *Brain*. It is a highly objective, quite scientific study, which quite ignores the personage of the patients involved. Wilder saw "The Frontal Lobe in Man: A Clinical Study of Maximum Removals" as a certain homage to Ruth because more than simply suffering her illness, she had also made a contribution because of it.

In the end, Penfield was no less disciplined with himself

than he had been with others. At eighty-five and with a malignant carcinoma of the stomach, Wilder feared that he might die some evening in their apartment where his beloved Helen would be shocked to find him the following morning. Having then decided to enter the hospital for the last time, he arranged the evening before a small party for just the two of them. Imagine that! They had—these two old and exceedingly frail lovers—a final dinner together with their favorite music and talked of fond memories. The following morning he left for the hospital where he died a few days later.

There is something extraordinary, something rarefied and mysterious about a brother and a sister. On the one hand they are flesh born of flesh, and yet there is a separateness within this extraordinary identity. When one dies, the other yet lives, but never as fully, never as completely, never as absolutely as before. Flesh of flesh is heavy with its burdens and carries far more than mere memories to the grave. Twisted somewhere within, somewhere about the silent, unbeating heart is a mystery and a covenant which cannot seem to rest content until they are whole and complete again. Flesh of flesh that is torn unto itself and cannot heal until it is reunited with its wholeness is a flesh discontent, furious, and frustrated with itself. Ruth and Wilder, who once were two, are once again one in a union that resolves all contradictions, resentments, guilt, self-doubts, and insecurities. Such reconciliation alone can transform our failures into splendid, glowing, and immortal successes.

6

Brother Damian

In these deep solitudes and awful cells,
Where heav'nly-pensive, contemplation dwells,
And ever-musing melancholy reigns;
What means this tumult in a Vestal's veins?
Why rove my thoughts beyond this last retreat?
Why feels my heart its long forgotten heat?

Relentless walls? whose darksom round contains
Repentant sighs, and voluntary pains;
Ye rugged rocks! which holy knees have worn;
Ye grots and caverns shagg'd with horrid thorn!
Shrines! where their vigils pale-ey'd virgins keep,
And pitying saints, whose statues learn to weep!
Tho' cold like you, unmov'd and silent grown,
I have not yet forgot my self to stone.

Alexander Pope
"Eloise to Abelard"

DISSEMINATED SCLEROSIS: Disseminated, or multiple sclerosis is one of the commonest nervous diseases. It is characterized by the widespread occurrence of patches of demyelination followed by gliosis in the white matter of the nervous system. A striking feature is the tendency to remissions and relapses, so that the course of the disease may be prolonged for many years. The early symptoms are those of focal lesions of the nervous system, while the later clinical picture is one of progressive dissemination. The cause of the disorder is unknown.

There are two chief modes of onset. In most cases the disease begins with the symptoms of a single focal lesion or sometimes of several such lesions occurring within a short time. Unilateral acute retrobulbar neuritis is often the first symptom. Other such symptoms include numbness of some part of the body, usually part of a limb or one side of the face or both lower limbs, or double vision, or weakness of a limb, particularly of a lower limb with dragging of the foot, or precipitancy or micturation. The other mode of onset is an insidious and slowly progressive weakness of one or both lower limbs.

In the insidiously progressive type of case, the abnormal physical signs are usually predominantly spinal, consisting of spastic paraplegia with some degree of superficial sensory loss over the lower limbs and trunk, or of impairment of postural sensibility and vibrations sense or sometimes of both combined, the patient exhibiting a spastic and ataxic gait. In such cases, it may be difficult to be sure that the symptoms are due to disseminated sclerosis unless there is a history or there are physical signs of lesions within the territory of the cranial nerves, or characteristic changes in the cerebrospinal fluid.

In a typical advanced case, the patients will be bedridden with scanning or staccato speech and slurring of individual syllables, pallor of both optic discs, nystagmus, and a dissociation of conjugate lateral movement of the eyes, the abducting eye moving outwards further than the adducting eye moves inwards. The upper limbs will be weak and grossly ataxic. There will be severe paraplegia, either in extension interrupted by flexor spasms, or in flexion. Cutaneous or deep sensory loss, or both, may be present in upper and lower limbs, and there is likely to be incontinence of urine and feces.

Roger Bannister
Brain's Clinical Neurology

I

It is three o'clock in the morning and Brother Damian is already awake. Outside, deep within the lavender darkness of

June, there is the soft rustle of night creatures for whom dawn brings danger. They seek the absence of light, ever retreating into darkness and from the day, for herein their appointment, their destiny lies. And here too lies the destiny of Brother Damian, who has come to regard the night as friend and ally. Slowly, ever so slowly, and with the cautiousness of the wild that surrounds and is also within him, Brother Damian arrests the night with the lamp beside his bed. And yet the night is not destroyed; it is not evaporated but only pierced and penetrated by the flowing arc of illumination. Cautiously then, as if in contrapuntal harmony with the slow and liquid movements of the man himself, the dark does not flee but only withdraws to safer havens. Outside, the inhabitants of the night listen with quickened ear and pulse to this invasion of their sanctuary and plan their escape accordingly. But Brother Damian has become in these final months himself one of them, himself a creature of the night and now consults the day only for the necessary longitude and latitude of his initial bearings. He too has inherited the night even as once he inhabited the day, and time constantly beckons him further into the purples, lavenders, and ebonies of itself. For herein there is room, space, openness, and the mercy of sanctification. But the day—ah, the day has become too heavy and thick for claustrophobics such as he. Rather, he prefers the endless lavender of night with its amnesia for details, its forgetfulness, its myopia and deafness of fine distinctions. The night cares only for distance, freedom, space, and expansion and keeps far more secrets than it reveals. Thus, Brother Damian quickly extinguishes the light, having now done with it, and returns to the sanctuary that he has chosen.

In darkness he grasps the fluted ridge of railing and guides himself by its uncomprehending sense of direction. The hallway is all cobble-stoned and rough-hewned rock punctuated occasionally by the height of casement window. Here there is neither softness nor warmth but only a cool texture of stone which invites the touch but shuns the eye. He prefers this tactile world to the visual, having long ago discovered the cruelty of the latter. By now, he has cautiously worked his way to the center of his journey and is joined by shadowed figures in hooded vestments like his own. They expand and contract the distance between them while now weaving closer and now weaving farther from one another. Darkness has melted their flesh and forms into each other so that one cannot discern their numbers but only the unity that dilates and constricts the space surrounding them. From behind they are a protoplasmic ocean of hooded figures in stark collaboration with one another, joined by a common destination which is barely illuminated in the distance. Now a single candle flame comes into view as the swarm of hoods and vestments silently turns the corner; it casts the shadow of a twenty-foot cross across these strange figures. It is frightful, indeed unnerving to see the brutality of this crucified light illuminate them in defiance of the utter silence they maintain. One feels that they are guided—or perhaps led—by this symbol of suffering, and yet they have freely chosen such enslavement and such misery as if it were a peculiar joy, a happiness more treasured, surely more rarefied than one could imagine. Now they funnel themselves together through the open doorway and in so doing engulf, enrapture the cross even as the center of a bow binds its circumference around. As the funnel empties itself only to reexpand its wholeness on the doorway's other side, one loses sight of Brother Damian, whose darkness is absorbed by a lesser light no greater than a candle's single flame. Who are these hooded figures, and whence begins and whence ends this strange, dark journey of theirs?

By 4:00 A.M. the morning vigil is ended and Brother Damian will need to wind his weary and most tormented way back among the twisted halls. This will not be easily done nor can time be wasted, for the 5:45 lauds will come all too soon for his languid and unhurried movements. The painful desperation of bathing, dressing, and preparing for the day will take every ounce of time and every minute of energy. Still, he will do it, for that is, after all, his obligation and every bit a part of his suffering. Brother Michael may help somewhat but not much, for his burden is his burden and not another's. Night is so much kinder, so much gentler than he had ever imagined. It makes no demands upon us and grants us space, circumference within which to expand our suffocating limbs and trembling hands. Neither does it embarrass us with the voyeurism of light nor humiliate us with spectacles of ourselves. The night is to be preferred, yes, it is definitely to be preferred to the hazards of the day.

Thirty-five years ago, when he was only a fifteen-year-old boy, Michael Winfield Strawson entered the Abbey of Geth-semani. He had been raised on a farm and knew nothing of the world, only of God and of hard work. He was divinely prepared for this sanctuary that awaited him, for here he was expected only to glorify God and work to His benefit. This he did not because it was easy but because he had never known anything else. Upon entering the monastery, he gave up his worldly identity by giving up both his belongings and his name. From now on he would be called Brother Damian and would own nothing, for while he was yet in the world, he was nonetheless no longer of it, and this transformation was in need of a sym-bolic reformulation. He was—how shall we say?—dead of the world but born again in Christ. All of this seems so strange, so utterly maniacal, mad, mysterious, and incredibly tortured to anyone who had not seen the things that Brother Damian had seen. For he had experienced visions—perhaps they were dreams—of such a splendid sort that he thought the remainder of his life to be but a recovery of slow degree. His true reasons and what could have possessed him, what could have so trans formed and empowered him were so absolutely remote from the daily world as to break like brittle glass upon the hard sur-face of rational explanation.

Seven years ago, the Lord saw fit to add another burden to the cross he already bore. He was diagnosed as suffering from multiple sclerosis. This punishment might seem too harsh for such a devoted servant who had given his life to God, and in-deed the thought had crossed Brother Damian's mind more than once. It seemed cruel, unjust, unfair, even demonic, to curse the very soul that blesses. And yet the spiritual world is not governed by the same gravitational forces that enslave the physical one. In the latter, a cause must precede its effect, whereas in the former the reverse is frequently the case. In the latter, A equals A and identity is never the same as difference; whereas in the former difference is precisely identical to itself. In the latter, up is up, down is down, right is right, and left is left, and there is an end to it. But in the former, in the spiritual

113

world, there is neither space nor time nor difference nor identity, and thus anything can happen since all laws are in a constant state of reformulation. It is all so very confusing when one attempts exact translations, for the delicate subtleties of the spirit are simply heavy weights upon reentering this dense atmosphere. Suffice it to say that all of it made perfect sense to Brother Damian and that he thought his affliction neither fair nor unfair, just nor unjust, but only another aspect of his journey and another dimension of a continuous sphere in which he had learned to travel at ease.

II

Brother Damian was first taken to Louisville for diagnosis, but it was some time before it could be determined what was causing his symptoms. There were so many possible explanations, and to sort each of them out was an exasperating, frustrating, and time-consuming ordeal. Multiple sclerosis is a chameleon which delights in assuming the coloration of other diseases such as syringomyelia, cervical spondylosis, amyotrophic lateral sclerosis, and even some of the hereditary ataxias. In order to interrupt its games of imitation, one must surprise and startle the illness when it is least aware of being watched. But this is not easy, for the clever eye of this tormenting snake watches from its hiding place to discern the exact moment of innocence at which to sink its fangs.

Unpredictable, ironic reversals and remissions are the armaments of its arsenal. An episodic explosion of paresthesias may one day punctuate the languor of healthiness, issuing pronouncements of doom and disaster. Confused, frightened, and filled with denials and affirmations, the victim finally consults his physician only to discover that the symptoms which first alarmed him have transformed themselves into seemingly harmless artifacts. The initial attack is a masquerade of discordant and disconnected symptoms that refuse to integrate or unify themselves into a clear and recognizable pattern—weakness in the extremities, a palsy in the hands, perhaps some stiffness here, some awkwardness there, or a clumsiness where precision was needed, or even an inarticulateness where eloquence was required, or finally just a simple tiredness of leg, arm, face, finger, foot, or even of one's whole being. There is nothing honest, nothing clean or precise about this illness, for it enjoys deception far more than truth and would much rather parade as another than surface as itself.

Brother Damian became aware one day last April during evening vespers of a dull, throbbing ache in his left eye. It was not exactly painful but instead rather irritating and even distracting from the careful meditation he sought to achieve each day at this time. When it disappeared the following day, he thought no further of it, but the day thereafter it returned. Moreover, he now found it hard to focus on the scriptural passages before him; he finally decided by Friday afternoon that he should mention the problem to Brother Michael, who was in charge of the infirmary. They got him glasses. Eyestrain, they all agreed, was the sum and substance of the whole problem, and glasses were the cure. But it was neither the cure nor the problem, and Brother Damian's retrobulbar optic neuritis only worsened over the months as it continued to play a game of hide-and-seek with him.

In the kitchen one day last May he was surprised to find that he had cut himself very badly paring potatoes and yet felt little pain. But by that afternoon he was relieved, or rather retraumatized, to feel an intensity of pain all the greater precisely because of its delayed arrival. As the weeks went by, he discovered more and more occasions of the same sort. On Wednesday, for example, he burned himself badly when his hand suddenly let go of a pot of boiling water. Again, on Thursday morning, his right hand was numb upon waking, especially the fingertips, and it was midmorning before all of the feeling returned. That evening, his hand began to shake during compline and continued to do so until nearly bedtime. It was nothing in particular, it was everything in general that alerted him to the danger from within. Naturally, neither he nor Brother Michael perceived any organization or pattern to these shutdowns and start-ups of his nervous system, nor would they have understood the subtleties of neuritis, diplopia, or hemianesthesia had they been explained. But both knew, in-

115

deed both sensed a profound and distressing evolution within Brother Damian which would announce itself within the next few months.

On and off, off and on, Charcot's triad played a kind of hopscotch with his nervous system over the following months. As the disease organized and reasserted itself, so did it also seek subtle and exceptional modes of manifestation. By the time his cerebellar symptoms appeared, Brother Damian had become the property of a disease process whose territorial boundaries included his entire nervous system. However, before it demanded this full respect and recognition, it enjoyed taunting and pestering him with coy suggestions of itself. For example, the numbness in Brother Damian's fingertips soon disappeared only to be replaced by a dull ache on the left side of his face, and when that finally resolved itself he discovered that his leg had become partially insensitive. It was this or that, here or there, and never anything definite or permanent, clear or precise. One day he could not speak without slurring; on another he could not walk without stumbling. And as the one aspect of himself recovered so did another worsen, so that he felt himself to be a sort of rubber band in which one end tightened the moment the other loosened. It was puzzling, strange, and altogether unsettling to feel these tremors and earthquakes of the body gather storm throughout the night and then explode with violence throughout the day. On his right side he would seem to have no reflexes whatsoever, whereas on his left everything was hyperreflexic. It seemed that one part of him was in a hurry, whereas the other was not; one part of him was lazy, whereas the other was anxious; one degree of him was depressed, whereas the other was hysterical. It all happened so unpredictably and suddenly that there could be no preparation or warning to brace against the attacks, and no doubt it would have been fruitless to do so anyway.

Far worse than the shudders and tremors that dissolved his posture and stability, however, were the visual apparitions and evaporations that both horrified and isolated him. His eyes shook! They actually shook and rotated in their sockets as if they immersed in a medium of quivering Jell-O. And as they shook, they also rocked with a continuous, cyclical nystagmoid rhythm. The visual world, after all, is our primary anchor and support for all that is real and palpable about us; and therefore to have this foundation quiver is to lose more than sight, it is also to lose substance, support, and the concreteness of reality itself. But quiver his visual field did, and as it quivered it also blackened with scotoma whose visual interruptions were seen more as fragmentations than actual absences or vacuoles.

As these things happened both to him and about him, Brother Damian withdrew further and further into a self-imposed exile which was born as profoundly of his impoverished physical state as it was of his enriched spiritual condition. The contemplative realm of prayer and meditation became more substantive, indeed more concrete than did this shaking, palsied, quivering world of apparitions and evaporations about him. More than prefer, he came to adore night and the absence of light wherein darkness consolidated these fragmentary bodies into solid, unmoving structures. It did not hurt to look; it did not alarm or frighten to see; and the thick vacuity of night seemed to devour everything extraordinary into the singularity of its unified indivisibility.

Lying now with the density of the darkness about him, Brother Damian feels at one and fully accepted by it. Light accentuates and individuates everything and in so doing harshly judges it. The curvature here is smoother, longer, and more delicate than that surface over there. These colors are more saturated than those pastels, and ocher yellow complements cobalt blue in such a way that green or red could neither imagine nor even imitate. It is all so arbitrary and artificial this cruel business of division, distinction, and difference. In the light Brother Damian is the exceptional monk. In the light he is the sick, diseased, and handicapped monk with all the motor disturbances and pathologies that translate themselves into stumbles and stutters. However, in the night he is ordinary, common, quite unexceptional, and just like every other monk. For the night accepts everything that is its own and reduces it to one; it reduces division to unity, difference to similarity, and the unusual to the usual. There is something comforting in that. Indeed, there is also something profoundly holy. For in the night there is neither a Brother Damian nor a Brother Michael nor a Brother Jacob but rather one assembled, integrated body of monastic brothers in communal union with one another. And in the night neither is there multiple sclerosis nor skin ulcers nor neurofibromatosis nor a dozen other disfigurations that individuated their owners. No, in the dark such things do not exist. They come into being only with the light, and so Brother Damian had come to love the night as one loves . . . well, as one loves . . . a Father or another brother.

Eventually, the disorganization of these disconnected symptoms begins to arrange and integrate itself into a characteristic pattern. The game of hide-and-seek, punctuated by remissions and readmissions, comes to an end, and the masquerader finally unveils himself. So ends the inaugural stage of disseminated sclerosis, and so begins the advanced stage.

Just as isolated iron filings assume a pattern through magnetization, so also do these symptoms constitute a syndrome with laws, rules, and principles of predictability. Before this stage, there appeared to be neither order nor continuity to the episodic eruption of one truncated and half-completed symptom after another. Thus, it was impossible to predict or forecast what would happen next or even whether what had happened before would ever happen again. But now all of that has changed as the disease process turns the corner from innocence to malevolence.

Incrementally, gradually, but most systematically Brother Damian will become totally incapacitated and bedridden. It will take time, of course, but as spinal paraplegia sweeps oceanically across his lower limbs and trunk, all of the corresponding muscles will weaken and atrophy, but first they will announce their eventual destination through spasticity and hyperreflexia. Silently, the process of demyelination will produce thick plaque whose dense accumulation will finally choke delicate parts of the cervical area and thereby anesthetize all comprehension of postural attitude or equilibrium. His least and his greatest movements will shake as intention tremors from cerebellar lesions accentuate and exacerbate the unsteadiness of his composure. His head will shake; his eyes will rock; his hands will tremble; even his clothes will produce violent spasms from the least irritation while the greatest intention will be impotent to inaugurate a single movement.

A storm is gathering somewhere; a tide of tremendous power and force is assembling itself; a hurricane of movement is creating a small silent center about itself. In the midst of this cyclone of erratic motion, Brother Damian lies huddled in a secret center of his own making. Now there will be no remissions but rather a steady and relentless course of decline and disintegrations. As spastic paraplegia transforms him into quivering stone, decubitus ulcers will feed and feast upon his trembling flesh. Some days he will be incontinent and some days he will be enuretic; some days he will shake and some days he will be still; some days he will curse his lot in life and some days he will be hysterical beyond measure.

Whether it be the mockery or whether it be the mercy of the disease, the final aspects of this demise will be little noticed by Brother Damian. In euphoria, he will celebrate his disintegration with an ignorance born of innocence and suffering. Others alone will see what he has become while he will be blinded by the very forces that daily destroy him. He will little comprehend his passing, for the demotorized and desensitized vessel that he has become confounds the subtle difference between life and death, between what he was and what he is. Does the disease, by these bizarre measures, only further scorn the one it has tortured, or is this hysteria in fact an end to past suffering and a celebration of new freedom?

III

The nervous system is a network, a maze of entanglements whose logic is geometric and axiomatic in complexity. Warren McCulloch referred to this system as a "logical calculus of ideas" in order to emphasize its essentially mathematical structure as well as the rule-governed nature of its operations. Such descriptions have inspired comparison of the nervous system with computers, electrical transformers, and other devices whose internal organization is dependent upon a highly specialized wiring schematic. It is neither inappropriate nor misleading to draw such comparisons, for, indeed, the specificity of neural connection patterns bears much in common with electrical circuits. Moreover, the proper and efficient operation of these circuits also depends upon a natural insulation system which prevents the messages of one circuit from distorting or contaminating the messages of another.

It is the function of the myelin sheath—generated by Schwann cells and deposited as an insulating envelope around the axon—to insulate each nerve fiber from the noise around it. The lipid substance sphingomyelin prevents the flow of ions from one nerve fiber to the other and thus insures that order rather than anarchy reigns supreme within the individual monarchies of the nervous system.

However, several metabolic disorders disturb this insulating fiber by a disintegrative process which demyelinates the nerve fiber. Multiple sclerosis—as the very name itself implies—is one of these disorders, but there are others. Niemann-Pick disease, metachromatic leukodystrophy, and Tay-Sachs disease are but a few. The loss of the myelin sheath is usually followed by degeneration of the nerve axon—and sometimes of the nerve body itself—which is an irreversible process. As demyelination continues, plaques and scarring appear throughout the inflamed and damaged areas. In particular, the optic nerves, the cerebellum, and large tracts in the pons and cerebrum are affected. A fibrous gliosis soon covers these long tracts whose multiple and sclerotic appearance gives the disease its name.

Disseminated sclerosis is a systemic disease whose global universality produces harmonies of an apparently disconnected but actually well-integrated symphonic orchestration. Much as the individual horns, fiddles, and flutes of a musical composition must be melded together, so also the full measure and decibel of multiple sclerosis cannot be discerned until the music masters transform these solos into symphonies. The prodromal stage is actually only a practice session for the full concert to be held at a later date. The disease takes its time and exercises its infinite patience by performing only a few notes at a time and in the most isolated wings of its eventual theater. But as time goes by, the individual harmonies are tested, the compositional range increases both in tone and tex-

ture, and finally the baton master establishes a rhythmic cadence which will identify the thematics of the disease from that
point on.

Some patients complain of optic neuritis and others of ataxia
or of sensory disturbances. Each is but a signature of the disease written in a different ink but penned by the selfsame
hand. Occasionally, however, remyelination will occur, and
even regeneration of the neural substance; this may well explain the bizarre and episodic remissions that are so puzzling
and resistant to diagnosis. Noise is the absence of harmony, and
precisely unorganized notes characterize the early stages of
this disease process. It seems as if the disease experiments with
itself by testing different strategies, tactics, and harmonizations
in diverse and separate keys. But finally the proper tempo and
concentration of force are discovered as the disease assembles
and reassembles the results of its several auditions in separate
halls. As the full orchestration is gathered together, and unity
achieved, the disease ceases to be an alarming irritation and
instead becomes a deadly, sinister force of decomposition and
degeneration.

Naturally, Brother Damian was quite unaware of these
chemical and physical transformations within him. He knew
nothing of segmental demyelination, peripheral neuropathies,
or lipoprotein layers secreted by oligodendroglia and undone
by myelin degeneration. He knew instead that he hurt!
Brother Damian, for all his spiritual sophistication, little knew
and little cared that Babinski's reflex was present in him and
that his pyramidal tracts were decomposing. Rather, he knew
only that he couldn't feel, couldn't speak, couldn't walk,
couldn't see as well—not nearly as well—as before. Charcot's
triad could have been explained to him, and certainly the effects of retrobulbar optic neuritis might have been brought
down to his level, but frankly he would not have cared. Brother
Damian—as is so true of all multiple sclerosis patients—was
little concerned with details; he wanted generalities such as
would he live or would he die, would he suffer or would he
hasten to the end, would he be conscious or would he be bless-
edly amnesic? Nor would he have been reassured by the information that hydroxocobalamin or corticotrophin is often

121

helpful in relieving symptoms, for anything that did not cure him would not help him. No, these medical niceties were of interest only to the historian and curator of diseases, and of no help whatsoever to the sufferer.

Rather, Brother Damian wondered whether he would be in pain and whether he would degrade or humiliate or further embarrass himself. It was important to him that his dignity be left untouched by this sinister disease and that his death be an honorable, a suitable, and a humble—but not a humiliated—one.

When he realized—fully and completely realized—that he would die, then the power and majesty of the physician suddenly lost all its importance and significance for him. Never mind that they could save others; they could not save him, and so they became fallen angels who were thereby reduced from divinity to humanity. To Brother Damian—and to many of his brothers and sisters alike—doctors had often appeared as arrogant and highly self-interested people who had overinvested confidence in themselves. They were, in so many ways, unpleasant to be around. With a self-importance bordering on adulation of a narcissistic sort, they often were impossible to reach as persons, as people, as ordinary fellows, or simply as friends. Rather, it was always a power game of one-upmanship with them in which the urgency of their lives had to take precedence over everything else. Some people—Brother Damian was not one of them—tolerated and actually applauded this investiture of self-celebration. Perhaps they did so in the hope that one of these gods or goddesses would actually turn out to be divine. But when they did not, when they proved themselves human, then even their enraptured audience deserted them. After all, they had glorified physicians only in the hope that thereby they would be protected from the jaws of death, but now it became clear that they possessed no such powers and were simply magicians with tricks of a limited kind.

It is always cruel to idolize another and especially cruel when that other is yourself. To believe that one is glorified, that one is omnipotent and empowered for acts of salvation is self-destructive not simply because it is false but, worse, because it is hubristic. There is a wanton, a somewhat depraved spectacle of such self-love that offends us precisely because it is a misbegotten love which finally destroys both the lover as well as the beloved. Brother Damian had come to pity such star-crossed lovers even more than he now pitied himself.

IV

Along the corridor he limped by slow degrees guided by the night whose friendship he had now come to treasure more fully than the light. His room and therein his bed had become a sanctuary of meditative repose. Here he was free to consult the heavens and the stars and request direction and guidance for his future journey. With only the lavender umbrella of night surrounding him, punctuated with ocher stars and silver beams of light, Brother Damian could peacefully pray, meditate, counsel and console, glorify and adore, beseech and beget the powers, forces, and spirits that ruled his slender earthly life. This life, this life of substance rather than of spirit, of flesh slowly becoming stone was surely overrated in his judgment. He did not regret its loss since in forsaking it there was still so much left to him. To this degree, Brother Damian was, of course, unusual. Most people cling with tenacious and frenzied claws to their lives in terror that the void and nothingness await them. Thus, in their desperation to survive at any cost, they will accept a cheapened, degraded existence in favor of death and the freedom it brings. Brother Damian thought not at all in such terms and believed—in fact, was utterly convinced— that life itself was a degraded imitation of a far richer, far more profound existence. Thus, he did not at all fear death but rather welcomed and adored it. In this respect, and to this degree, he was different from most people.

Pain did affront and offend him. But still, even here it was not a physical but a spiritual concern which motivated him. Pain in itself was neither good nor bad. Rather, it was entirely a question of how well and how properly one suffered and endured one's pain. Different illnesses produce different types, different geometries of pain, and this is a certain fact that anyone who has suffered at all understands well. The pain of angina is right-angled and sharp in its intensity, whereas the pain of a brain tumor is diffuse, nonlocalized, and more a curvature than a flat surface. Brother Damian had endured pains of every degree and sort in his fifty years of earthy life and had come to terms with most of them. But not with the pain of multiple sclerosis, which was, for him at least, an unmanageable and unwieldy sort of pain. The painful spasms in the midst of insensitivity were confusing; the aching, gnawing thud of ocular neuritis was confusing; the full, bloated tight sensation of his face was an oily, dirty, and hot sort of pain. In short, pain that assumed a form and remained faithful to it, Brother Damian had learned to tolerate. But pain that refused all structure and contour was unmanageable because it was unorganized and unpredictable. Such pain haunted, taunted, and toyed with him to such a great degree that he was distracted and disabled by it. He fought this gravitational force of his body's misery constantly, seeking to free himself from its seduction in order to attend the more fully to his meditation. And yet, it seemed the greatest challenge and temptation of his entire spiritual life.

Is this clear? Or does this strange paradox perhaps confuse? It was not death that disturbed Brother Damian. No, he had long ago made his amends on that issue. It was not debilitation or invalidism that bothered this noble brother, for he was an expert—even a connoisseur—when it came to suffering. Neither was it pain that terrified him, for pain was a blessing when it permitted suffering. No, it was none of these that disturbed Brother Damian's tranquillity and peace. Rather, it was the amorphous and unstructured nature of this kind of pain, this sort of misery that distracted and drove him nearly mad with misgivings, self-doubts, and grievous misunderstandings of his own substance and direction. Why could he not handle it? Why did he, of all people, feel weighted down and burdened by this physical cross which he could neither surrender to nor fully abandon? His main fear was that his illness would undo in a single moment of agony all the spiritual work that it had taken him years to accomplish. The question before Brother Damian, and the one that he could not seem to answer, was how does one spiritually die a physical death?

It had, of course, occurred to him that satanic forces were busy at work to unravel all the spiritual substance that he had become. How ironic and utterly cruel it would be should he fail at this point and after all this labor! He had entered the monastery at the age of fifteen; he had given his life to God and obeyed all the rules and commandments required of him. He had traveled so far and so long to prepare himself for God's blessing, and then to be defeated by an illness, by pain, by hellish fires, and at the very last moment. It seemed so unfair, so impossible but also so very real and so very certain.

So was the sanctuary of his thoughts haunted by the incubus of his disease. Sequestered by the night and meditation and prayer, he witnessed a constant battle between gods and demons for the possession of his slender, delicate soul. While positive forces drew him deeper and deeper into his contemplative prayer, there were also correspondingly negative forces which eroded and distracted each advance with a contrapuntal retreat. There was a spiritual significance to his disease that could not simply be reduced to the biological and that was certainly more complex than the demyelination of nerve fibers. His physicians in Louisville had entirely misdiagnosed his malady as one of the body whereas it was actually one of the soul. And diseases of the soul are neither recognized nor cured by the instruments of scientific medicine. One dies of a broken heart, of a wounded soul, of a twisted mind, and for modern medicine it is simply a metabolic disorder expressing itself in psychosomatic ways. One dies of nostalgia, of loneliness, of bitterness, and of regret; but for modern medicine it is all the same, for one has only died of biological disturbances expressed in psychological ways. But there are true spiritual diseases, and they will kill you, and Brother Damian was just now dying of such a one. It was, therefore, spiritual pain and spiritual death that Brother Damian constantly battled each evening under that lavender umbrella of night with its ocher trim of silver moons and stars.

He remembered first entering the monastery and the final, silent thud of the gatehouse door that sealed him in while sealing the world out. In many ways his illness is just like the physical enclosure of the monastery, for it also seals him up within his soul and may just as quickly suffocate him. Flesh no longer flesh, flesh become stone, flesh paralyzed and insensitive to outside stimulations, his disintegrating nervous system has formed a hermitage in which he is forced to reside in loneliness and isolation. He remembers now his friend and mentor Thomas Merton, who was his brother in the monastery for many years. Merton constantly sought out enclosures, hermitages, retreats, but always with the intention of being locked up in order that he could break out again. Merton wanted to lose his freedom precisely in order that he could constantly rediscover and reassert it. But Brother Damian is not certain whether he has lost his freedom or is being suffocated by it. He remembers once having said to Merton: "You do not seem like much of a hermit," and Merton agreed, with only the explanation that "I need a lot of time to myself."

For Brother Damian, death is not an enemy but a friend. Last December, when Brother Casper died, the community held a celebration in his honor and in thanksgiving for his eternal liberation. They will do the same for Brother Damian. All of life is suffering, and all of suffering is growth, renewal, and strength. Brother Damian is, therefore, not afraid of suffering, for it is the very geography of his salvation. Pain is neither hideous nor monstrous but only an aspect of one's humanity in transformation to divinity. Brother Damian does not fear pain, for in understanding it he therefore also transforms it.

And yet there are frightful, monstrous, and dangerous demons in this world which can devour and deform you in an instant. Neither death nor pain nor suffering is among these; they are innocent by comparison. Rather, it is the loss of spiritual energy, the decomposition of one's divinity, and the erosion of the eternal within the mortal that occupy Brother Damian's nightmares and greatest fears. Will he die a spiritual death before he dies a physical one? Will these twisting, contorting, cold, and insensitive muscles so taunt and tempt him into such seizures of despair that he will abandon his faith? So close, so very close to the treasured moment, will he lose it all in one desperate lunge for a humanity which he neither desires nor can ever hope to possess? His fear—perhaps it should be the fear of us all—is that some visceral and unguarded aspect of ourselves will at the very last moment make a frantic lunge toward the flesh and away from the spirit. Weakened, distracted, frightened, he constantly seeks to guard against this human frailty which clings to the earth rather than reaching for the sky, which in some crazed and human madness embraces death rather than life. This is what he fears, and all that he fears, that at the last moment when courage is called for, he will respond with weakness. While overhead, the lavender night falls like a curtain, and Brother Damian meditates on what he is and what he shall become.

II

Metabolic Furnaces

Imagine God as tailor. His shelves are lined with rolls of skin, each with its subtleties of texture and hue. Six days a week He cuts lengths with which to wrap those small piles of flesh and bone into the clever parcels we call babies. Now engage the irreverence to consider that, either out of the tedium born of infinity, or out of mere sly parsimony, He uses the occasional handicraft a remnant of yard goods, the last of an otherwise perfect bolt, dusty, soiled, perhaps a bit too small or too large, one whose woof is warped or that is cut on the bias. I have received many such people in my examination room. Like imperfect postage stamps, they are the collector's items of the human race.

Richard Selzer
Mortal Lessons

7

The Face of a Wolf

As a dare-gale skylark scanted in a dull cage
Man's mounting spirit in his bone-house, mean
    house, dwells—
That bird beyond the remembering his free fells;
This in drudgery, day-labouring-out life's age.

Though aloft on turf or perch or poor low stage,
Both sing sometimes the sweetest, sweetest spells,
Yet both droop deadly sometimes in their cells
Or wring their barriers in bursts of fear or rage.

Not that the sweet-fowl, song-fowl, needs no rest—
Why, hear him, hear him babble and drop down to
    his nest
But his own nest, wild nest, no prison.

Man's spirit will be flesh-bound when found at
    best,
But uncumbered: meadow-down is not distressed
For a rainbow footing it nor he for his bones risen.

Gerard Manley Hopkins
"The Caged Skylark"

DISSEMINATED LUPUS ERYTHEMATOSIS: Systemic lupus erythematosus (SLE) is a chronic, inflammatory disease of unknown cause which may affect the skin, joints, kidneys, nervous system, serous membranes, or other organs of the body. The classic facial "butterfly rash", when present, facilitates diagnosis. The clinical course may be fulminant or indolent, but generally is characterized by periods of remissions and relapses. Patients with SLE develop distinct immunologic abnormalities, especially antinuclear antibodies, which facilitate diagnosis.

Lupus, which is the Latin for wolf, has been used since about 1230 to describe cutaneous conditions which resemble the malar erythema of a wolf. . . . Osler described the systemic complications of lupus and noted that they could occur in the absence of skin disease. The clinical recognition of SLE has changed greatly since Hargraves first described the LE cell test in 1948 and since the development of the immunoflourescent antinuclear factor test by Friou in 1957.

Lupus erythematosus is characterized particularly by autoimmune phenomena. Patients develop antibodies to many of their own cells, cell constituents and proteins, representing a loss of tolerance to self antigens. This may be due in part to a loss of suppressor T lymphocytes. This defect in turn may be due in part to antibodies to these cells.

The classic picture of a patient with well-advanced lupus is one of a young woman with fever, weight loss, arthralgia, a butterfly rash, pleural effusion, and nephritis. With better methods of detection (the antinuclear antibody tests), many more patients with less obvious and more varied symptoms and signs are being recognized. Most patients complain of some fatigue, arthralgia, rashes, and fever. This chronic disease is best characterized by periods of remission and activity.

Wyngaarden and Smith
Cecil's Textbook of Medicine

I

Flannery O'Connor's illness started with a fever and an odd butterfly rash across her face. She was staying with Bob and Sally Fitzgerald in the Connecticut woods, and everyone thought she had the flu or perhaps, when her joints began to ache, a touch of arthritis. She feared it might be rheumatic fever or even some sort of female trouble. At first she only felt a little out of sorts, but then the rash worsened into dense erythematous lesions that covered her breasts, the back of her neck, and even across the bridge of her nose. With the swirl of coloration and maculopapular spotting, she looked something like a wolf. Within a few days, small painful ulcers began to punctuate her lips and soft palate, and still the hot debilitating fever continued. She knew now—indeed, she sensed now in some visceral and instinctual way—that she was desperately ill. It was in late December 1950, and the Fitzgeralds drove her that afternoon to the train station where she boarded the express to Milledgeville, Georgia.

That was almost fourteen years ago, and now the hot July heat of Georgia only added to her suffering as she lay dying in the Baldwin Memorial Hospital of systemic lupus erythematosus. It is awful to die in such heat, to suffocate in the summer sun of a raging fever which consumes and consumes. Your hair is wet and matted together in a slime of oily perspiration, your toes and fingers stick to one another, and the skin underneath your arms and in your crotch and between your buttocks is raw with damp, itching infections. It is enough to drive you mad. It seems the summer heat only further inflames the fever, or does the fever only serve to further inflame the summer heat? Whether the one or the other, they conspire to make of you a metabolic furnace of such intense temperatures and flame that your every organ is devoured by the suffocating heat. Her nights were seized with hysterical and confused dreams; she could not sleep. Her days were unimaginable agonies of sweat and oil and fever and the evil smells of her own disease; she could not rest. And so she would suffer day in and day out for another two weeks until August 3, 1964, when life—frightful and fearful life—fled in terror from the rotting corpse she had become.

There are two types of lupus. One is playful and shy; one is sober and deadly. Discoid lupus erythematosus is the delicate one whose retiring ways are usually private and rarely public. A lesion underneath the hair, upon the nose, or within the ear will announce its quiet presence, but it also rather likes the breasts, the back, or even the rich mucosa of the mouth. It is far too gentle, far too bashful to do any real harm, but it does enjoy teasing the skin with its round scaling papules that scar and tattoo the face like the markings of a wolf.

However, there is nothing gentle or kind about systemic lupus erythematosus. Indeed, one wonders how the malevolent and the innocent could possibly spring from such common loins, and why the one craves death whereas the other seeks only recognition of itself. Disseminated SLE is a cruel, territorial glutton which marches with its deranged immunoglobulins of death and destruction throughout the system, leaving fibrinoid necrosis and hematoxylin bodies in its wake. Its special delight is to prey upon young women in their twenties and thirties whose lives are just beginning and whose minds are filled with plans of loving husbands, babies, and homes of their own. The tough, muscled tissue of men is far too sinewy for its greedy palate; it prefers soft, young, tender victims with delicate organs—such as heart and liver—that become its gourmet delight. Therein it feasts and fasts in contradictory relish while devouring and resting, gorging and dieting in endless crises and remissions of itself. Neither does this thoughtless, malevolent cell factor hold itself in custody to guilt or remorse for its transformation of normal nuclei into disturbed, homogeneous globular bodies that are phagocytized and thereby become the signature of itself. Nor does this glutton regret the pericarditis, the hyperglobulinemia, the thrombocytopenic purpura, or the dozens of other histological changes it inflicts upon its unwilling victim. It is a rape, a mutilation of cells and tissues which disregards the agony of its host in preference to the pleasure of itself.

Fulminant SLE expresses itself in fourteen clinically characteristic ways according to the American Rheumatism Association. It is hard to make sense of these fragmented and disconnected symptoms, for there seems to be no singular interface that unites them all. They are simply a confusing jumble of butterfly rashes, alopecia, cellular casts, proteinuria, photosensitivity, arthritis, oral ulcers, certain hematologic changes, LE cells, discoid lupus, false-positive STS, serositis, Raynaud's sign, and central nervous system disorders. They are signs without a referent, streets without a city, whose meaning is to be found both everywhere and nowhere. How puzzling and paradoxical is this disease which affects everything in general and nothing in particular.

For example, some patients have splenomegaly while others have only lymphadenopathy, and some have neither and some have both; some have pericarditis while others have myocarditis; some have basilar atelectatic pneumonitis and some do not; some have peritonitis, ileocolitis, or ulcerative colitis but others don't. Most have myalgia and arthralgia, but not all! Some are anemic and some have thrombocytopenia purpura, but then, in turn, some don't. Some go into remission and some do not; some lose their hair but gain pigmentation everywhere; others have ulcers, erythematous rashes, and lesions everywhere and some do not. Some die in a year and some die in thirty. It doesn't make any sense.

But then, again, it does make sense! It makes sense because disseminated lupus erythematosus is, after all, a systemic disease which recognizes no individual territorial boundaries precisely because it demands sovereign and universal domination over everything. Everything is invaded and nothing is spared; all circumferences are dilated to their farthest extension, and conquest is therefore unmerciful and absolute.

Perhaps Novalis was right that "every sickness is a musical problem; every cure a musical solution." But what then is the harmony, the melody, pitch, and timbre of lupus erythematosus? Does the disease have a characteristic signature of its own, or is it simply a clever forger writing checks on the accounts of others but never drawing on its own? Kidney, heart, muscle, gut, joint, brain, blood, liver, spleen, bone, lung, and skin—it dominates and enslaves them all. Everywhere the LE cell factor insinuates itself, and yet nowhere does it give a clear accounting of itself. Even the sophisticated Coombs test is frequently negative; and while the presence and discovery of the LE cell is certainly of diagnostic importance, its absence does not thereby rule out the presence of systemic lupus erythematosus. Nothing in particular is pathognomonic while everything in general seems to be. Even the LE cell factor—the product of an antibody reaction—is a peculiar and often misleading signature whose significance is difficult to discern. Its structure is that of polymorphonuclear leukocyte whose contents stain purple with Wright's stain. But the LE cell factor is also found in other diseases, and so even its presence is not definitive.

Perhaps the best diagnostic instrument is experience itself. Should a young lady in her late twenties or early thirties present herself to you one day with a recurrent fever, leukopenia, and hyperglobulinemia, with a deep red skin rash across the bridge of her nose, complaints of pleurisy, and generalized arthritic pains, you should suspect systemic lupus erythematosus. Moreover, should you discover the LE cell factor as well as other indicators such as thrombocytopenia purpura, you may be further confirmed in your diagnosis. Of course, none of this is conclusive, for everything with SLE is circumstantial, but such evidence finally does arrange itself like iron filings in the presence of an unseen magnetic field whose influence is silent and invisible.

Dr. Arthur Merrill correctly diagnosed Flannery O'Connor's condition at once; in fact, he had suspected lupus when her mother first described the symptoms to him over the phone that day in December 1950. Flannery was immediately placed in the Baldwin Memorial Hospital on a salt-free diet, with daily injections of ACTH and total bedrest. It was nearly a year and a half—not really until the summer of 1952—that she sufficiently recovered from the crisis that first announced her lupus erythematosus.

Her symptoms began in late November 1950 with fainting spells, weakness, and a general malaise accompanied by a fever. She would suffer for almost fourteen years from this disease with countless stays in the hospital, innumerable infections, and many transfusions. Frequently, her hemoglobin would drop to 8 and she might require six or seven or as many as ten transfusions to become restabilized. Even when her lupus was in remission and inactive, she constantly fought daily scrimmages with fever, minor infections, and a general debilitating weariness. In the end, this crafty and cunning enemy won; and it won through sheer patience and a relentless but silent attention to detail.

II

Mary Flannery O'Connor was born in Savannah, Georgia, on March 25, 1925. She was the only child of Edward Francis and Regina Cline O'Connor. When she was twelve years old, her father fell ill with systemic lupus erythematosus and the family moved back to her mother's birthplace, Milledgeville, and into the Cline family residence. Her father's condition grew worse, and he died when Flannery was fifteen and enrolled in Peabody High School. She lived at home while attending the Georgia State College in Milledgeville and graduated with a B.A. degree in 1945. There she continued to live—except for brief periods in Iowa and the North and time spent at her beloved Andalusia outside of town—for the rest of her life.

The Writers' Workshop at the University of Iowa was the most outstanding academic facility in the country at which to study creative writing. The atmosphere, the collegiality, the opportunities provided were a nourishment beyond measure to the young writer, and Flannery grew quickly under these influences. In 1946 she published "The Geranium," her first short story, in the literary magazine *Accent*. The following year she won the Rinehart-Iowa Fiction Award for a novel which was later published as *Wise Blood*. It appeared that her literary career was well under way. She was recommended for a term of residence at Yaddo, the writers' retreat in Saratoga Springs, New York, but by March 1948 Yaddo had fallen into such political turmoil that Flannery and everyone else left and went their separate ways. She first journeyed to New York City where she met Bob and Sally Fitzgerald and then, after spending part of the summer in Milledgeville with her mother, moved to the Fitzgeralds' home in Ridgefield, Connecticut, during the month of August 1949. Here she lived and wrote until the first symptoms of lupus appeared near the middle of November and she was forced to return permanently to Milledgeville. Her career had just begun; she was not yet twenty-five years old; and lupus had already taken hold of her life and was in the process of gradually transforming it.

She did her best work during the course of her invalidism; far from being debilitated by her illness, she seemed to be nourished and enriched by it. The manuscript of *Wise Blood*, partially revised and rewritten during her confinement at the Baldwin Memorial Hospital and then at the Emory University Hospital, was completed and mailed to her publisher Robert Giroux on March 10, 1951. During the past three months, she had been in and out of two hospitals, undergone countless transfusions, battled fevers, withstood cortisone treatment, tolerated special diets, and still she wrote. She thought that she was being incapacitated by rheumatoid arthritis—her mother, however, knew that she was dying of lupus—and every swelling in every joint reacted painfully to the least movement, and still she wrote. In fact, she wrote every day for the next fourteen years, beginning in the mornings when her strength was at its peak and continuing until noon when she was too exhausted to continue. The combined and consummate result was incredible.

In thirteen and a half years, she wrote thirty-one short stories, the novel *Wise Blood*, and a collection of essays later published as *Mystery and Manners*. It would be an impressive amount of work—especially given the amount she revised—even if she had been in excellent health. But she was not, and each and every day was a painful, exhausting agony which she endured through sheer self-discipline, courage, and, of course, her personal faith. But what was her faith, and was it important to her?

Often in reading these stories—such as "Good Country People" or "A Temple of the Holy Ghost"—one cannot at all be certain where their author stands on questions of faith. At times it seems that she is certainly a believer; whereas at other times it seems certain that she is not. The whole matter is quite confusing. Consider, for example, the following exchange in "Good Country People" between Hulga, a Ph.D. in philosophy, and a Bible salesman.

Her face was almost purple. "You're a Christian," she hissed. "You're a fine Christian! You're just like them all—say one thing and do another. You're a perfect Christian, you're . . ."

The boy's mouth was set angrily. "I hope you don't think," he said in a lofty indignant tone, "that I believe in that crap! I may sell Bibles but I know which end is up and I wasn't born yesterday and I know where I'm going!" [*The Complete Stories*, p. 290]

And yet she was, in fact, a Christian, and not merely a Christian but also a Catholic Christian in the very Baptist state of Georgia. She knew—she must have known—of the mystery that surrounded her, and perhaps she herself even helped to perpetuate it. A reader once wrote to tell his distress that all the characters in her books always lost their faith; how peculiar, thought she, since her belief was precisely that they always found it. This personal faith of hers was so constant and all encompassing that she lost sight of it herself precisely because she never saw anything without it. "I once wrote a story called 'Good Country People' in which a lady Ph.D. has her wooden leg stolen by a Bible salesman whom she has tried to seduce. . . . Early in the story, we're presented with the fact that the Ph.D. is spiritually as well as physically crippled. She believes in nothing but her own belief in nothing, and we perceive that there is a wooden part of her soul which corresponds to her wooden leg" (*Mystery and Manners*, pp. 98–99). How peculiar and even grotesque, it might be said, to write such stories. Flannery would no doubt have agreed, but she then added her own characteristic apology. "When people have told me that because I am a Catholic, I cannot be an artist, I have had to reply ruefully, that because I am a Catholic I cannot afford to be less than an artist" (ibid., p. 146).

Perhaps *Mystery and Manners* is a most appropriate title for her collected essays since beneath her southern manners there was a mystery—even a gothic mystery—about her. Religious but not pious, self-determined but not obstinate, frightened but not cowardly, dying but very much alive, she was in so any ways a mass of contradictions.

And yet somehow beneath the thick webbing of these contradictions there was a tough gristle which kept her alive throughout all the transfusions, loneliness, pain, and disappointments. She survived; in fact, she excelled and even flourished and might well have even triumphed had it not been for the appearance of a fibroid tumor in February 1964. Within six months it would be all over. Quiet, silent, cunning as a fox, the lupus had patiently waited in keen anticipation of just such an opportunity. It coiled and recoiled upon itself in relaxed elaboration of its powers and poisons. Why not, since it had waited so long already in expectation of this delightful moment. When the jaws finally snapped shut and she was absolutely and relentlessly within its deadly grasp, this devourer of collagen and bone began to consume everything within its reach: heart, liver, kidney, lung, and brain. It was a marriage of life and death, of sickness and of health, and she became the finalization, the realization of a disease whose thirteen-year growth had now rendered it giddy with its promises and possibilities.

III

Mary Flannery O'Connor—a slender and rather pretty single woman of thirty-eight—began the elaborate and complex process of dying her death during the Christmas holidays of 1963; she was slow and meticulous in her efforts, as, indeed, she was at everything, and therefore did not finish her labor until August 3, 1964. Was she frightened? Of course, but also she was expectant, for death is so much like birth that it is often difficult to distinguish the one from the other. The delivery of a death is a labor no less solemn and certainly no less serious than the delivery of a birth. Both are works of love, and each is a passage from enslavement to freedom. For Flannery, pregnant with the promise of time and eternity, the entire period of gestation was nearly the same length of time for death as it would have been for life. From the beginning to the end of her final crisis, she lived a total of eight months and ten days, the sum accumulation of 253 sleepless nights or 6,072 painful hours. Perhaps such statistics seem quite meaningless to the living, but to the dying they are vital and urgent coordinates that fix the exact longitude and latitude of one's navigation from life to death, first by the day and then by the hour. They are numbers only, to be sure, and yet they serve to record the minute and incremental etchings of the slow disintegration upon the integrity and unity of one's life. For Flannery did not die all at once but by gradual, precise degrees, and the agony of the whole must have been keenly felt within the particularity of each moment.

This whole business of dying is so completely misunderstood by the living. The assorted visitors, well-wishers, bereaved family members, curious doctors, distracted nurses, angry attendants that one receives throughout the day are but travelers in a foreign country. They enter the court and kingdom of the patient but only on official business of import and export; they tarry not nor do they adopt the local customs of the country within which they find themselves. Indeed, there is an arrogance, even an insolence to these tourists which is the insulation by which they protect themselves against the contamination of death. After all, what do they know of pain, sweat, incontinence, putrefaction of rotting flesh, and the sheer humiliation of not being able to control your bladder and bowels? They measure your fever, but they do not suffer it. They study your blood, but they do not bleed it. They palpate your liver, your spleen, your guts; but they do not feel them. They hear your heart and yet cannot feel its weakened beat; they measure your blood pressure and yet cannot feel its intensity; they peer, with curious abandon, into the various interstices, holes, canyons, craters of your body and yet are never part of the great cavern you have become. They are guests, not residents, of this house of death which you inhabit. How then could they possibly understand?

In the evenings, they go home to husbands, wives, friends, or lovers. Cool and comfortable in their freedom from pain and disease, they lounge in languid, lazy luxury and finally curl up in front of the television or in one another's arms. And later, in their beds and surrounded by darkness, they drink freely and deeply from one another's flesh. Their strong, muscled loins arch and twist with intense pleasures far beyond your own diminished recall while yours instead quiver with an agony born of death rather than orgasms issuing from life. Later, lying in one another's arms, they are renewed while you are depleted; they sleep well and soundly while you dream dreams of death and frightful, hideous sights. In the morning they enter once again into the ever diminishing circumference of your dying light.

They ask you how you slept without waiting for the answer. They hope that you are feeling better today although they know that you are not. It is small talk, simply chatter intended to break the boredom and monotony of their required and enforced visit. You, in turn, are polite, casual, and self-effacing. They already know of your pain, of your dying, of your fear, and of your agony. And so why mention it? They know already that you are worse today than you were yesterday and worse yesterday than the day before. And so why mention it? When asked how you are feeling, why not simply agree that you are fine? Does it matter; could it make a difference? It is a game, an elaborate series of gestures and half-truths intended to make the visitor feel comfortable in the presence of death. After all, it is the privilege and the obligation of the dying not to alarm or unduly frighten the living. Thus, the entrance of every visitor for whatever reason must be handled delicately and precisely. After all, you are dying and they are busy. Be careful not to disarm them with stark realities, truths too cruel for the light of day, or hysterical scenes of fear and remorse. They have come into your room, specifically to your room and to no other, to be entertained! Do not forsake your obligations as host and guestmaster.

The living will inquire of the dying about their conditions of living. "Are you comfortable; do you have enough to eat and is it good?" Perhaps they will even make a little joke about the hospital food. Laugh along with them and agree that it is not so very good. They will, of course, tell you that you look good—much too good to be sick—and that they wished they looked half as well. Do not become angry; it is an innocent little game and you should, out of respect and obligation, play along with them. Soon now they will depart, for the atmosphere is becoming oppressive and they have discharged their obligations, and you should thank them very much for coming, confess that you actually feel better after their visit, and invite them back again. Out in the hallway you will hear their rushed and whispering voices disappearing down the corridor, and you cannot avoid the fragmentations of meaning that float like nuclear fallout back to your room. "Dying . . . God, she looks so bad . . . only a few days left they say . . . did you see her eyes? . . . Myra says that she is . . ."

IV

Flannery's lupus had been in remission for some time now, and although she never forgot its constant presence, neither did she precisely remember its exact details and particulars. You adjust, and in adjusting you tend to accept less rather than yearn for more. You know that you will never feel good, and so you adjust to feeling bad. You limit what you can do and how it can be done until it seems that there are no limitations imposed because you never strive to reach beyond your grasp. You no longer expect to be cured, and so you are not surprised that you are sick. Having lost—or at least forgotten and misplaced—the parameters of feeling good, of excellent health, of having strength, you no longer have standards with which to judge your present state of being or condition. Thus, what would have been a very bad day at the beginning of your illness is now a good or even an excellent day. It is strange, but one can adjust to anything, and in so doing the footprints of your past are obliterated by the imprints of your daily living. And so, to put the matter quite simply, having forgotten what it was like to be well, Flannery also nearly forgot that she was sick.

But life despises all stability, permanence, and the arrogance of anything that resists change; rather, it demands either growth or diminution, either maximization or minimization, either hypertrophy or atrophy. These—all of these and any of these—it will tolerate in whatever combination is prescribed, but it will not tolerate, will not suffer the sterility of obstinate endurance. Things had to change. And so they did.

Near the middle of December 1963, Flannery began to feel weaker and weaker with each passing day. She awoke each morning even more weary than when she went to bed. By January she was so weak and anemic that denial was no longer an adequate antidote. She confided to her friend Maryat Lee that "I've been sick. Fainted a few days before Christmas and was in bed about 10 days and not up to much thereafter. Blood count had gone down to 8 and you can't operate on that" (*The Habit of Being*, p. 562). By February the trouble was diagnosed as a fibroid tumor, and she was scheduled for operation on Tuesday, February 25, 1964. Her internist was extremely nervous about performing surgery on a lupus patient, but he felt there was little alternative. The tumor was uneventfully removed, however, and by March 7 she was writing to her publisher Bob Giroux to say that she was out of the hospital but still not feeling very well.

March was somewhat uneventful, but a serious kidney infection developed near the end of the month, and by April 2 she had been placed on five different antibiotics without successful results. In fact, she confided in a letter to Janet McKane that the medication has "torn up my stomach and swollen shut my eyes. Then the cortisone comes along and undoes the swollen eyes but gives you a moon-like face" (ibid., p. 561). By the middle of May it was clear that the lupus had returned with full force, and she was confined to the Baldwin Memorial Hospital. She had a blood transfusion on May 11 and felt much better afterwards, but she still expected to remain in bed for the rest of the summer. Four days later, on May 15, she needed another transfusion, but she still continued to work at least an hour a day on the short story "Revelation." That day, she wrote to Maryat Lee and recalled the ten transfusions she needed in 1951 when her lupus was last active while mentioning that her hemoglobin level remained at 8.

There were three stories that occupied Flannery's time during these final days of her life: "Revelation," "Parker's Back," and "Judgment Day." They were the last stories she wrote, and one, "Judgment Day," is a careful rewriting of her very first short story, "The Geranium." It is, no doubt, coincidental that she should appear so intent to finish what she had begun and seek thereby to arrive at such an absolute completion of her life. Still, her friend Sally Fitzgerald observed that from the time the lupus first reappeared "there was probably never much doubt of the outcome, and I find it hard to believe that Flannery didn't know it" (ibid., p. 559). In addition, there is a certain irony to these stories, not only in their titles but also that she should begin the last one with the following words:

"Tanner was conserving all his strength for the time home." She tells us that Tanner wants to get home and he does not care how he does it: "the next day or the morning after, dead or alive, he would be home. Dead or alive, it was being there that mattered; the dead or alive did not." Coincidental or not, it is a fair description of Flannery's own situation, for she also was conserving her strength in order to get home dead or alive.

By June 9 she had already been in the Piedmont Hospital in Atlanta for three weeks, and it was not until Saturday, June 20, that she was allowed to go home to Milledgeville. The night before, she got another transfusion and two more the following morning. On June 24 she wrote Cecil Dawkins from home and mentioned that "I've had four blood transfusions in the last month. The trouble is mostly kidneys—they don't refine poisons out of the proteins and therefore you don't make blood like you should or you lose it like you shouldn't or something. As far as I am concerned, as long as I can get at that typewriter, I have enough. They expect me to improve, or so they say, I expect anything that happens" (ibid., p. 587).

She felt somewhat better on June 27 and was working about two hours a day by June 28. By July 1 her prednisone dosage had been reduced by half in order to counteract a blood nitrogen increase of over one-third. Four days later, in a letter to Sister Mariella Gable, she said, "the wolf, I'm afraid, is inside tearing up the place" (ibid., p. 591). A week later, on July 8, her parish priest administered extreme unction or the sacrament of the sick to her, and another week later she sent Janet McKane a copy of "The Prayer to Saint Raphael" written by Ernest Hello:

O Raphael, lead us toward those we are waiting for; Raphael, Angel of happy meeting, lead us by the hand toward those we are looking for. May all our movements be guided by your light and transfigured with your joy.

Angel, guide of Tobias, lay the request we now address to you at the feet of Him on whose unveiled Face you are privileged to gaze. Lonely and tired, crushed by the separations and sorrows of life, we feel the need of calling you and pleading for the protection of your wings, so that we may not be as strangers in the province of joy, all ignorant of the concerns of our country. Remember the weak, you who are strong, you whose home lies beyond the region of thunder, in a land that is always peaceful, always serene and bright with the resplendent glory of God. [Ibid., pp. 592–93]

On July 21 her hemoglobin was down to 8 again, and she spent the following day at the Baldwin County Hospital receiving another blood transfusion. A few days later she required another transfusion, and by July 26, she was still battling a resistant kidney infection with double doses of antibiotics; the complications with her cortisone also continued to compound matters. On July 28 she wrote the last letter she would ever write and addressed it to her friend Maryat Lee (ibid., p. 596).

Dear Raybat,   28 July 64
     Cowards can be just as vicious as those who declare themselves—more so. Don't take any romantic attitude toward that call. Be properly scared and go on doing what you have to do, but take the necessary precautions. And call the police. That might be a lead for them.
     Don't know when I'll send those stories. I've felt too bad to type them.
                                                                    Cheers,
                                                                    Tarfunk

She was worried about her friend in New York City, who had recently received a disturbing phone call. In less than a week's time, Flannery would slip into a coma and die on August 3, 1964. The letter to Maryat Lee would be found on her bedside table a few days later and dropped into the mailbox by Flannery's mother.

V

Monday, August 3, 1964, was a hot, muggy day in Milledgeville, Georgia. Flannery had received Holy Eucharist the day before and immediately felt the familiar sense of secure calm and serenity that always engulfed her after communion. Still, she was unprepared for the crisis that was to come within hours and unaware that by the following evening she would herself be transformed from body to spirit even as bread and wine are also transubstantiated.

By late Sunday afternoon—had Eucharist that morning already been a fortuitous preparation for this migration?—her body began to assemble its instruments of transfer from what she was to what she would become. A weariness came upon her, a profound and deep fatigue which was far more than the mere heaviness of bone and blood and brain of physical illness but rather a sheer and utter exhaustion of the soul. She was too weak to resist its gentle beckoning and far too uncaring even to protest. Therefore, she embraced, nurtured, and even welcomed it.

Life becomes a burden. Life with all its tortures, temptations, false promises, and seductions finally becomes a burden which is far too heavy to bear. After all, she had endured its agony for thirty-nine years, suffered its thin and empty hopes, and sought for substance behind its fragility for too long, for far, far too long. So she was ready that Sunday afternoon in August and well prepared to receive that for which she had spent her entire life in hopeful searching. Christians are an odd sort when it comes to this matter of death, for rather than damnation they see liberation, rather than an end it is for them a beginning, rather than running from it, they run toward it. They are a strange and an odd lot.

She said no goodbyes, neither to her mother nor to herself. Rather, she suddenly felt a door open somewhere in the distance; she heard a wind of powerful and magnificent proportions approaching as if on winged heels; and she surrendered herself to it without regret! The wind rushed toward her—and even through her—with urgency and then surrounded her at once as if with delicate fingers it sought to caress her most invisible flesh. She felt herself fall, even swirl and spiral through immeasurable depths. Down, down, spiraling down into deeper and darker recesses, gentle, fragile Mary Flannery falls. Far in the distance, she hears the hardened sounds of reality beckoning. But within these greater depths there are soft groves, sounds of hushed seduction, and the gentlest down. Within that softness, these voices are so much stronger than those of reality. Turning now upon the pivots of her own thoughts, she dreams; she floats and follows lights of intense coloration, hues of cobalt blue and ocher yellows. Here too are the reds and lavenders, so delicious in their crimson array, and also all the emerald greens and delicate pastels, the whites and grays, the shades and lights of everything. It is as if she has penetrated beneath the surface of coloration to the very architecture that makes it all possible. So too can the very texture, design, saturation, and structural equation of light itself be found herein. They are all here and so entwined, so enmeshed, and so bleeding into one another. Here also are currents, flows, and eddies of immeasurable force that seem to pull and draw her poor broken body along their corridors. But as they flow—these fluid avenues of light and sound—so also do they cleanse and refresh. So Mary Flannery follows in innocence and naïveté; she is not afraid but rather curious and inquiring. For here everything is richer, stronger, more saturated than what she left behind. Even had she wished to return, she, of course, could not! Indeed, the effort would be far too great, far too demanding for brittle tissues such as hers had now become.

Suddenly there—over there—is it not a doorway, an opening through which she might pass? She hesitates and turns— half turns while remaining still—to look behind to what she has left. Above the pounding oceanic pulse of reality beats like a hardened drum of recall and retreat. Should she return, and if so, what awaits her? The hammering of a strained and arrhythmic heart, the labored effort to pull clean air through thickened pus already green in its diseased mucus are the sounds that greet her. The wasted bones eroded through and through with pockets of decay and decomposition, the swollen, tight face mooned into an oval by an avalanche of cortisone, the bleeding vessels, the anemic, white, and wasted tissues, and the awful stinking smell of it all hover above her as the tides upon a ocean. She turns to one; she turns to the other. She turns once more again toward the open door, toward its silence, toward its tranquillity, toward its gentle, soft, and beckoning benevolence. May she walk through? Dare she? Can she? Yes! She does.

It is early morning, August 3, 1964. All that can be seen from the bedside are the eyes, which turn once in their sockets and then . . . and then . . . are forever still. Her left hand, still surrounded by a delicate band of gold, clutches at the metal bars of the hospital bed. And then relaxes. The nostrils constrict once and then slowly, infinitely, languidly, and eternally dilate. They are forever still. Her heart grips itself around, shudders once, and relaxes into utter oblivion. A visitor, an attendant, a passerby might observe all of this, but nothing more.

For what cannot be seen from this angle of intense earthly light are the tiny feet running with happiness and abandon through fields of succulent green. What cannot be seen from that cold steel bedside is the smile of recognition and expectation that floods her gentle, hopeful, and most relieved face. What cannot be seen from that observatory of steel and glass which she has left behind is the falling away, the evaporation of gray hairs, parched skin, muddy unseeing eyes. For now, herein and within this place, youth renews and resplendors itself as powerful equatorial winds grasp round her slender self and flow with speeds far too intense to measure and far too languid to register.

8

The Fear of Light

I have sensed that somewhere about the premises
which
    I inhabit,
        probably in its storm-wracked attic,
There lives a dark and cunning old creature
    whom I know as the spider,
        obsessively industrious, adaptable to
    whatever conditions
have thus far assailed him in his secluded corner,
    And so I think of him as the loom of my
        heart,
    This creature receives assignments that shake
        him,
        that make his ancient web tremble,
but he rarely, if ever declines them,
    knowing what's left of his craft,
        and what's still expected of it.

Tennessee Williams
"Wolf's Hour"

CONGENITAL ERYTHROPOIETIC PORPHYRIA: Fewer than 100 patients with this condition have been described. Pink urine and cutaneous photosensitivity are the principal manifestations and, classically, are present from early childhood. While the diagnosis usually is made at this time, a first presentation has been described also in adults, whose clinical state resembled that of relatively severe porphyria cutanea tarda. Acute attacks of abdominal pain with neurologic manifestations do not occur. Cutaneous lesions consist of bullae, vesicles, and shallow ulcers on light-exposed skin. Repeated injuries are accompanied by hypertrichosis and, in patients surviving beyond childhood, may cause disfiguring scars with loss of portions of the nose, ears, eyelids, and digits. Erythrodontia, reflecting accumulation of porphyrins in teeth and bones, and spenomegaly also have been present in a high proportion of cases, associated with a compensated hemolytic anemia, which may be intermittent. The chemical abnormality that characterizes this disease is overproduction of uroporphyrin and also of coproporphyrin, predominantly of the isomer I type; this is consistent with a defect in the formation of uroporphyrinogen III, although the inherited enzymatic lesion remains to be defined. Blood and urine both exhibit striking—and often massive—increases in these porphyrins, whereas urinary ALA and PBG are present in normal amounts. Circulating normoblasts and, to a lesser extent, reticulocytes exhibit intense fluorescence owing to their high content of uroporphyrin. The feces also contains excess uroporphyrin and co prophyrin with a minimal increase in protoporphyrin. Treatment relies on avoidance of sunlight; topical sunscreens and A-carotene (the latter useful in protoporphyria) are of no proven value. In patients with hemolysis, splenectomy may lead to prolongation of red cell life span and diminished porphyrin excretion.

Wyngaarden and Smith
Cecil's Textbook of Medicine

I

Henry Atkins had few pleasures in life, but he did enjoy the evening newspaper. This evening, however, he read a piece that truly disturbed him:

Los Angeles—There's strong medical evidence that werewolves and vampires really existed—that they were victims of a rare disease that still exists, a Canadian biochemist said Thursday.

Two related blood defects, according to David Dolphin of the University of British Columbia, give their victims a hideous collection of symptoms that are familiar to any fan of late-night movies. Some people have excessive hair, prominent teeth and skin damage; others have a painful aversion to sunlight that could be fatal if they ate garlic.

"It seems more than likely that such people might well have been considered werewolves," Dolphin told a gathering of the American Association for the Advancement of Science meeting here. "Imagine . . . the manner in which an individual in the Middle Ages would have been received if they only went out at night and when they were seen they would have an animal look about them—being hairy, large of tooth and badly disfigured."

Today, these diseases are known as porphyria. The few people who have them—Dolphin estimates 1,000 in the United States—usually are protected from disfigurement with injections of a blood component.

But there were no blood banks in the Middle Ages.

"The next best thing would be to drink a lot of blood," Dolphin said.

"It's a cute idea," was the response of Dr. Sidney Schrier, who heads the hematology department at Stanford University Medical Center. Hematology is the study of blood and its diseases.

But Schrier is skeptical of the idea that drinking blood would relieve the disease. "It's not at all clear to me" that it would work, he said.

Schrier said Dolphin's description of the blood diseases matches those in the medical literature, but he added that he can't speak from experience.

"They are so rare that I can tell you that in 26 years I have seen no cases at Stanford," Schrier said.

According to Dolphin, if these diseases are the origin of the old folklore, the tales have been twisted slightly in the telling. He finds nothing special about silver bullets or wooden stakes. Also, a werewolf—supposedly a manwolf that could change forms—could not revert to normal, he said. And animal blood would have done just as well as human blood. And both diseases' victims could be women, not just men.

However, the tales that say a vampire's victim also would turn into a victim make sense, Dolphin says.

The diseases, which are inherited, can lie hidden in their victims until they are triggered by some strain on the body, such as puberty, too many drugs, too much alcohol—or a sudden loss of blood.

In the close, inbred communities of the Middle Ages, Dolphin said he believed it would not be unusual for a vampire to have neighbors, apparently normal, who were relatives harboring the same disease.

"Inbreeding could increase the likelihood of the disease in Transylvania perhaps," he said.

Porphyria ailments are caused by defects in a substance called heme, the pigment that gives blood its red color. Several porphyria diseases are more common and less serious than the two that Dolphin described.

The disease he linked to werewolves causes its victims to be extremely sensitive to any light, not just sunlight.

The light causes an intense chemical reaction that can begin destroying skin and extremities in a few days, he said. Victims lose their fingers and noses and their lips and gums recede, leaving their teeth prominently displayed. Another chemical reaction causes heavy hair growth.

The other disease, the one he associated with vampires, is less disfiguring, but sunlight is still very painful for the victims. "You learn very quickly that when the sun comes up, you go in," he said.

Another effect of the disease is that a certain chemical in garlic, which healthy people process in their livers, would increase production of the faulty heme in the victims and possibly kill them, Dolphin said. [Ansley, May 31, 1985]

His hands trembled to realize that he had, in fact, just read a perfect description of himself.

Henry Atkins put the paper down and crossed the room swiftly to reach the telephone. As he walked, one could see that he was a short man but with fine features and a strong, powerful body. He had always been proud of his good biceps, thick arms, and barrel chest. He looked dangerous—although, of course, he was not—and perhaps he had never been challenged to fight only because he looked as if he would always win. Even his manner of walking and moving was intimidating since he had adopted an attitude of slow, purposeful steps while also holding himself low and close to the ground. From a distance he presented a somewhat ominous vision to the casual observer. And yet all of this was only an appearance, for he was really a very gentle, kind man who was often misunderstood by those around him, and occasionally by himself as well! The truth was that he disliked physical violence and would have retreated more suddenly than he would have advanced. Unless, of course, he was cornered. Yes, if he was cornered, he would have to fight, wouldn't he? But then any animal—a dog, a rabbit, a wolf—would do the same. Fortunately, Henry had never been cornered . . . at least, not yet. Reaching the telephone, he immediately dialed the number: 555–2591. At first, there was no answer, and then the familiar recording: "Hello. This is Esther in Dr. Harris's office. I am sorry, we are out of the office, but we do care about your call. Please call 555–2233, and our answering service will take your message. If you are having a physical emergency, please go to the nearest emergency room."

He was angry—and yes, somewhat frightened—by the newspaper article because he knew that he had had porphyria cutanea tarda for the past year. But his doctor had said nothing about any of this werewolf nonsense. After all, that's all it was, wasn't it?—stupid nonsense? Harris had told him only that he was suffering from a very serious disease which was something like Gunther's disease but wasn't it, and that nobody knew what caused it, and that it was incurable but that he wouldn't die of it. He had been terrified, of course, and Harris had done little to reassure him. But Henry had gone to the library later in the week and looked up his disease—it was his disease now, wasn't it?—in the fourteenth edition of *The Merck Manual*. And there it was on page 962 along with a very complex chart showing the heme biosynthetic pathway, but this only confused and alarmed him. On the following page were a list of the symptoms, and Henry knew that he had the disease—or it had him—as soon as he finished the page.

> The cutaneous manifestations begin as areas of erythema with vesicles or bullae that occur on exposed portions of the body, usually following minor trauma. Crusts and scabs develop, following by scarring. Hirsutism, areas of pigmentation and depigmentation, and sclerodermoid changes may be evident as chronic lesions. The vesicles and bullae are usually most evident in sunny weather, par-

ticularly in late summer and autumn. Acute photosensitivity reactions are not uncommon in this disease. In severe untreated cases, disfiguring changes can occur in the ears, nose, and fingers. [Berkow, p. 963]

He had it! He didn't understand all the words at first—such as "sclerodermoid" and "hirsutism"—but he looked them up, and he knew he had it. Why did he have it? Why did he have to have it? He had never done anything wrong; he believed in God; he took care of himself and had quit smoking a few years ago and watched his diet and got enough sleep and didn't fool around on his wife and did his damn job and was a good guy and . . . and why the hell did he have to have it? But he did, and he had come to accept that fact over the past year and even learned to live with the disease. And then this stupid newspaper reporter had written an article and made Henry Atkins feel like some kind of an animal. He wasn't an animal! Was he? The writer was wrong. Or Harris, his doctor, was wrong! One of them was wrong, and Henry was angry because now he didn't know exactly which one to believe. If Harris had told him the truth right away—the whole truth—he would have had no doubts whatsoever. But he hadn't, and Henry had found things out in that *Merck Manual* that the doctor had never mentioned, such as the part about cirrhosis of the liver, and since that time he had never had complete confidence in Harris. But, on the other hand, newspaper reporters are always looking for a sensational story because they have their careers to worry about and they need to make a buck. So that was really it, wasn't it, here was a stupid journalist just trying to make a buck. Except . . . except that newspapers don't let these guys print whatever they want to; Henry knew that! They have all this stuff checked and rechecked, and they talk to doctors and nurses before they print these stories so they won't be sued. Maybe the newspaper was right; maybe they knew more than his doctor; maybe his doctor knew more than he was telling Henry. Maybe Henry Atkins was a werewolf.

II

Where ends man and where begins the beast in us? We are divine; we are rational; and having souls, we are therefore human. And yet grace is built upon nature, and all that is human about us is fed and nourished by the animal within us. Are we gods or demons, men or monsters, or are we rather spiritual and physical hermaphrodites whose ambiguity is precisely that in being both we are therefore neither?

Domesticated throughout the centuries, man has learned to replace violence with negotiation, brutality with controlled restraint, and destruction with reconstruction. He is reasonable, rational, and cerebral in his dealings with enemies, competitors, and aggressors. The husked fangs that once tore flesh and devoured entrails have long softened and decayed from neglect and a diet of cooked meats, tender vegetables, and stewed grains. They are tough and dangerous no longer. The claws with tufted, pointed nails that once eviscerated the enemy in a single lunge have now lost their sharp edge in exchange for the rounded manicure of civilized man. They are a weapon and a threat no longer! The barbed stinger, fanged tooth, poisoned tongue with deadly venom are reabsorbed by brutal tissue and regenerated to the delicate but cunning eye, the twice-forked, thrice-forked tongue, and the invisible ether that kills with a deadly certainty even in the absence of the viper. Man is transformed; he is a metamorphosis become death; he is a deadly creature of the night with the beautiful manners of a bird in flight and the brutal savagery of a thing that crawls upon the ground.

And yet man is man and not an animal. He has no hair upon his body save that which celebrates his sex and decorates his face. His claws are fingers; they cannot hurt. His hoofs are feet shod in Gucci loafers; they are ill equipped for rapid flight. His teeth are brittle, fragile, missing, and often simply false; they cannot devour or digest the unprocessed ingredients of nature any longer. His skin is thin with blue veins and transparencies that reveal the gentleness beneath; it is protective no longer. His eyes are occulted and myopic as they squint and blink to focus; no longer can they discern the enemy from afar but only the enemy within. His ears are tuned only to hear harmonies, contrapuntal rhapsodies, and civilized symphonies; they filter out all other sounds of danger, warning, and approaching disaster. His nose is anosmic to the smell of death, blood, and the thick heavy smell of mating sex; rather he perfumes himself with fragrances not to be found anywhere in nature.

Behold—*ecce homo*—the civilized man! No longer beast but fully divine. His jungle of survival is transformed from the dense vegetative coves of equatorial Africa to the three-dimensional topographical map in Manhattan that illuminates enemy target areas in red and friendly allied reserve silos of radioactive weapons in greens and yellows. But it is still with the color of blood that he marks his enemy and still with forest greens that he recognizes his friends. Civilized man—the prideful product of evolutionary history—no longer brutalizes and scourges the body of his victim or drinks his liquified brains from a cup fashioned of a broken skull. Instead, he charms, negotiates, and seduces the hostile force with alliances, treaties, and covenants of devilish design and thereby ensnares him within traps of international legal jargon and reciprocal inspection contracts. But it is still the enslavement of the one by the other that motivates these most refined, most delicate, and most cerebral rituals of charm and brutality, of manners and morals, of peace and war. Civilized man is no longer a hawk but a dove whose gliding flight is well disguised as a ballet rather than a hunt. But is it really so, that man has changed from beast to god, from monster to miracle of evolution, from animal to human? Or rather, has he not changed so often and so much—turned and twisted in so many different and in so many contradictory ways throughout history—that having transformed himself once too often, the complex chemistry of the whole process finally failed and he ironically metamorphosed back into what he originally was?

The beast within the divine lies buried deep and awakens from its restive slumbers only occasionally. Most often, man feeds his hungry, comforts his sick, ministers to his dying, and offers fellowship to his enemies. Only occasionally does he rape, murder, defile, humiliate, and destroy, but when he does it is with a vengeance born of anger over injustices forgiven but never forgotten. Most often he tries to compromise, arbitrate, and negotiate a settlement which avoids bloodshed and death. Only occasionally does he find it necessary to brutalize his enemy by such measures of degradation that even he must

157

shudder to behold what he has done. Most often he uses reason rather than force, love rather than hate, and seduction rather than destruction to gain his advantage. But occasionally he denounces a nation, defiles an entire race, degrades a whole people out of sheer frustration, anger, and sometimes even boredom. Such departures from the divine are rare, and yet when they do occur, so also is revealed a beast of such deadly poison—but such incredibly elegant plumage—that one knows not whether it be a beast from the jungle or a god from the starry heavens.

It all happens in a flash; as quick as quicksilver seeks distribution of its constrained shape so quickly does the god become beast and just as quickly return to itself again. There, over there, do you see the glint in the eye, the nostrils flare and flange upon the scent of death within the wind? The slender, manicured fingers thicken into jagged claws, and just as suddenly those rounded teeth now reassemble their solid, punctured points. The jaws swell from the maxillary shelf to sphenoid ridge as the powerful sternocleidomastoid muscles reassert themselves and test their rediscovered strength. Those jaws, those teeth, those muscles which once fed upon softened foods and weakened as they feed are now sufficiently powerful once again to break bone, crush and pulverize skull and rib in order to feast upon the brain and heart within. It is all so sudden and unexpected that one is perplexed by a metamorphosis so clean as not to leave a trace of itself. In a moment the civilized eye turns murderous and turns civilized once again. Was it an illusion? In an instant—or so it seems—the claws glisten in the sunlight and return again to a soft but firm handshake. For just a second, the nostrils flare, the eyes explode upon the air, the ears peak, and the body lunges forward . . . in a warm embrace of fellowship, peace, and humanitarian brotherhood. What does it all mean, and who is this hermaphroditic monster who poisons itself, anoints and baptizes, impregnates and destroys itself with quivering genitals that smell of both life and death? Behold—*ecce homo*—it is the man himself who is both divine and damned, monstrous and magnificent, mighty and small, anointed and cursed, deadly and dangerous, and so very kind and cunning in his benevolence.

Naturally, Henry Eliot Atkins saw none of this within himself. By self-analysis he viewed himself as far too gentle, forgiving, and kind for his own good. Neither aggressive nor malicious, he suffered the indignities of the world in patient anticipation that ultimately there is a justice to things that rewards the good and punishes the bad. He was, of course, one of the good, and so he waited in patient anticipation for his reward. It did not arrive.

Instead, he had fallen ill with a rare disease whose name he could not pronounce, whose suffering he could not reconcile with the good life that he had led, and whose cure, cause, and natural course was unknown to the doctors who treated him. Why him? he asked, why did he need to endure this monstrous, painful, disfiguring disease? He had never raped, murdered, stolen, or transgressed against anyone; neither had he lied, been unfaithful to his wife, engaged in strange and unnatural practices, or blasphemed his God. No, his life had always been rooted in reason, patience, diligence, and the doing of good works. He had cared for his body and neither smoked nor drank to excess. He worked hard and always paid his bills and went to church almost every Sunday. And yet for all of that, in spite of and even in defiance of all of that, he had a disease— or rather it had him—of such incredible dimensions that it was incomprehensible to Henry Eliot Atkins what it might all mean and why it had chosen him.

Henry neither liked nor trusted doctors. Or rather, he did not trust them, and therefore he did not like them. In the past thirty-seven years of his life, he had visited doctors as infrequently as possible. But in January of this year—right after his birthday—he began having terrible and intolerable headaches. At first, he thought it tension, stress, or eyestrain, and then he finally realized that it was none of these but instead the sun! Yes, it was the sun; whenever he went outside into the bright light his eyes burned and his head ached the rest of the day. At first, it was simply an avoidance of the light, but his shunning of the light became a fear, and the fear became a phobia, and the phobia drove him to the sanctuary of night. Here, in these filaments of lavender and deep purples and comforting shades upon deeper shades, he found sanctuary. The arrival of spring and then of summer increased his hatred of the light; the intensity of the sun during June and July drove him into hiding throughout the day, and only after sundown did he feel safe. This compromise in life-style was so obviously necessary to his well-being that Henry barely regretted the requirements so imposed upon him. He began to sleep through the day and therefore regarded the night as day and the day as night. It was a simple biconditional and bilateral equation which once calculated was balanced in perfect parity on both sides. And yet, notwithstanding this major concession, his discomfort continued. For after all, he could not avoid the light entirely, and any natural sunlight brought sores and blisters to whatever skin it touched. For him, the light was like a fire which burned and boiled his skin into ulcers and rashes that crusted with thick pussy scabs. It took days, even weeks, for these to heal, and they always thickened into scars and welts that drew the attention of everyone. And yet still his resistance to doctors was greater than his resistance to pain and disfigurement until the day when he discovered blood in his urine. It was a Sunday, and he had felt nauseated and feverish since Friday afternoon; when he urinated and found the toilet bowl dripping in blood as if from a massacre, he was revolted both with himself and his disease. It turned out after all not to be blood but the excretion of uroporphyrin, but it looked like blood to Henry, and he was terrified. Just last week, he had been reading an article on cancer, and his greatest fears were exactly confirmed by this unpredictable revolt of his body against itself.

There had already been countless signs and symptoms, both minor and major revolts of his body against itself, that he had negotiated with reason and convinced himself thereby of their innocence. The nausea, the headaches, the stomach pains as well as the scars and scabs and rashes he had all integrated into a rational explanation which minimized their malevolence and maximized their innocuousness. "It'll go away," he thought of the rash. "It's just that the sun is too bright today," he argued with himself. "My stomach is just upset today but it will be better tomorrow," his brain reasoned with his body. But they did not go away, and neither did the more subtle and silent signs of his disease disappear. For example, he noticed that he seemed to be getting hairy and was even getting hair where it had never been before. His chest and arms were much hairier than they had been a few months ago, but so also were his hands and fingers and even his feet. This was not the fine, thin kind of hair that grew upon his head but a tough, wiry, and altogether unruly sort which was coarser and much heavier than he had ever known before. It seemed to grow everywhere and even appeared on his brow, the palms of his hands, and the soles of his feet. But finally it was the blood—or what he thought was blood—that drove him to a doctor.

He had made an appointment with Dr. Harris on Tuesday afternoon at 2:30, and Harris had given him a thorough examination. Of course, he also took tests—all kinds of tests including his blood and his urine and who knows what else—and it took days to get the final results. Finally the results were in, and Harris told him what they meant.

"Mr. Atkins, we finally know what is causing your symptoms."

Henry said nothing, for he did not trust doctors.

"You are suffering from a rare and chronic disorder called porphyria cutanea tarda."

Henry did not ask what it was but rather would it kill him?

"No, probably not if we treat it. But the problem, Mr. Atkins, is that while we can treat it we can't cure it. There is an element—a very important element in human blood—that you seem to be missing. It is called heme, and while we can treat the deficiency, we can't treat the cause. Do you understand? In other words, we can't cure you, but we can medicate you for the symptoms."

Henry understood enough—he was not going to die—to be satisfied for the time being. Actually, if he didn't know more about his disease—and learned of it only through the newspaper—it was in part his own fault for not asking more. But there it was, and here he was standing by the phone, listening to a recording from his doctor's office, angry and frightened by a newspaper article that carried the headline: "Werewolves Might Be Real."

III

The human body is a prismatic structure of oblique angles, intertwined dimensions, surface reflections, and complex refractions whose total constitution is often rendered invisible by the very brilliance of the individual parts that compose it. Even as the transparency of light humbly effaces itself in order to proudly promote the blues, yellows, greens, and reds that compose it, so also does the metabolism of the body insinuate itself everywhere in general while never appearing anywhere in particular. Kidneys, heart, lungs, and liver; bone and brain and blood; gut and gizzard are each a celebration of a metabolic power which feeds everything while starving itself.

The body is an oven; it is a stove, a metabolic furnace whose fuels are in a state of continual combustion as wastes are diminished by its constant flames. The temperatures must, of course, be exact, for degrees either too intense or too shallow will produce an uneven burning which consumes or fails to consume the contents of this biological flame. There is an order, then, to this vast and highly complex metabolic furnace in which several flames burn in synchronistic individuality only in order to unify their combustion in a symphonic and unified flame.

Within the crucible of flame, there is forged and fashioned heme, which is a metalloporphyrin whose alloys include compositions as remote as chlorophyll and vitamin B_{12}. The heme biosynthetic pathway is a network of exceeding transparency whose very invisibility insures the efficiency of the products it designs. Heme is one of these complex products fashioned by invisible hands from the chelation of ferrous iron by protoporphyrin, which in turn combines with other substances to ultimately produce hemoglobin. It is an exceptionally complex process whose very delicacy is a compliment to the mastery of the whole metabolic process. One is hardly surprised to learn that something might go wrong; the far more relevant question in matters as complex as these is why does anything ever go right?

Porphyria cutanea tarda is precisely a metabolic misfiring—a thermostatic rupture in the regulation of this metabolic furnace—in which uroporphyrin excretion is accelerated while coproporphyrin is exaggerated and porphobilinogen is either decreased or totally absent in urine excretion. Recently, a group of tetracarboxylated porphyrins—the isocoproporphyrins—have been discovered in the stools of some patients. Precisely what happens within this strange furnace is not at all clear, and whether one flame burns exceedingly bright while another dulls into embers remains a carefully guarded secret of the pyrotechny itself. But it is certain that the smoke and ash seen on the surface are a clear indication of a monumental volcanic disturbance within.

With the presence of a heme deficiency—either from an increase in the formation of heme proteins or an impairment of the heme synthesis—a feedforward-feedback series of indicators is activated by the enzyme aminolevulinic acid (ALA). Acting as a governor over the provinces of tissues requiring heme, ALA synthetase determines the rate production for the entire biosynthetic pathway. Aberrant porphyrinogenesis produces a spectrum of symptoms including photosensitivity, hirsutism, and neurological problems. There are several types of porphyrias—about seven in all depending upon the person counting—and these are customarily divided into the erythropoietic and the hepatic. The former include congenital erythropoietic porphyria (or Gunther's disease) and protoporphyria, whereas the latter include coproporphyria, variegate porphyria, porphyria cutanea tarda, and toxic porphyria. It is porphyria cutanea tarda that has been called the werewolf disease.

Porphyria cutanea tarda may lie dormant within the genetic constitution for years or even forever. Transmitted as an autosomal dominant defect, the disorder patiently waits for the proper occasion before announcing itself as a decrease in uroporphyrinogen decarboxylase activity. Several factors can instigate its activity, from severe stress through alcoholism to excessive iron ingestion. Oddly enough, the disease was almost unheard of in menstruating women until modern health consciousness insisted upon iron supplementation; the disease then began to claim more and more young women among its victims. In men, occurrence is usually after the age of thirty-five and frequently follows a drinking problem.

The first symptoms are often seen as a blistering and erosion of exposed skin areas after exposure to the sun. The blade of the nose and the pinna of the ear are particularly affected. The tiny vesicles coalesce and rupture to an open sore which gradually crusts over to heal with heavy scar formation. Repeated episodes are erosive, and the disfigurement of the face becomes evident after a period of time.

The second collection of symptoms is an increase in skin pigmentation and hirsutism. The unprecedented growth of hair is not just confined to the usual growth areas but may also involve the soles of the feet, the palms of the hands, and the brow of the face. Uneven and spotted pigmentation may alternate with areas of depigmentation and alopecia to produce a severe disfigurement which is further exacerbated by the lesions of photosensitivity.

Erythrodontia combined with recession of the alveolar bone often elevates the teeth into prominence by retracting the gum line. Ulcers within the tonsillar crypts and dental alveoli are not uncommon, and loss of teeth or even gangrene of the maxilla and soft tissues may occur.

The combinatory product of these several pathological equations produces a most disturbing set of characteristics that appear descriptive of classic lycanthropy. In darkness, the hunched and shrouded form seeks the sanctuary of night in a desperate flight from the awful, ulcerating light. His pain from kidney and abdominal disorders has doubled him over, and he perhaps staggers, rather than walks, from the delirium of his untreated agony. Everywhere there is hair to be found upon him; it covers him as a thick and violent wrap about his shoulders, back, hands, feet, and brow. His teeth have been elevated into prominence by the recession of the gum line, and ulcers irritate the mucosal lining of his tongue, lips, and palate. The scabbed lesions have left a mosaic of scars and deformations upon his face, while aspects of his nose, lips, ears, and brow are puckered into pockets and craters of misalignment. His body craves a release from the intensity of this continual misery and seeks out the heme in human blood without knowing the whys or wherefores of its insane logic. With a genius all its own, our physiology seems to know what it needs; it seems to desire and quest for precisely those ingredients which will quench its thirsts and satisfy its acute impoverishments. It is well known, for example, that children in low-income tenant buildings will chew flaking paint chips to supply the calcium missing from a proper diet of milk, or that wild animals will identify precisely the grasses necessary for their dietary supplementation during times of stress or illness. So too, it appears to be intuitively understood that the missing heme resides within the redness of fresh blood and that its ingestion is an elixir which quenches the agonizing pain of lesions, nausea, and hypertrichosis.

IV

In anger and desperation, he slammed the phone back into its cradle and called the number of Harris's answering service, 555–2233.

"Good evening, this is Dr. Harris's office, may we help you?"

"Yes, yes, this is Henry Atkins, and I have to get hold of Dr. Harris."

"Are you one of Dr. Harris's patients?"

"Yes, of course, it's an emergency."

"If you have a physical emergency, Dr. Harris recommends that you go to the nearest emergency room."

"It's not that kind of an emergency." Henry had grown so impatient that he was barely making sense and even starting to slur his words. "It's an emotional emergency, not a physical one."

"I beg your pardon, sir." The voice had turned cold and suspicious at such pronouncements.

"Never mind," Henry shouted, "just tell the doctor to call me as soon as possible. My number is 555–3906. It's important; tell him that it is very, very important! Will you do that?"

"I'll give him the message, sir."

Henry was frantic; in fact, he was hysterical. He knew that he was probably overreacting, but this whole business had set his imagination to working in the most hideous and terrifying of ways. Was he a werewolf? Was that newspaper right? Was the doctor telling him the truth? Strange things did happen in this strange world, and you never knew who or what to believe.

He remembered reading a story once in German class about a man who woke up one morning to discover that he had become an *Ungeziefer*, an insect. And he hadn't even been sick the night before. Henry was sick; he was definitely and decidedly sick, and if it could happen in a story, it could happen in life, in real life. Couldn't it? Yes! It could, couldn't it? The story was by Kafka, and Henry remembered the title, *Die Verwandlung*, or *The Metamorphosis*, which means to turn into or to be changed from one thing into something else. And that was exactly what was happening to him: he was being changed from a human being into a wolf. He knew that he was; he had seen the effects for the past year, and that son-of-a-bitch Harris had lied to him. He had found out about himself by reading the paper. Now isn't that a hell of a note when you have to find out about yourself by reading the paper because your own doctor won't tell you the truth? By this time Henry had worked himself up into such a confused and frightened state that he didn't know what he believed because he believed everything and anything. He had lost his reason, his sense of logic, and now he was running on pure instinct without thinking any of it out in a reasonable way. But just then the phone rang.

"Hello?"

"Mr. Atkins, this is Dr. Harris."

"Harris, you rotten bastard, you lied to me. You told me that I was going to be all right when you knew I was turning into an animal."

Now Edgar Harris, M.D., was a seasoned veteran at handling emotional crises. He had been in practice for almost forty years and during that period of time had, as he himself expressed it, "seen it all." In addition, his wife Dorothy and his two children had also given him plenty of opportunities to practice his techniques and strategies with frightened and disconcerted people. Accordingly, he always began in the same way. First, he lowered his voice to a soft, melodious pitch and spoke very, very slowly. This tended to reduce hysteria and return the person to reason. Second, he never—not ever—responded to charges, insults, or accusations. Rather, he asked questions, and he continued to do so until he felt in control of the situation once again. For Edgar Harris, control was everything, and he never permitted himself to lose control or be manipulated by angry people. Once you capitulate to a demand, Harris had discovered, the demands only escalate and that was a very good way to end up in a malpractice suit. Therefore, he asked and continued to ask questions even if the person demanded a direct explanation.

"Are you in pain, Mr. Atkins?"

"You're damned right I'm in pain. I read in the newspaper that people like me—with my kind of disease—turn into werewolves."

"Which newspaper did you read that in, Mr. Atkins?"

It was, of course, a preposterous question, and even Harris wished he hadn't asked it. But at the moment he was standing in the hallway foyer wearing his pajamas and holding half a glass of beer. In short, he really did not need this kind of grief at this hour of the evening, and after all, where in heaven's name do patients get these ideas anyway?

"What the hell difference does it make where I read it? Is it true?"

Of course, Edgar had to admit that it made no difference at all, but he was careful not to give an answer to either question.

"Do you think it's true?"

"No! I think it's a damn lie, and that's why I called you so that you would tell me it was nothing but a lie."

"I'm very glad that you did call, Mr. Atkins. Now, I want you to calm down, get a good night's sleep, and call Esther tomorrow morning for an appointment. Goodnight."

Henry felt a little better. After all, Harris had definitely told him that it was all a bunch of lies and that he had nothing to worry about. He trusted that because who can you trust if you can't trust your doctor?

Already he could feel himself calming down and becoming

rational, reasonable, and sensible again. Just moments ago, he had been so angry at Harris that he could have killed him in an instant and no doubt would have, given the opportunity. He would have squeezed the life out of that lying, cunning bastard with his bare hands and not regretted a moment of it. But now, everything looked all different and in proper perspective again. It was odd; in fact, it was unsettling! This sudden transition from fear to calm, from instinct to reason, from brutality to civility had occurred so abruptly that Henry now sensed acutely the profound divisions and ruptures within himself. In so many ways, he was a mindless abyss of endlessly empty corridors and chambers, each holding secrets too dark and fragile for the light of day. Immediately, they evaporated into mist upon the first exposure to sunlight, and therefore they could never actually be seen but only sensed, felt, and smelled in some distinctly animal fashion. To that degree, they were the inner surface of his outer structure; they were the depth to the flat dimension of his reality, and just as his skin was ulcerated by the sun, so also were these secrets and fragile depths evaporated by the light of reason. They dwelt secure only among the darker instincts and forces that lay buried deep within him. He sought to look longingly within those labyrinthian chambers which divided—by quite invisible lines of demarcation—all that was emotional and all that was rational within him, all of him that was animal and all of him that was divine. His transformation complete, his metaphorphosis finished, Henry was reassured to know that he could never become an animal as long as he remained human. The two were simply incompatible. Weren't they?

III

Diseases of the Heart

Oh, heart, my heart, what does this mean?
What is it that so besets you?
What strange new life!
I no longer recognize you.
Gone is all you used to love,
Gone is all that used to grieve you;
Gone is work and peace of mind;
Oh, how can this come about?

Johann Wolfgang Goethe
New Love, New Life

9

I Grow Old before My Time!

I grow old . . . I grow old . . .
I shall wear the bottoms of my trousers rolled.

Shall I part my hair behind? Do I dare to eat a
peach?
I shall wear white flannel trousers, and walk upon
the beach.
I have heard the mermaids singing, each to each.

I do not think that they will sing to me.

T. S. Eliot
"The Love Song of J. Alfred Prufrock"

PROGERIA: The Hutchinson-Gilford progeria syndrome has been reported in 71 patients since first described in 1886. Data are insufficient to verify either an autosomal recessive or autosomal dominant mode of inheritance. It has frequently been erroneously diagnosed in conditions resembling it (e.g. Cockayne syndrome, Hallermann-Streiff syndrome) despite remarkably constant phenotype.

Children with progeria are usually considered to be normal in early infancy, but there may be such manifestations as "scleroderma", midfacial cyanosis and "sculptured nose" to suggest the existence of the syndrome at birth. Profound growth failure develops during the first year of life. The characteristic facies, alopecia, loss of subcutaneous fat, abnormal posture, stiffness of joints, and bone and skin changes become apparent during the second year. Motor and mental development are normal.

Features always present when the condition has become apparent are: short stature, weight distinctly low for height, failure to complete sexual maturation, diminished subcutaneous fat, head disproportionately large for face, micrognathia, prominent scalp veins, generalized alopecia, prominent eyes, "plucked-bird appearance", delayed and abnormal dentition, pyriform thorax, short, dystrophic clavicles, "horse-riding" stance, widebased shuffling gait, and coxa valga and thin limbs with prominent stiff joints.

Features frequently present are: skin which may be thin, taut, dry, wrinkled, brown-spotted in various areas, or "schlerodermatous" over lower abdomen, proximal thighs, and buttocks, prominent superficial veins; loss of eyebrows and eyelashes, persistent patent anterior fontanel, "sculptured" beaked nasal tip, faint cyanosis in the nasolabial area, thin lips, protruding ears, absence of ear lobes, thin, high-pitched voice, dystrophic nails, and progressive radiolucency of terminal phalanges.

There are no demonstrable abnormalities of thyroid, parathyroid, pituitary, or adrenal function. There are insulin resistance, abnormal collagen, increased metabolic rate, and variable abnormalities of serum lipids. Growth hormone responses are normal.

Progeric patients ordinarily develop athero-sclerosis and die of cardiac or cerebral vascular disease between 7 and 27 years of age, with a median age of 13.4 years at death. Other features associated with aging such as cataracts, presbyacusis, presbyopia, arcus senilis, osteoarthritis, or senile personality changes, are not found.

Waldo Nelson
Textbook of Pediatrics

I

What of youth and what of age? Are they divisible, in any way distinct, or rather one unto the other even as the continuous aspects of a circle complete itself? Time alone—the passage of time—is powerful enough to separate the magnificent hopes of the one from the terrible anxiety of the other. Youth hopes; it yearns, believes, and so renews itself; while age despairs; it suffers, turns bitter, and so destroys itself. And thus, a slender interval of time becomes the final circumference that encapsulates the first in promise and isolates the latter in hopelessness. And yet . . . what more can be said? . . . except that we all grow old sooner or later.

Birth is the metaphysical explosion and exfoliation of every promise and every possibility. Indeed, each and every chance for good or for evil, for triumph or defeat, for greatness or smallness, for glory or for failure, for a useful life or a wasted one, for happiness or despair, for light or for darkness resides within these few freshly formed tissues. Remarkable! All the hope, promise, joy, and sanctity of this new life is germinally enriched with freedom and unbounded choice. One can do anything; one can become anyone; one is free! That, after all, is what it means to be young. Of course, youth is smiles and laughter, fresh taunt skin and damp hair drying in the wind; of course, it is the discovery of romance, of love, and of the first delicious taste of sex; of course, youth is being happy, carefree, and independent and also new friends, new places to see, and new experiences to undergo. But before it is any of these, long before youth is anointed by such hopes and such joys, it is first of all the freedom of choice and a staggering horizon of geometrically endless possibilities and opportunities. This is youth; and it is precious; and it is all yours when you are young.

When you are old it is altogether different. Part of being old is being "out-of-sorts," having aches and pains, and feeling poorly in the morning and tired before half the day is over. It is also knowing that cancer, heart disease, liver and kidney malfunctions are enemies that await you at every twist, corner, and bend of each new year. It is frightening to realize your vulnerability and your fragile, delicate nature. And yet, the physical discomforts, bad as they are, are not nearly the worst part of growing old; nor is it the loss of friends who die before you do, visiting hospitals, going to funerals, and losing relationships of fifty and sixty years. No! It is none of these; it is not the gray hair and wrinkled skin; it is not the sickness, death, and fear of becoming feeble; it is not being alone, isolated, and friendless or the dozen other disruptions of life that terrify and taunt the old. Rather—and most exactly—it is the simple realization that all of one's possibilities have disappeared and that whatever hope or promise there was in one's life has now become concrete and actual. One is a failure or a success; one is a saint or a sinner; one has led a good life or a wretched one, and now it is over. You are no longer free but are decreed to be what you have become. That is the stain upon old age which disfigures and deforms more surely than supple bones turned brittle or smooth fresh skin turned dry and wrinkled. It is over! It is simply over! All the possibilities have been used up. There are no new beginnings and indeed no beginnings now at all. There is only the end and terminus of a life used up, smoked out, and exhausted. Old age is this completion, this finalization, and this total actualization of what was once pure freedom and innocent hope. But one is innocent no more.

Where did it all go? Once one was twenty—not so very long ago—and passionately in love with life. A blink, and instantly one is twenty no longer but now forty. A sudden wind from somewhere, and one is sixty and then seventy, and one has devoured his youth in the process of planning his life. It isn't fair! It isn't fair! In fact, it is unreasonable and even unjust that once one was twenty and now has become eighty. Moreover, it makes no sense! Where did the years go, for they seemed to be no more than the passage of slender months and delicate, deceptive weeks? A day passed—a Monday perhaps—and it was Tuesday, and Tuesday evaporated into the week, and the week became a month, and soon the month passed into the following year, and the year became a decade, and the decade became a passage from youth to old age without division and without difference. After all, one still feels young and still remembers the springtime and the vivid smells of a quarter century ago, and yet time—that evil, malicious demon—has slid through our fingertips with such velocity that we are transformed and bewildered by its speed.

Youth and age are thinly separated from one another by a slender envelope of time so invisible that its presence cannot be seen and only occasionally felt. One day one is young; the next day one is old! The evaporation of possibilities is like the drip of water upon a hot stove, and each day the lightness of the future is suddenly being replaced with the heaviness of the past.

Nonetheless, there was warning; there were signs and symbols of our passing and we could have heeded them. But we did not. We simply chose not to do so. Nature was neither false nor brutal to us because well in advance of our demise it was announced through our wrinkled skin, clouding eyes, falling hair, and aching bones. We knew that youth was gone; we knew even if we refused to believe.

But what can be said of a nature which gives no warning whatsoever and instead amuses itself with endless deceptions and mirrored reflections of youth that both deceive and mislead? What shall we say of a nature which turns youth into old age more quickly than a blink of an aging eye and more absolutely than the passage of time? What name can be given to a nature whose time operates by such accelerated velocities that a day passes like a second and a year like a moment? For in this case youth has no possibilities and not even the grace of distant eventualities that require the passage of time for their realization. Rather, time explodes and youth instantly becomes death, so suddenly that neither the whys nor the wherefores of its becoming can be measured or informed.

II

The developmental disorder progeria is so rare that there are less than a hundred known cases. Indeed, in the eighty years following Hutchinson's first confirmed case in 1886, there were less than fifty additional discoveries of such patients. In 1904 Gilford coined the term "pro-geria" to denote a kind of senile dwarfism and advanced aging "in which death takes place from old age long before it is due." Whether the disease is inherited or whether it is acquired, whether it is curable or whether it is not, whether it is indeed accelerated senility or only appears to be so are all shrouded in a mystery as dark and foreboding as the disorder itself. What is certain is that a child suffering from this disease is unmistakably grotesque and unmistakably hastened in its aging. How sad that youth should become death without passing through experience.

It is most common for babies with progeria to appear perfectly normal at birth—a smiling, laughing, happy child with pink, taut skin and eyes as clear blue as the sea on a calm summer's day. With no storm in sight but only clear and innocent weather, you plan for your baby's future. Will she be a doctor; will he be an artist; will she be beautiful, witty, and gay or sad, solemn, and meditative? Will he always be your sweet baby, or will he grow cold and hard with the ice of brittle experience? Will she come home to Mama with her friends, her lovers, her own children; will he still be your own little boy even at twenty and thirty? They are silly questions, perhaps. But they are the thoughts of a mother or a father whose hopes and fears and expectations are born again in that tender promise of the future. Throughout the first year, you plan and organize the future as an accomplished and experienced maestro harmonizes the symphony that he conducts. Your plans are endless; your attention to detail is precise; and each day and week and month you carefully watch the slow development of your baby's future.

But comes the second year, and something—although it is not at all clear what or why—is wrong. It is nothing specific at first, and indeed—or so you think—perhaps it is only your imagination. Within weeks, however, you know that a transformation has occurred and that the steady, vertical development of your baby has become lateral and transverse. It is not exactly a reversal of growth, but then neither is it a continuance, for something has profoundly altered and redirected the dimensions and parameters of the normal and the natural.

One has the sense—without quite knowing why—that the essential diagrams and blueprints of normal development have been suddenly abandoned and in their place has been substituted a prototype of an entirely different measure and moment. If there actually are genetic formulas and equations that direct and guide the unilaterality of normal development, then in progeria it is as if a rut has been hit or a snag encountered which dislodges normal orders and issues instead a set of bizarre and insane commands guiding this entire process from deep within the genetic lighthouse. And yet, at first it is only a hunch as the beacon lights flicker briefly and then seem to resume their steady burning. But that interrupted incandescence was the subtle announcement of a power failure brought about by a redirection of circuits. New commands are now being issued—although it will take time for their effects to be noticed—and these are not the coordinates of a planned navigation but an insane and disturbed set of orders proclaimed by a drunken first mate whose incompetence will dash the ship against the distant shore far sooner than it was booked to arrive.

By the beginning of the second year, it is clear that development is slowing down, stabilizing, and then beginning to reverse itself. It is as if one is climbing up a steadily increasing incline which finally becomes too steep for normal ascent. Therefore, one must crawl rather than climb and finally creep rather than crawl until only descent is at last possible. During the next decade—if your child lives this long—his growth rate will continue to decelerate and retard itself until at the age of ten his height and weight is only that of a five-year-old.

In your heart, you will have understood the truth of these things long ago. But it will break your heart to know, and so you will believe what you like rather than understand what you must, suffer lies rather than withstand the truth, and see your baby as normal rather than not. But now the truth insists upon recognition by you as well as by others. In the street they will stare and gawk at you and your child; in the supermarket or the department store they will make cruel comments and whisper to one another. Yes, people are like that! You cannot be proud of your child as a mother should be, for they will not permit it, and their penetrating eyes and knowing smiles are candid, yes, all too candid, to be easily dismissed or disregarded.

Your baby—God forgive us—looks like a plucked bird! His face is small and pointed, but his skull is large and completely out of proportion to the rest of his head. Crisscrossing the prematurely balding scalp here and there are huge, prominent blue veins that swell like pulsating welts upon a whipped and tortured back. So much suffering, why is there so much suffering in such a small and fragile creature? His eyes have lost that deep blue luster of early innocence and are now clouded over with a dull and vacant stare which is accentuated by the pressurized bulging of his eyes in their miniature sockets. His tongue is thin and pointed like an internalized beak, and his long, swanlike neck only adds to the high-pitched scream or cry or call that issues from his mouth. A delicate, undernourished, and wasted body is attached to the bird's head and resembles wings and a trunk far more than arms and a torso.

He moves, or trots, like a horse or a donkey or some kind of four-legged animal and seems to wobble rather than walk. Legs held apart, as if they won't come together, he bends his knees and hips while straining forward with his head elongated out from the neck. As arthritis comes to complicate his motions, he resembles an aged workhorse intently pursuing a carrot on a stick which guides him forward in this hunched position while constantly escaping his grasp.

Fortunately—or is it unfortunately?—he is not retarded but even bright and perhaps precocious. He knows well what is happening to him, and he fears for himself just as much as you fear for him. He has seen your love turn from soft to brittle, your pride transform itself from embarrassment to humiliation, and he is ashamed first of himself and then of you and then of the two of you. For he is yours and you are his and no amount of rationalization can dissolve this inexorable causal nexus. The two of you belong to one another as mother to son, and your face is superimposed everywhere upon those bluish veins and balding skull. You cannot deny him, and your efforts to do so are not merely in vain but also on record in his undisturbed and undeformed consciousness. He knows and he sees and he is frightfully humiliated to be what he is.

What is this thing, this "creature"—yes, you can say it for it will be better to get it out—this "monster" that has issued from your body? What crazed and perverted twist of genetic messages has spawned this darkened vulture, fashioned its tallowed wings, forged its hideous beak, and sculptured its aberrant and unnatural form? Did it feed upon some foul and evil food while still deep within you? Did some perversion of sex or flesh recoil back upon the pleasure it provided and poison instead? Was there some deep sin, some awful crime, some unspeakable thought within you that longed for the light of day and sought its expression in this twisted and maimed manner?

Or was this monster of the night born in innocence and purity? Is it therefore all the more grotesque precisely because it is all the more undeserved and unwarranted? Were you a good and decent woman who loved her husband, nurtured her child, and committed no evil, and desecrated her body with no forbidden pleasures, but nonetheless was chosen as the site and entrance into the world for this creature? Are you therefore not punished but rather martyred and thus soiled but stainless, cursed but strangely blessed?

And what of your baby, your child, your monster? What does he think of this? Are the thoughts within his sore and aching head as wounded as he is? What is it like to be a monster, a vermin, a viper that people stare at and point at and laugh at and are also terrified of? You cannot, of course, rescue him from this, but rather you must let him bear his terrible pain in isolation and loneliness. He will never know what it is to have friends, buddies, or chums, for his burden must be suffered alone. He will never hold a girl or a woman in his arms; he will never feel the fertility of her ripe body or enter her taut flesh with swollen seeds for fear that another like himself would issue forth. Neither will he ever have a job, own a home, drive a car, buy a new suit, go to the beach, walk down the street alone, or walk unattended. He is in this world, but he truly is not and shall never, never be of it. He is a freak; he is a monster that frightened everyone around him and has therefore come to regard himself as frightful and hideous.

Does he frighten himself? At night, when he lies down with himself alone, does he fear for his own safety? As if . . . well, as if there is some beast caged within his birdlike body—like a hawk or a condor—that will use the subtle occasion of sleep to sneak past the post guard, bend the bars apart, and fly to freedom? Circling then in ever widening and ever increasing arcs of youth and age, will it seek to complete itself and so suffer incineration in this doomed flight? Rising out of the ashes— even as a phoenix is said to rise—will the birth of this new bird of paradise require the destruction of the oiled, blackened vulture that hovers with taloned feet above the bed in order to devour the sleeping form beneath? It is a dream, a fantasy of colored lights and symbols too rich to reside for long within this world, a dream such as sufferers and those cursed dream when they meditate upon the elixirs that might bring cure and surcease to their agony. In short, why should he not hate and loathe himself sufficiently to wish the ultimate metamorphosis upon himself: death by self-destruction, in which the bird of paradise within devours the vulture that resides without? But these are only speculations, for how could one ever know what thoughts reside within that tortured skull?

III

All this pain, all this suffering and humiliation. Who is to blame? Who is the responsible party whose irresponsibility has brought about this immense disaster and degradation? Can he be found and brought to justice for his treachery? Somewhere, within the shadows of the night and the darkness of diseased tissues, he lurks and waits with invisible hand to crush the skull, twist the brain, pull the hair, taunt the skin, and break the body of another victim. And yet where lurks this traitor, for all efforts so far to capture and arrest the sinister villain have failed. Progeria seems a crime without a criminal; it is a homicide without a murder weapon.

We cannot blame the parents, for they are innocent in what they do. It would be easy—and most convenient—to believe that somewhere within their dark and brooding genes lies a chromosomal accident which explodes and destroys the very life which they have created. But it is not true. In fact, there has only been one reported case of parental consanguinity (Gabr et al., "Progeria, a Pathologic Study"), and it is shrouded in some ambiguity.

We cannot blame the chemistry, the organs, the glands, or the metabolism of the body. Everything in progeria seems perfectly normal including the thyroid, adrenal functions, metabolic rates, and even the growth hormone responses. It was thought for a while that the eosinophilic cells of the pituitary's anterior lobe were responsible, but research has not upheld even this possibility.

We cannot blame the child himself, for he among all of us mourns the most for his own tragedy. He has not sinned, done evil, committed crimes punishable by gods or men, or failed to obey the laws of nature. Indeed, he is at the same time both the most innocent as well as the most accountable of us all. And yet while he is not the cause of his agony, he is certainly the consequence of it.

Who then can we blame? Who, finally, is responsible for both these present sufferings and the continual, eternal grieving of men? Perhaps it is God! If we cannot blame God, then who can we blame? But why should God willingly grieve the hearts of men through the bodies of babies?

And yet this entire thesis is uncontrollable and false, for we are not really seeking an explanation but restitution, redress, and revenge. And since it is not reasons that we want but apologies, we therefore stand ready to blame anyone in satisfaction of our frustration and suffering. God is convenient only because He refuses to defend himself, but then it is not explanation that we wish but condemnation. Why, in short, do any of us suffer?

John and Marilyn McRae were in their late thirties when they first met, near forty when they wed, and perhaps well past the proper age for children when their first child was expected. It seems that nature has established a biological time clock which ticks continuously from sixteen to thirty-six and then falls silent. Whatever is privileged and special about these slender, delicate childbearing years cannot presently be ascertained, but our biology demands obedience to its established timetable. The incidence of malformations, deviations, deformations, and defects rises geometrically when these parameters are insulted through disobedience. It was not, of course, maliciousness but only pride and self-indulgence that made the McRaes criminals in violation of laws that they did not even discern. And yet ignorance of the law is no exception, and despite all their good intentions, the McRaes had transgressed eternal and immutable laws whose recoil would demand recompense and justice.

As early as her first trimester, she sensed that something was wrong. It was not a pain or even a discomfort but a deep maternal shudder. There was silence within her where there should have been joy. To John—who saw only what he wanted to see—she was unnecessarily worrying. After all, her doctor had reassured her; her family and friends had reassured her; and, for God's sake, even he had reassured her. Was that not enough? But for her, for the mother who can see far beyond what she can actually see, there were dreams, disturbances, and ominous forewarnings of a most remarkable degree. Something was definitely wrong with the fruit within her womb, which rotted even as it ripened.

A mother knows. She knows—not in a cognitive and rational sense but in a primal and altogether primitive way—when her baby is diseased, deformed, or a sickness unto death. And this was, indeed, a sickness unto death which would destroy rather than recover, would atrophy rather than grow, and would expel a fruit of doom rather than a promise of a normal and healthy baby. What could she have thought, during all this time, to know that harbored within her belly was death itself? It is, is it not, as if all the topographical coordinates of gestation and creation have gone haywire, and one is thereby producing a monster which stands in stark contradiction to all that is normal, sane, and healthy.

Both her doctor and her husband, however, found extreme fault with her constant complaints, miseries, and worries. After all, she was fine, her baby was fine! She had been assured and reassured countless times, and now her hysterical ministrations were simply irritating and no longer beseeching in any way whatsoever.

Still she worried, and added to the burden of this worry was the rising impatience of her husband and her doctor. She felt, quite frankly, trapped between the horns of a terrible metaphysical dilemma. On the one hand, her worry was physical rather than metaphysical, as her tortured body seemed constantly to remind her of what she constantly sought to forget. On the other hand, her husband and physician constantly reminded her that, in fact, she was failing to forget. Accordingly, poor Marilyn was caught in a vicious circle which permitted neither exit nor entrance. What was she to do?

She pretended, she imagined, and she fantasized that her body was normal, well, and healthy. We often do the same when truths too grotesque to confront openly are given proper attire in masks, disguises, and masquerades. Thus, every shudder, convulsion, spasm, and ache within her belly was immediately transformed from a cry of agony to a measure of joy and healthy expectation. Every twist and torsion became a healthy kick; every bend, turn, or movement became a sign of new growth and strength. Every degree of increasing weakness became instead a measure of greater power just as fragility became strength and illness became health.

Behind these outward and apparent signs of growth and development, there lay coiled and hidden like a snake the genetic circuits and transformers that controlled the entire process. Invisible, inscrutable, and mysterious, these minute messengers direct and determine the entire mosaic of development. The neural tube invaginates to form a hollow sleeve inside which the spinal column is eventually housed and outside which the characteristics of flesh, cartilage, and skin are layered.

The entire development process is articulated into eight stages. With fertilization of the ovum by the sperm, the first stage begins with the formation of a pronucleus and the first mitotic divisions. In the second stage, the embryo develops from a two-cell to a multiple-cell blastocystic cavity. In stage three, the blastocyst begins the necessary preparations for implantation and attachment to the endometrium, and in stage four, actual attachment takes place. In stage five, a number of important events occur: the amniotic cavity develops, the primary yolk sac develops from the hypoblast of the bilaminar embryonic disk, and the foundations of uteroplacental circulation are constructed. In stage six, chorionic villi develop as cytotrophoblastic clumps, and the entire embryo begins to assume shape and polarities such as a rostral and caudal end as well as a left and right alignment. In stage seven, the notochordal process occurs, which will later become the axial skeleton. In stage eight, the neural groove develops, to become the spinal cord in later stages of development. Much more refinement and development must happen, of course, before this million-celled, rapidly dividing embryo becomes a human being. But it is somewhere within these first eight stages that developmental and genetic disorders first insinuate and establish themselves. Buried deep within the imprinted diagram and schematic of these early stages are to be found the outlines of progeria.

The entire process is so mysterious and complex, so subtle and delicate that even the most slender miscalculations will radiate throughout the entire physiological process. Errors seem to produce and reproduce themselves logarithmetically according to a set of mathematical formulas that proportionately increase into divisions of a dozen, a hundred, hundreds of thousands, and so on throughout infinite subdivisions. It is precisely here—within these incredible combinations where the slightest deviation may produce the greatest consequences—that disorders such as progeria begin. One looks for causes, guilty parties, and responsible agents, and one finds only the anonymity of blind genetic forces combining and recombining in an odd sort of mathematical biochemistry. It seems hopeless, bizarre, and even totally unfair that all these agonies have been devised by stupid, uncomprehending, and absolutely mechanical processes. Imagine a terrible traffic accident in which the injured parties seek out the drunken driver for retribution only to discover that there was no driver but only a slipped emergency brake.

Nature does not punish, and neither does it reward. Rather, it obeys—in a blind and unconscious fashion—laws that it does not comprehend and cannot change. A malignant tumor does not seek out the unjust nor does it purposely avoid the worthy when seeking a site of implantation. Rather, it randomly and arbitrarily selects the first available passerby. The order in nature, the unfailing logic of its constancy rest exactly in its blind adherence to biological laws without regard. In right or wrong, good or evil. It is not surprising, therefore, that the working of these biological laws and the daily workings of the McRaes' life should one day meet head-on and collide.

By the end of her second trimester, Marilyn McRae had started to read and research developmental disorders. She did not know what she was looking for, but she knew most certainly that she was in search of something. The list of possible and probable dysfunctions of the growing embryo was frightening and overwhelming: Down's syndrome, spina bifida, progeria, and a host of others. Would she recognize her disease—her

184

baby's disease, their disease—when she found it? Somewhere within that long and complex list of things that can go wrong with a baby she would find the one thing that had in fact gone wrong with her baby. And when she did, what would she do? What could she do? It would make little difference to have a label or tag of identification, for that could change nothing. But still—realizing all of this to be true—she needed to find out what was happening within her and what Latin or medical name had been given to it.

When we name things—thrombocytopenia, leukodystrophy, hydrocephalus—we give them a place in the world. Before the act of naming, they were merely abstract entities with neither sense nor significance. Thus, a disconnected and utterly fragmented set of symptoms is shattered in meaning by its disunity. But given a name, its disharmony is synthesized and its disorder polarized by magnetic fields of meaning. A disease exists only when it is named; before that it remains merely a collection of complaints or pains or irritations. She therefore had to find a name—that is, a meaning—to what was occurring within her.

It was understandable, therefore, that she should go to the library and look up the word *pregnancy* in a medical book. As it happened, the book was the *Oxford Textbook of Medicine*, and there was her present state of being, pregnancy, clearly named and discussed in Section II on Reproductive Medicine. It was alarming to discover the different things that can go wrong in what seems like the most natural of events. There are, for example, thyroid disorders, diabetic and blood disorders, and a host of metabolic dysfunctions. But these were of little interest, for she was not concerned with herself but with her baby. She returned to the index and began her search again through the strange sounding words: pregnancy, prekallikrein, presbyacusis, primidone, proctocolectomy, proctosigmoiditis, progeria.

There remain forces, instincts, and powers within us that science has yet to understand. Why does a mother dog smell and nuzzle each of her newborn and by that means alone select the healthy from the diseased? And why is she always right in knowing that this pup cannot live—because of a heart defect or a missing ingredient in its constitution—and why is she correct in refusing therefore to nurse and tend to its care? We do not know the answers to such questions, of course, but we recognize powerful instincts at work that we do not understand. Such powers were operative at this moment within her when the strange word *progeria* seemed to leap from the page and yet she knew not why.

"Progeria," the text read, "is associated with alopecia and birdlike facies as well as artereosclerosis." She had to look up some of the words—such as *alopecia*, which simply means baldness—but she was certain that she had found what she was looking for. Still, she had to be certain, and the librarian directed her to another textbook in medicine, Nelson's *Textbook of Pediatrics*. There, on page 1987, figure 26–3-c, was a photograph of the chemical and genetic disturbance she harbored within her.

It was a bird or like a bird. Not a dove or a swan or any bird of paradise but a vulture of doom and despair. The head was large and cumbersome like a pot too big for its base, and the crown was devoid of all hair, even down, with a hard, shiny circumference interrupted by large blue veins that swelled and pulsated with each passage of blood. The eyes were dull and dim and stared rather than saw in the uncomprehending way they had about them. The textbook dismissed the full misery of this vulture's blight as a "craniofacial disproportion with thin nose and visible cartilage contours," but for Marilyn McRae, mother and fellow sufferer, it was the look of a dying animal slowly humiliating itself. The body was short—it was, in fact, an abbreviation of what it ought to be—with short, stubby legs that bowed out like a crippled pony's. None of these features was human or even drawn from the anatomical reservoir of human forms and possibilities. Rather, the monster seemed to be a disharmonious synthesis of different animal parts. Here was the beak of a bird molded upon the head of a giant with the legs of a horse and the body of a malnourished bear. Nature had simply chosen indiscriminately the spare parts of its anatomical inventory and thrown them together without regard for sense or significance or aesthetics. And in its confusion—

whether deliberate or not—it had produced a hideous monster masquerading as a child.

Was it necessary to love such a thing? Because it grew within her body, fed upon her tissues, and nestled about her heart and belly, was she therefore obligated to love it? Indeed, and more to the point, was it even possible to love or adore or even tolerate such a thing. She thought not, and now that she realized exactly the fullness and enormity of her burden, she was revulsed and disgusted by it. She felt cursed, even singled out, as an unwilling recipient of death and destruction.

It would not be long, just a few days into her last trimester, when her doctor would confirm what she as a mother already knew. Then they would counsel and coerce her judgments in just the opposite direction from the way they had formerly been encouraged. What should she do? Did she have a right to destroy this life? No one had such a right, did one? Or was it the case that only a mother enjoyed the privilege of electing death since only a mother had the privilege of promoting life?

What constitutes life? If life is an assemblage of organic units held in causal juxtaposition with one another, then anything is life that lives. Anything that lives is life, but does any such thing also deserve life? Are there not things—even persons—who have so abused the privilege of life that they should therefore forfeit it? Or is it true that we can make no such value judgments at all? Must we instead agree that survival is the only accreditation that life needs to justify and certify itself? If this is so, then we must treat monsters as just another miracle of life.

God forgive her, but how she hated this cruel and disgusting viper that nourished itself within her. She felt as if she had been impregnated by the very devil himself, and the thought of feeding this child of Lucifer's at her breast disgusted her. She knew that she was obligated to its well-being and bound to feed and support its growing existence, but she could not bring herself to love or cherish it. If she could expel this rotted fruit from her womb, she would have done so, but now it had grown too large and fed itself too fully. She must rather deliver it into the light of day and then endure the sight of it until it died.

Her baby was born on Saturday morning at 3:00 A.M. As with all progeria babies, it looked perfectly normal and would continue so until the first or second year. But then the biological time clock would demand its justification, and rapidly the symptoms would begin to appear. And as they appeared, the baby would age, grow senile, and die by age eleven or twelve. Strange to say, it was as if a day becomes a month and a month becomes a year of aging. The process of growing old is so accelerated and advanced that what had once been a healthy baby would soon become an aged and decrepit old man. All the aspects of aging would compound themselves, and by the age of five or six the child would already show arteriosclerotic changes; death often occurs from coronary occlusion or stroke.

So there it was. She had conceived, nurtured, and delivered a monster in order that it might die in misery while she continued to live in sorrow at its memory. What was the point of it all? Who was to gain and who was to profit from this misery? Surely not the baby and surely not the parents. One must wonder at the majesty of a universe whose biological experiments can be performed in the absence of all mercy. Is, perhaps, life simply overrated?

10

Fox-Teeth

Winter smoke is blue and bitter:
women comfort you in winter.

Scent of thyme is cool and tender:
girls are music to remember.

Men are made of rock and thunder:
threat of storm to labor under.

Cypress woods are demon-dark:
boys are fox-teeth in your heart.

Tennessee Williams
"Winter Smoke Is Blue and Bitter"

AIDS: The acquired immunodeficiency syndrome (AIDS) was originally defined empirically by the Centers of Disease Control (CDC)
as the presence of a reliably diagnosed disease that is at least moderately indicative of an underlying defect in cell-mediated immunity. Typical examples of such diseases are Kaposi's sarcoma in an
individual less than 60 years old or a life-threatening opportunistic
infection such as pneumocystis carinii pneumonia. These disorders
must occur in the absence of known causes of underlying immune
defects, such as iatrogenic immunosuppression or malignant neo-

plasms. This surveillance definition was used for national reporting and was formulated prior to the recognition of human T lympho-trophic virus type III (HTLV III) or lymphadenopathy-associated virus (LAV) as the etiologic agent of the disease. Since tests for HTLV III/LAV antibody and virus are now available, the CDC has refined the case definition. The diagnosis is now excluded if tests for serum antibody to HTLV III/LAV are negative, all other types of HTLV III/LAV tests are negative and the number of thymus-derived (T) helper lymphocytes is normal. Furthermore, in the ab-sence of a classic opportunistic disease required by the original case definition in the presence of a positive serologic or virologic test for HTLV III/LAV, any of the following diseases are considered indi-catie of AIDS: disseminated histoplasmosis; isosporosis causing chronic diarrhea; bronchial or pulmonary candidiasis; non-Hodgkin's lymphocytic lymphoma of high-grade pathologic type and of B-cell or unknown immunologic phenotype; and Kaposi's sarcoma diagnosed by biopsy in patients who are 60 years or older when diagnosed.

Braunwald et al.
Harrison's Principles of Internal Medicine

I

Martin looked at his leg. He was standing in the middle of the bathroom where the light was brightest to reveal the slightest detail. He looked again and then put on his reading glasses to look even more closely. The red, pulsating lesion was still there and somewhat larger and more painful than the day before. A cool shiver of icy terror touched his spine and melted down the long, slow distance to his groin. Only moments before his hard-ened genitals had been warmed and liquified by the sweet ca-resses of his lover Christopher, but now Martin felt the warmth evaporate as cold, icy drops rained down upon his shivering loins.

He looked again but this time tried to assume the anony-mous indifference of the clinician. The small purplish lesion had appeared nearly a week ago as a brown, discolored blotch and had gradually granulated its edges to erupt finally into a painful, bleeding ulcer, growing from a spot to a dime-sized circle. It was frightful and terrifying because it first appeared so innocent and benign as if insidiously seeking to take him off guard with gentle reassurances. At first he really wasn't worried because the limpid discoloration of the bruise appeared perfectly ordinary and nonthreatening. But as the treachery of the betrayal became obvious, Martin grew more confused and disoriented. What should he do? Should he see a doctor or forget it? Should he watch it or ignore it? Should he ask a friend or keep it to himself? Should he warn his lover Christopher or was there nothing to warn him about? Every answer was the wrong one, and every solution was a trap. A doctor would call for a blood test; his friends would grow suspicious and begin to gossip; Christopher would flee in terror from the touch that had both loved and cursed him; and finally, to do nothing at all was simply to bury his head in the sand while this storm of fire burned his body raw but spared his brain. There were no right answers because this disease offered only lonely, isolated, painful degeneration, despair, humiliation, damnation, degradation, and certain death. Martin shut off the light, reapplied a bandage to the lesion, and returned to the sorrowful amnesia of Christopher's arms.

II

Martin loved men. He loved men as a woman loves a man, and often he loved them for the same reasons and in the same ways. He loved the smooth, porcelain surface of their skin and the taunt, amber length of their decorative bodies. He loved them strong, and he loved them weak; he loved them bold, and he loved them shy; he loved them tall, and he loved them short; he loved them old, and he loved them young; he loved them soft, and he loved them hard; he loved them whatever or wherever they were or came to be because he loved men more than anything else on earth. Why he was this way, he did not know.

So many times he had wished it was otherwise, but then there were so many times he was delighted that it was not. He knew that others disapproved, even hated and despised him for what he was, and he had tried to hate himself as well. Oh, how he had tried. Perhaps, he reasoned, with enough self-revulsion and self-disgust he could free himself of this curse that had brought him so much pleasure. But then another young man with tight jeans, blond pepper-colored hair, and smiling eyes would come along, and his resolve would crumble once again to dust, just as it had so many times before.

The next morning he always hoped that he would be disgusted or feel guilty at the indecent things done throughout the night, and this would be his salvation and benediction to a cure. But it never happened. It never happened once. Instead he always felt the opposite. Looking at the soft, naked flesh of his sleeping lover, Martin would suddenly be filled with a profound sense of joy, rejuvenation, and even fulfillment, as if all of this had been right and was exactly as it should be.

Why couldn't he feel what other men felt? Why did the long, limber legs of perfumed women or the full nectar honey of their breasts, hips, thighs, and loins leave him distracted and wanting? What charm, grace, magic, and madness did men find in their women that he failed to find? There had been several women in his life and more than one or two affairs but never any passion or lust for them. Lying in bed, he was content to talk or toy the night away, and when sexual demands were made upon him, he felt angry and resentful at needing to pretend what he did not feel. In the end, they always wondered whether they had done something wrong but then suddenly would realize that it was nothing about them and everything about him. He was gay, and they confronted him with anger and revulsion in their voices. He was gay, wasn't he? He was a homosexual. He had heard it all and been called every name as she gathered up her clothes and raced from the apartment in disgust or ordered him out of her place like some wretched creature that had befouled its own nest.

Finally, the day came when he discovered gay bars with all their strange, glittering forms and soft, anonymous lights, secret entrances, muted voices, aliases, and disgusted identities. It was a strange, bizarre world unlike anything he had ever encountered before, and Martin loved it. He felt at home here and knew at once that he belonged. Here men came—men like Martin—to find someone for the night who would not object to the strangeness within them. Having made your selection, you disappeared into the lavender night to sin against decency in sweet, secret delight with one another's bodies.

The long, dark bar held a paradise of lean and passionate bodies offering a variety of different charms. Some were tall, muscular men with bulging biceps and flat carved stomachs who dressed in leather, metal, and chains. These were the rough trade who took control immediately and used you like a woman. Their brutal domination could ignite passion like sparkling flames in the most subservient and obsequious. Then there were the soft, puffy queens who pranced and postured in the most theatrical ways. Their lips were crimson, their faces sometimes lightly rouged, and each eyebrow was plucked to a clean, straight line. With eyes narrowed to snakelike slits, they flirted their seductive talents in exaggerated and queenly fashion. A royalty among the ordinary, they were proud of their effeminate ways and swung their puffy hips and pulpy loins with invitational abandon. Finally, there were the gays pretending to be straight—or were they straights pretending to be gay?—who moved with easy anonymity from one world to the next and back again. There was nothing about their behavior to even suggest the abhorrent lives they led, and they looked exactly like husbands, fathers, respectable businessmen, and well-adjusted straights to the untrained eye. Ah, the untrained eye! The eye of the heterosexual world that judged tough, macho men as normal and labeled the slightest effeminacy as queer. How little they knew. How very little they really knew. The most conservative, masculine-looking Don Juan was often but a clever disguise for a gay. They had learned to be experts at camouflage, and when you least expected it, they would draw their pale and trembling lips to yours and reveal their true identity. It was all a question of "knowing how to read their beads," and Martin had learned very well indeed "how to read beads."

Having made your selection, you arranged to leave separately and then met somewhere else down the street. Walking to your apartment or his, it was important to maintain this elaborate pretense and never touch or show affection. Finally, however, the doors were closed, the curtains drawn, and as your clothes fell in liquid puddles upon the floor, there were no secrets left. Pale lips drew warmth from one another, arms and thighs caressed and teased the other, loins locked in tight embrace, and the night held secret the curse of your sexual lives. In the morning you still ached from the fervor of your lust, but there was splendor in the surrender with which you entered one another. It was so delicious, so wicked, so glorious, so depraved, so magnificent, so malevolent, so wrong, so right that none of it made any sense at all.

Neither did Martin ever feel guilty, remorseful, or disgusted at his own lusts and longings. In fact, to him it all seemed quite natural and perfectly normal. One falls in love; one seeks the warmth of human flesh; one wants to hold and be held; one needs a little human affection in this cruel and unforgiving world. Is that so wrong? Is that so strange? Whether it be man or woman, whether it be common or extraordinary, whether it be favored or forbidden, whether it be right or wrong, whether it be saintly or sinful, whether it be depraved or exalted, whether it be within the law or without, and whether it be dangerous or safe, the fact remains that love is love and cares not for reasons, excuses, explanations, justifications, and sanctification. Love is love.

III

Christopher turned in bed and reached out with blind, sleepy limbs to encircle Martin, just as an octopus draws the sea within him. And Martin? He reached back. During the past several years each had many affairs with many different men. Martin was older than Christopher by seven years, but Christopher, although younger, was the wiser of the two. He had known all of his life that he was gay; whereas, it had taken Martin years to arrive at the same knowledge. In high school, when other boys were beginning to take an interest in girls, Christopher was already well advanced with his interest in boys. His first experience was with an uncle who fondled him to orgasm and then proceeded to initiate the young nephew into all the secret rites and rituals of gay love. Christopher loved all of it, and not once did he look back with longing or regrets at what he had become. He was what he was and accepted this truth with the innocence of a child.

Martin, on the other hand, had spent the majority of his life in doubtful despair and anguish. For years he had resisted essential truths about himself, and much of his adult life was an elaborate denial of who and what he really was. But then an act of fate occurred several years ago which made further denials impossible. While hitchhiking through Indiana, he was picked up by two workmen in a farm truck and raped. Even as it happened, he was overcome with a wild, erotic joy that he had never experienced before. "Somehow they must have known"—he later confessed to himself—"what I did not even know about myself." It was not a brutal rape; it was hardly even a rape; it was rather a seduction of the unwilling by the very willing, and it changed his life. From that moment on he dreamed and fantasized, thought and daydreamed about his pleasure, again and again, until finally he could stand the tension no longer and made contact in a public restroom. It was wonderful; it was just as perfect, just as beautiful as he thought it would be, and from that moment on he was transformed. But the soul runs far behind the body in these matters, and for years he paid for his pleasure with guilt and self-disgust. Always hating himself for not being what he ought to be and loathing himself for simply being what he was, Martin continually taunted his self-esteem with the unforgiving malice of a parent who beats his child. Then he met Christopher.

They worked together in the same office complex and quickly became friends. At first Martin was uneasy in Christopher's company because he felt vulnerable, almost naked, as if all his secrets were obvious and exposed to public view. And indeed he should, for Christopher had accurately "read Martin's beads" the first moment he saw him. They had coffee together and then, more frequently, lunch until finally they seduced one another over dinner one evening in Christopher's apartment. They had been together ever since. The following year Martin found an old Victorian house, and working together, they restored the mansion to a semblance of its former elegance.

It was a beautiful home with high vaulted ceilings, hardwood floors, rich wood paneling, and accents of emerald green that contrasted richly with the antique furnishings. Everything was sharp, clean, spotless, and luxurious throughout the glass and stainless steel kitchen. The dining room was an opulent, oval enclave with velvet cushions in the bay window seats and burled oak furnishings that could easily accommodate ten guests for dinner. And guests they often had, for during these years the house hummed and buzzed with parties, cocktail hours, and all that makes for warm friendship with others. After a rich and succulent meal prepared by Christopher, the entourage of guests would repair to the book-lined library or sit by a roaring fire in the large living room. Their friends included lawyers, doctors, business men and women, realtors, executives, artists, professors, and anyone else they happened to meet and befriend. These were still the days when being gay was not quite the sin it used to be and not nearly the disease it was soon to become. Of course, their straight friends knew that Martin and Christopher were "simply that way," but they didn't seem to care. Well, perhaps they did care, but at least they accepted the way things were even if they did so reluctantly. "After all, Christopher is so handsome;" they would say, "what a pity that he's that way because some nice girl would be happy to have him." "Martin is nice," they would say, "and you would never guess that he's that way, would you?" Behind their backs there would be giggles and laughs, and everyone knew that they slept in the same bed together.

While it lasted, it was Camelot—even if it was Camelot with a flaw—for these were the olden, magic days before AIDS turned everything rotten and foul. There was music in the air, touch of gold upon the sun, and Martin was in love. He was in love, and suddenly life had meaning, substance, and purpose. For the first time in a long time he was content as only those who have found love can truly be content. In the evening, there was someone waiting for him at home. At night there was a warm body to hold and make love to and find beside you the next morning. Was it a deception? Perhaps it was, for things simply seemed too good to be true, and Martin had come to distrust fortune as much as he dreaded disaster. When he discovered the strawberry mark upon his calf, he knew that it was over and that Camelot had fallen into ruin. Now there were dozens of the crimson, purple Kaposi's sarcomas erupting everywhere on his body. Face and neck, arms and legs, belly and back were crisscrossed with the multiple scarlet stigmata of this curse. As one would heal, another would appear, and each was impossible to hide. It seemed as if an underground well-spring of sewage rumbled through his veins erupting here and there in small cesspools of stinking death. A blood test taken a week ago came back positive for the AIDS virus, and Martin had been counseled by his doctor that the five-year survival rate was less than 8 percent. Camelot was no more, and everything was decaying into ruin around him. Why? What had he done? Who was to blame? There were endless questions without answers, sorrowful pains without pleasures, terrible fears without reassurances, and Martin prepared himself to suffer death in painful, humiliated isolation. Meanwhile, the straight world smiled back with the justified benediction of the blessed. After all, the queers were finally getting what they deserved, and we'd soon be rid of them all. Government officials turned a bored and disinterested ear to the moanful pleas for help, and religious leaders took the opportunity to reaffirm that God punishes the unrighteous and unjust. Meanwhile, the AIDS virus sought out its victims with the accuracy of a heat-seeking missile, looking for the warmth of human blood, and found its target in sick children, drug users, pregnant mothers, bisexual lovers, hemophiliacs, surgery patients, lab technicians, teenagers, and anyone else who offered a safe, warm haven of rest.

IV

By February 1988, 52,256 clinical cases of AIDS had been reported to the Centers for Disease Control in Atlanta. These were diagnosed clinical cases reported by health care professionals across the United and States to the CDC and represent cumulative figures since AIDS statistics were first started in the early 1980s. The year before, in February 1987, the number of cases that had been reported was 30,396, and in 1986 the number was 17,001. The numerical increase of 21,860 new cases from February 1987 to February 1988 represents a 72 percent increase in new AIDS cases. From February 1986 to February 1987 there were 13,396 new cases, or an increase of 79 percent. The incidence of cases does not seem to be decreasing despite the beneficial measures of safe sex, AIDS testing, condom use, New York City's experimental program of sterile needle distribution to drug users, and a variety of other prophylactic measures. In fact, the CDC's projections for the next three years continue to show numerical increases (table 10.1).

Even more alarming than the number of new clinical cases reported, however, is the ratio of seropositive cases to actual clinical cases. The CDC calculates that the number of people in the United States carrying the AIDS virus but not yet showing symptoms is about 1.5 million. Of those untested but suspected of being infected, the CDC has calculated a figure of 30:1 to 50:1. In short, for every person presently diagnosed with AIDS, there are thirty to fifty who will begin to show symptoms in the next five years. The population of the United States is about 250 million. At present, the number of clinical cases represents about .0209 percent of the population, with an estimated .073 percent of the population infected with HTLV but showing no symptoms. Using the CDC's ratio of 50:1, the percentage of the population that shows clinical symptoms of AIDS will continue to increase over the next five years from .0209 percent to 5.2 percent in 1991. This steady increase in clinical cases will not be a simple arithmetic progression but a geometric increase (table 10.2). Furthermore, if we presume that each one of these infected persons manages to infect five more people each year, then the increase is proportionately affected.

Table 10.1. Centers for Disease Control clinical case projections

Year	New cases	Total cases	Increase
1988	33,000	85,256	66%
1989	45,000	130,256	73%
1990	58,000	188,256	77%
1991	74,000	262,256	78%

Table 10.2. Centers for Disease Control seropositive / clinical case projections

Year	Total cases	Seropositives	Increase
1988	85,256	4,262,800	1.7%
1989	130,256	6,512,800	2.6%
1990	188,256	9,412,800	3.7%
1991	262,256	13,112,800	5.2%

There is so much gossip woven between threads of truth that it is impossible to tell where the one ends and the other begins. For example, it has been argued that the real truth about the spread of AIDS is actually far worse than the media's exaggeration of that truth. But how can one determine the validity of such claims? Some health officials have claimed that AIDS will behave precisely like bubonic plague did during the Middle Ages and essentially kill everyone who is susceptible to the virus, sparing only those who are immune by some genetic fortune. Secretary of Health and Human Services Otis Bowen made just such a claim in the winter of 1987 when he compared AIDS to the black plague that destroyed nearly half the population of Europe during the 1300s. One year later, in January 1988, Bowen had revised his judgment considerably and said that the disease will probably remain within the gay community and not "explode into the heterosexual population." What is truth and what is fancy? In truth, we do not even know if anyone is genetically immune, and it may well be that everyone will succumb to the disease. At present, the disease is believed to be 100 percent fatal in those who have shown symptoms or have AIDS-related-complex syndrome (ARC). Moreover, it is believed that everyone infected with the virus will eventually demonstrate symptoms whether the incubation period be two years or twenty. Indeed, there could be a span of sixty years or more before the symptoms of an infection caught in youth manifests itself in old age. On the other hand, such assertions are merely speculations without the benefit of informed data and research statistics. It does seem clear that the gay population will continue to suffer the major burden of this disease for the immediate future and that cities such as New York and San Francisco will be among the hardest hit. The total health care cost during 1988 for AIDS patients in New York City was $385 million, and this figure has been projected to exceed $1 billion in 1991. *Science* magazine estimated in its February 5, 1988, issue that health care costs for the 270,000 cases anticipated to occur between 1981 and 1991 will be about $22 billion. It is very difficult, however, to assess the meaning of these statistics accurately and to determine what significance they bear for lives lost and dollars spent.

To begin with, consider the incidence of AIDS reported by February 1988 to the CDC. Of the 52,256 clinical cases in the United States, 91.2 percent were male, and of this figure, 98 percent were either homosexual or drug users or both (table 10.3).

It is noteworthy that 7 percent of the AIDS cases affect heterosexual females while less than 1.9 percent affect heterosexual males. These infections may have come from drug use, transfusion, or bisexual intercourse several times removed. For example, a woman may have a bisexual lover and contract the virus, which she in turn passes on to a heterosexual partner who may pass it on to other heterosexual lovers. The whole pattern of transmission is complex and depends upon many factors. Open sores or herpetic lesions can increase transmission, as can anal intercourse or even oral intercourse under some conditions. Since anal intercourse appears to be the major risk factor in contracting AIDS, the actual sexual practices of the parties, whether they be male or female, may be just as important as whether they be homosexual or heterosexual. In short, AIDS does not have a preference for homosexuals but rather for those who engage in anal intercourse and especially for those who have open lesions while doing so. The incidence of AIDS among children is usually the result of blood transfusions or intrauterine transmission by a mother already infected. There was a somewhat higher incidence of AIDS in male children (426) than in female children (363) for the 1987–88 period, but whether this difference is actually significant remains to be seen.

On February 14, 1988, the *New York Times* reported another interesting set of statistics of infection rates within the

Table 10.3. 1987–88 Clinical cases by sex

Clinical cases	Male	Female	Children
52,256	47,676	3,791	789

1987–88 Clinical cases by sexual preference

	Male	Female
Heterosexual cases:	948	1,110
Homosexual cases:		46,728

American population. Taking approximate estimates based upon figures from the CDC, federal officials estimated that there are about 2.5 million men in the United States who are homosexuals and that nearly 25 percent of these are already infected with the AIDS virus, or roughly 625,000 individuals. Counting bisexual men and those with only occasional homosexual contact, it was estimated that of the 2.5 to 7.5 million in this population, only about 5 percent, or between 125,000 to 375,000 persons, are infected. There are nearly 900,000 intravenous drug users in this country, and 25 percent, or 225,000, are probably infected with AIDS. Hemophilia A patients account for another 12,400 persons, and ironically almost 70 percent, or 8,700, carry the virus, whereas only 35 percent of the 3,100 hemophilia B patients are infected, or about 1,100 persons. Finally, of the estimated 142 million heterosexuals, only .0021 percent, or 30,000, are infected. In New York City, AIDS is the leading cause of death in men from twenty-five to forty-four years of age and in women from twenty-five to thirty-four. Since 1981 there have been over thirteen thousand cases reported in New York City, and this number is expected to pass the fifty thousand mark by 1991.

As of February 1988, 29,206 people have died of AIDS in the United States. At present, AZT (azidothymidine) is the only effective drug approved for use in AIDS patients. It is marketed under the name Retrover by the Burrows-Wellcome Pharmaceutical Company, and while not a new drug—it was first synthesized in the 1960s by University of Michigan researchers as a cancer chemotherapeutic agent—it is antibacterial to gram-negative bacteria and, therefore, effective against many opportunistic infections that affect AIDS patients. From October 1986 to March 1987, 4,800 AIDS patients were administered the drug AZT over a forty-four week schedule. The survival rate during this period was an impressive 73 percent. For a period of time the demand for the drug far exceeded its availability, but it has been taken off the restricted list, and currently there are 9,000 patients on the AZT regimen in the United States. The drug, however, is not a cure and at best seems to provide temporary relief from pneumocystis carinii and Kaposi's sarcoma. The drug is taken in tablet form every four hours around the clock, and this regimen is so strict that users must carry an alarm device that sounds whenever their dosage is due.

In November 1987 the number of worldwide cases reported to the CDC was 68,217. This figure, however, is very misleading because many countries either do not keep accurate records or fail to provide honest and precise reports when correct information is available. Russia is a very good example, citing only four cases of AIDS and claiming that those were contracted in the United States by Soviets visiting abroad. Dr. Jonathan Mann, director of the United Nations' program on AIDS, places the worldwide figure much higher and estimates that over 150,000 cases of AIDS have occurred to date. Asia has the fewest number of cases, and the United States has the greatest number. There are 45,436 cases that have occurred in the United States, and the majority of these were in San Francisco and New York City. In short, the United States had 66.6 percent of the cases in the world. It has been projected by several agencies that the number of AIDS cases worldwide will exceed 300,000 by the year 1989. The World Health Organization (WHO) estimates that between five and ten million people in the world probably carry the AIDS virus.

The first case reported in the United States was in 1981. However, recent medical records have revealed the existence of a patient in St. Louis, Missouri, who died of the disease in 1969. Assuming that he actually contracted the disease two years earlier, it would appear that AIDS has been disseminating throughout the American population since 1967, or a period of almost twenty years. Given the geometric increases in seropositive and clinical cases, it has been suggested by several AIDS researchers that we are just beginning to see the tip of an enormous and dreadful iceberg floating toward our shores. In Haiti, for example, it is estimated that more than half of the heterosexual population is infected with Slim's disease, or AIDS, and that by the end of the century the population of that country will be decimated. One must be wary about the significance of such statistics, however, because the figures constantly change from one reporting center to another and there are many contradictions between local and national figures. It is sufficient to note that the disease is epidemic, incurable, and likely to become the leading cause of death in the next century unless a vaccine or cure is found. There is a growing suspicion, however, that this disease has the ability to mutate and, therefore, to change into different forms and patterns that could evade and avoid standard treatment and prophylactic procedures. If this is true—and it is a theory yet to be established—then AIDS could pose a Hydra's head of such enormous complexity that as soon as a cure is found for one form, another or several others appear to take its place.

v

The disease doesn't kill you, ironically, but the symptoms do. With a genius bordering on stupidity, AIDS discovered the delicate network of protective immunity that guards us all and found a way to sneak beneath it. Imagine being exposed to your enemies by a bodyguard that falls asleep at his post. A hole in a fence is the only apparent damage done, but through this hole climbs, crawls, and creeps every pest, pestilence, disease, disorder, virus, bacteria, and plague that endangers us. As you lie naked, alone, defenseless in your bed, these assailants and assassins tear you to pieces under the cover of secrecy and the night. In the morning the bodyguard awakens to find you festering with mortal wounds, but, of course, then it is too late. The opportunistic pathogens—so called because they wait for the ideal opportunity when the host is seriously compromised—include the pneumonias, various types of encephalitis, esophagitis, enteroclolitis, and a group of miscellaneous infections as well as the herpetic viruses of the mouth, genitals, and eyes. These infections are not new, nor are we inexperienced in their treatment. In fact, cancer patients, burn victims, and those suffering from metabolic disorders have always been the target for such opportunistic fungi, viruses, parasites, and bacteria. A partial list of these opportunistic infections, along with the treatment of choice, appear in table 10.4.

Pneumocystis carinii pneumonia is certainly one of the most deadly opportunistic infections and often becomes the angel of death for AIDS patients. One reads in the newspaper that such and such a person recently died of pneumonia, and it is apparent that some other disease was the underlying cause, such as cancer or AIDS. These are opportunistic infections that lay in wait for their victims because only the most compromised and impoverished of constitutions is susceptible to them. On occasion the first diagnosis of AIDS is actually made after the patient enters the emergency room of a local hospital for respiratory distress: A week or a few days before, a dry cough developed with moderate fever, and there was difficulty breathing. As the symptoms worsened, the patient rehearsed and rearranged his symptoms with greater and greater denial until hypoxemia made further denials impossible. Biopsy of lung tissue quickly identifies the trophozoites of pneumocystis that easily stain the Gomori methenamine silver. In retrospect, the crisis recalls a host of disorganized and disunified symptoms that prevailed over the past several months and were denied systematically by a bodyguard of falsehoods with which the patient reassured himself. But finally the truth emerges like a pattern of iron filings when a magic magnet is held upon them.

The first and even second bout with pneumocystis can usually be treated effectively, but additional infections will become more and more resistant to medication until finally the patient's defenses are entirely eroded away by the disease. The treatment itself elicits further discomfort because the high dosages of trimethoprim-sulfamethoxazole produce various joint and muscle pains along with fever and nausea. It seems that suffering never ceases with this disease as it finds new and

Table 10.4. Opportunistic infections and treatment of choice

Infection	Drug
Pneumocystic carinii	Trimethoprim-sulfamethoxazole
Toxoplasma encephalitis	Pyrimethamine and Sulfadiazine
Cryptosporidosis	Spiramycin
Cryptococcal meningitis	Amphotericin B and Flucytosine
Oral candidiasis	Amphotericin B
Candida esophagitis	Ketoconazole
Herpes virus	Acyclovir
Mycobacterium	Isoniazid

Adapted from Braunwald et al., *Harrison's Principles of Internal Medicine*, 11th ed. (New York: McGraw-Hill, 1987).

unique ways to martyr and humiliate its victim. In some cases the treatment can be worse than the pneumonia itself and even lead to blood disorders such as thrombocytopenia or megaloblastic anemia that are life threatening. Even minimal reactions to trimethoprim-sulfamethoxazole include projectile vomiting in which the patient defecates at the same time that he vomits or the more distressful Stevens-Johnson syndrome in which lesions appear in the mouth, eyes, anus, and genitals. In some cases these infections may be so severe that it is painful even to close the mouth, and eating or talking is impossible. The eyes may swell shut or become so impacted with pus that they cannot be opened, and vision is impaired through scarring.

AIDS creates a vicious cycle in which one opportunistic infection creates a crisis, and the very methods used to treat this crisis in turn create a different one. Thus, bouncing like a ball from one fatal infection to another, the patient quickly becomes so exhausted that a host of other pathogens seize the opportunity to reinfect him again. Toxoplasmosis, cryptosporidosis, and a variety of fungi infections, including cryptococcus neoformans, produce a rainbow of disorders from encephalitis to meningitis which produce such vast amounts of internal toxins that the entire cardiovascular system simply falters, fails, and collapses or bacterial infections, such as mycobacterium tuberculosis, seize the chance to infect the patient on his rebound from other disorders.

Tuberculosis has recently reached epidemic proportions once again in New York City, San Francisco, and parts of Texas. For years it was one of the most fatal and feared of all diseases until an adequate treatment was found in isoniazid and various other types of chemoprophylaxis. Now it is recurring with alarming frequency and is often the first opportunistic infection to present itself in AIDS patients, frequently months in advance of any others. Moreover, it is not merely a disease of the lungs but can infect any body system including bones, brain, eyes, ears, joints, heart, mouth, liver, urinary tract, and central nervous system.

In addition to bacterial infections there are a number of viruses which find a reluctant but unresisting host in AIDS

patients. In particular the herpetic viruses can either disseminate throughout the system or focus in specific areas such as
mouth, rectum, genitals, eyes, and other locales rich in mucus
membrane. Usually, infections from herpes are painful, inconvenient, and frightening but rarely life threatening. The one
exception, of course, is herpetic encephalitis, which may cause
irreparable brain damage. Lesions upon the genitals or within
the rectum sometimes cause discharge and bleeding but often
disappear within a week or so when treated with acyclovir. This
drug is available in oral or injectable form and can even be
applied as a topical ointment. The creams are applied every
three hours to the lesion; the oral form of acyclovir is taken in
a 200 mg tablet five times a day for two weeks.

The treatment of these herpetic lesions by acyclovir, however, is purely supportive and symptomatic medication that
does not address the more important immunosuppression
problem that underlies it. Therefore, the infections recur, and
recur, and recur once again. On occasion a number of multiple
lesions will lead to a polyneuritis with ocular, genital, oral, and
even varicella infections all happening at the same time. Intravenous medication with acyclovir at 5 mg per kg every eight
hours may control this hailstorm of sores, but it will only act as
a temporary measure.

At some time, most AIDS patients will show evidence of
infection from cytomegalovirus. This diffuse and disseminating
infection can affect each organ in particular and every organ in
general. Extreme fatigue and associated weight loss and fever
are global symptoms followed by specific infections in bowels,
brain, eyes, and lungs. Most of the antiviral agents are totally
useless against cytomegalovirus, and treatment usually consists
of supportive therapy that reduces the symptoms but does not
cure the disease; it simply waits for another opportunity to
reappear.

One of the most noticeable—and certainly one of the most
alarming—opportunistic infections is Kaposi's sarcoma, named
after the Austrian dermatologist Moritz Kaposi (1837–1902).
Xeroderma pigmentosum is a disease so rare that its precise
description alone earned Kaposi a place in medical history.
This disease, which may begin in childhood and then progres-

sively lead to death through multiple ulcerations and muscular atrophy, also appears in elderly Jews and Italians. The more aggressive and widespread form of Kaposi's sarcoma being seen in AIDS patients, however, consists of flat, pinkish or purple lesions that occur in clusters on the legs, back, and stomach and then rapidly disseminate to any part of the body including the face, neck, and arms. One or two lesions can quickly develop into several dozen neoplasms within a short period of time. Treatment with chemotherapeutic agents such as vincristine or etoposide can promote periods of remission from a month to a year or more.

The incubation period from exposure to infection is undetermined. Some experts have located this dormant phase between a few months and several years, with five years appearing to be the average or mean. There are, however, several prodromal symptoms that often appear months or even years before the actual appearance of the clinical disease itself. These include fatigue, fever, loss of appetite, diarrhea, enlarged and painful glands, weight loss, and a spectrum of opportunistic infections such as herpes zoster and oral candidiasis.

VI

Martin suffered much. Perhaps he even suffered too much. Certainly he suffered more than he ought in exchange for the full and sufficient discharge of his sins. Within a year's time he had paid the full martyrdom of six saints—Epipodius, Alexander, Elphege, Rogatian, Callistus, and Demetrius—as well as expatriating the vices and wiles of several hermits, doctors, and bishops of the church. By this time he should have been cleansed completely, but still it didn't seem to be enough. And so he suffered just a little more before he died.

He was wasted thin as a paper kite, and his ribs shown forth with the sharp, white edges of his disease. Brittle, delicate bones poked through the surface of his flesh in order to peer and peek about into foreign regions. A good anatomist could have counted his ribs like the hull of a ship and even discerned from a distance the outlines and ridges of the flat, puffy liver, the swollen, hardened spleen, the frightened heart beating like a captured bird, as well as every nodule and bump, every crest and valley of his wasted torso. It seemed as if this disease was slowly turning him inside out, as all his internal organs slowly floated to the surface while weakened skin and bone fell inward like hot, moistened jelly.

His skin was bleached clean of color save for dozens of red, weeping sores dotting the frosty surface like tiny drops of blood upon the snow. The tremendous fires that daily burned within had roasted his skin to a dusty parchment, just as the sun wrinkles and wastes fallen leaves to a dry, flaky crunch. Within he was cold as ice, as internal polar winds shook him daily with freezing chills. Outside he was hot and scalding to the touch, so much so that the heat evaporated from his body like steam on a winter's night. Now nearly blind, almost deaf, and hardly able to feel, touch, smell, or taste, he had become a solitary shaft of rotting flesh basting in its own foul juices. Whether his boiled brain understood the tragedy it had become, one cannot say. Certainly madness would have been a blessing because the euphoria of the insane can laugh at anything including its own pain and death. Sober sanity, clarity of thought, and lucidity would have added only another aching pain to the ones he already suffered.

Martin died of drowning. Floating in a sea of infected mucus, he simply inhaled the thick ropy slime until he could breathe no more. Wet as he was, he died in a dry bed with scaling skin cracked by ferocious fevers, with a brain baked dry and boiled away of its own juices, with a tongue so thick and limp that it turned to dusty parchment from the metabolic furnaces that consumed it.

Moreover, he died alone. Friends and lovers, family and relatives had long since ceased their polite and occasional visits. They found Martin to be a scornful humiliation which reminded them far too richly of their own vulnerability and of human flesh's peculiar damnation. Cautiously they came at first to see him but always went away with horror in their hearts, a foul odor upon their bodies, and a sense of soiled disfigurement which no amount of washing could remove. They worried about themselves, having seen what had become of Martin. Had they been infected merely by being in the same room with him? Should they discard the clothes they wore, abstain from sex, drink disinfectant from a glass, or bathe their polluted bodies in waters of purification? Could a doctor prescribe a cleansing rise, a healing balm, a protective vaccination, or would a priest offer some absolution and benediction? They left feeling contaminated because Martin was himself soiled with this terrible infection which actually seemed to hang in the air like suspended droplets of oil. Visitors to his room were almost certain they could feel death around them, even smell and taste the salty AIDS virus settle on their lips as it sprayed like blown sea mist into the air and tainted with mercurial death everything around it.

Doctors were clinically indifferent and examined his lesions with the cold calculation of anatomy professors preparing a lecture or pathologists completing a report. Nurses were often hostile, sometimes cruel, and always distant and aloof as they managed his body. Orderlies were vindictive and revengeful as they stood outside his room to gossip with laughing chatter.

His family in the Midwest was ashamed of him and especially of what he had become. Martin's father was a carpenter and his mother a simple, unpretentious women involved with her church groups. When they first learned that Martin was gay, it was the worst day of their lives. What had they done wrong? How had this malformed monster developed, and what happened to little Marty who used to go fishing with his father? Then when he got sick with AIDS, it was difficult not to believe that he only got what he deserved. After all, they had warned him, and it was not their fault if he ignored their warnings. Moreover, they had three other whole and healthy children— all married and having babies as they ought—and it was easy to abandon Martin, just as one leaves a stillborn fetus by the roadside. From that time on he simply ceased to exist for them. No one in their hometown ever asked what had become of Martin, and so the family found it convenient simply never to speak of him again.

Martin's lovers and then his friends began to disappear as soon as the diagnosis was confirmed. Suddenly, invitations to parties stopped; people avoided him on the streets; the phone fell silent; and he stayed at home for days without hearing a single knock upon the door. The mailman brought bills and brochures but no letters or cards. To his lovers, Martin was a monumental reminder of all that they might become, and it was a prophecy no one wished to contemplate. Finally, the circle of his acquaintances constricted to just the few friends he made in a gay support group, and then finally even those disappeared.

And what of Christopher? He moved out the day he heard the news. Christopher had yet to show any symptoms, and perhaps he didn't even have the disease. His behavior was understandable; he was afraid and probably angry and simply looking out for himself. Martin understood, or at least he thought he understood. Every now and then they might see each other on the street, but each would avoid the other's eyes and passed on by. So much had passed between them that cruel indifference came easy. Christopher's new lover was younger, bolder, and better looking than Martin. It was ironic, Martin often thought, that even as his own life was ending, Christopher's was simply starting over again. Just as a phoenix rises out of the ashes of its own destruction, so had Christopher been reborn. Perhaps someone must die so that someone else might live. There is death, and there is rebirth. There is renunciation, and there is resurrection. The past dies in order that the future may begin. But why did it have to be Martin who died, and by what fortune was it Christopher who was chosen to live?

There were those who said that Martin deserved everything he got and others who said that no one deserved as much as he received. Perhaps. Perhaps not. Who can say? Was it true that he had desecrated his own body and performed satanic rites with holy instruments intended to sanctify? Who knows about such matters? It could be true that being forewarned of the dangers that he courted, he should not be surprised to wed the very disaster he seduced. He knew the risks, understood the reasons, and took his chances nonetheless. Yes, it may be true that prophecy fulfilled itself in Martin's life and that his damnation was proper, even justified, and well deserved. As a matter of fact, Martin himself might well have agreed with such judgments.

Yet one wonders. After all these good reasons are given,

there still remains a doubt. Did Martin really deserve such a death—does anyone deserve such a death—and what kind of justice has been served? AIDS seeks out the young and the old, the gay and the straight, the beautiful and the ugly, the sick and the well, the good and the bad, the saint and the sinner without regard for their names, deeds, ages, sex, or race. It is an equal opportunity killer that is satisfied with a small pool of blood in which to bathe and with no regrets about the owner. Heart patients become infected through transfusions; children inherit the virus from their mothers; bleeders and hemophiliacs are cursed by the same elixir that saves them; lovers die by the same orgasmic ecstasy that unites them, and nurses, doctors, firemen, policemen, paramedics, orderlies, and technicians unwillingly lend their veins to death through an accidental scratch or cut.

The virus does not care. It is not a moralist or a metaphysician; it neither contemplates nor praises nor blames but simply seeks a haven of bloody rest in which to survive, to populate and reproduce itself in endless repetitions of a mindless, thoughtless genetic formula. This is not vengeance but the mere business of survival, and suffering is simply the price that must be paid. And it doesn't matter who pays that price— a pregnant mother, an old man, a young child, or a man who loves other men instead of women. It doesn't matter.

Life goes on. Martin dies. Christopher lives. In the ecstasy of night, bodies twist and turn into one another and through the medium of delicious orgasm deliver death and destruction to one another. To receive these seeds of deep despair within one's naked loins is to anticipate a pregnancy of death. For months or years the womb grows fertile with a sorrow more beautiful than love and more deadly than hate. Then one day there is birth with its bittersweet reminder that the old must pass away in order to make room for the new.

11

The Smoker

Sublime tobacco! which from east to west
Cheers the tar's labour or the Turkman's
*   rest;*
Which on the Moslem's ottoman divides
His hours, and rivals opium and his brides;
Magnificent in Stamboul, but less grand,
Though not less loved, in Wapping or the
*   Strand;*
Divine in hookas, glorious in a pipe,
When tipp'd with amber, mellow, rich and
*   ripe;*
Like other charmers, wooing the caress
More dazzling when daring in full dress;
Yet thy true lovers more admire by far
Thy naked beauties—Give me a cigar!

Lord Byron
"The Island"

LUNG CANCER: Embryologically, the laryngotracheobronchial tree
is a ventral endodermal foregut derivative lined with five or more
types of epithelial cells that form a pseudostratified mucosal sheath
resting on a basement membrane. Mucus-secreting goblet cells,

ciliated cells, brush border cells, short basal or reserve cells, and granular cells that rest on the basement membrane, giving the mucosa a pseudostratified appearance can be seen on electron microscopy. The granular basal cells are called Kulchitsky or K-type cells. They have neurosecretory granules that can synthesize polypeptide hormones or biogenic amines. Thus they are presumed to be the cell of origin of small cell carcinomas.

As the embryonic lung diverticulum branches to form bronchopulmonary buds, splanchnic mesenchyme surrounds these structures and gives rise to the fibroelastic, vascular, muscular, and cartilaginous components of the lung and forms the visceral pleura. The parietal pleura is derived from the corresponding somatic mesenchyme.

Lung cancer arises most often by segmental and subsegmental bronchi in response to repeated injury and chronic inflammation. At segmental bronchial bifurcations, bronchial epithelium is particularly susceptible to injury, and carcinogens may be deposited in these areas. Initially, basal cells respond to injury by proliferating to generate mucin-secreting goblet cells. When there is added injury, the columnar cells are replaced by orderly, arranged, metaplastic, stratified squamous epithelium. Finally, the epithelium becomes disorganized and nuclear atypia and mitoses are seen in the basal half of the mucosa (findings that are called atypical metaplasia or dysplasia). When this process occurs throughout the full thickness of the mucosa, a diagnosis of carcinoma "in situ" (intraepithelial carcinoma) is made. Finally, the basement membrane is violated by the neoplastic cells; frank infiltration of neoplastic cells into the underlying stroma follows. This process may take 10 to 20 years and represents the first phases of the natural history of lung cancer. The carcinogens implicated in this process include the constituents of tobacco smoke, radioisotopes, asbestos, polycyclic aromatic hydrocarbons, haloethers, nickel, chromium, inorganic arsenic, iron ore, printing inks, and other possible occupational and atmospheric pollutants. Several groups have performed bronchoscopy and bronchial biopsy on smokers and found a significant correlation of metaplasia with smoking. Of great interest, after treatment for 6 months with a retinoid (etretinate) the degree of metaplasia dropped significantly, thus indicating a potential prophylaxis against lung cancer.

DeVita and Rosenberg
Cancer: Principles and Practice of Oncology

I

Tuesday, March 6, 1978: Blood test today. A few snow flakes this a.m. So tired and my stomach feels like a drum. Tried to take a nap. First Sue Wilson called. Just when I got to sleep, Martha Fry called. Sam Holloway died this morning. 40 degrees today, some sun, some clouds. We stopped at Tom and Ann Steward's on the way home from my blood test. If it turns out the way I feel today, it won't be good.

Thursday, April 5, 1978: Gloomy this morning. Finally sun in the p.m. The O'Reileys came while I was taking a nap. Rose D'Oreo died this morning after a long session of cancer. I ironed five shirts, so Bob will have clean shirts if we can go on our trip. Did not feel good this morning. A lot of pain in my lung, but I didn't have to cough much last night. That was a relief.

Wednesday, April 25, 1978: Bad, bad day . . . Bob made an appt. with the Doctor for me. He said it was bronchitis and sinus. Gave me an antibiotic, shot and capsules. Voice coming back, ears still clogged. Then when we went out Mr. Sullivan across the street from the Dr.'s office backed into our car with his truck. Put a big dent in the left door and cracked the paint. He felt so bad he cried. I got a splitting headache along with my other problems. It rained all day.

Friday, May 11, 1978: I seem to cough all the time and my chest is so tight. I feel sorry for Bob. He tries so hard to make me feel better, but there is nothing that really helps. He painted the spouting today and it was so hot outside while he was working in the sun. He came in at noon white as a sheet, purple below his eyes clear to his cheeks. He flopped on the couch and broke out in a cold sweat. I was sure he was going to have a heart attack.

Saturday, May 12, 1978: I could not stand it if anything happened to Bob. I love him so much.

Wednesday, August 23, 1978: It was sunny and very pleasant today. I had an appt. with a tumor specialist. The tumor in my right lower lung is malignant and a small bit has crept up to the left side of the other lung. He put me on cytoxan and prednisone, which he says will control it. I have to have a blood test once a week for four weeks, then one in another three months, and then again a week

214

later. Bob bought me a new purse today; it is very pretty. We are both relieved that I can be on medication.

Sunday, October 1, 1978: I am 75 years old today. Bob's shoulders and joints hurt so bad that he can hardly move around. My bronchitis flared up and I had trouble breathing. Bob got so upset. He just won't let me have enough time alone to properly doctor myself up. He doesn't feel good but he says that I am in better shape than he is. I guess he's right.

Saturday, November 25, 1979: All of the news is about Jim Jones's religious settlement with over 900 suicides and murders. It happened just a year ago. Gruesome. How can one man influence so many people?

Thursday, November 29, 1979: I was worn out all day. I tried to rest but couldn't stop coughing, and I hurt all the time. What's the point of living when you feel this way? "Please, dear God, let it be over soon."

Erma Katherine Denbrook, a housewife and mother, died of respiratory failure at 11:23 A.M. on Thursday morning, December 6, 1979. She was alone at the time.

II

When Erma was sixteen years old, Aunt Edith gave her a diary. The diary quickly became more than a book for her; it became her best friend. She wrote in the evenings each day, and she wrote every day in that diary for the next sixty years. She wrote all kinds of things: private thoughts, personal messages, nonsense, important world events (such as the bombing of Pearl Harbor), recipes (such as for her brown stew), whether it rained or whether it shined, if she was sad or if she was not. It didn't matter what she wrote, for Erma—at least when it came to her diary—was governed by no rules save those which she willingly imposed upon herself.

At the age of thirty-eight, she married a divorced man slightly younger than herself. Almost at once she realized her mistake! But where does a woman of thirty-eight go—especially in the year 1941—when she decides to leave her husband of only a few weeks? Back home to her parents? Certainly not! Well then, back to the same single life she had so recently abandoned? No! She could not leave. She was caught like a rat in a trap with neither the power to withdraw nor the ability to advance. Therefore, she made the only movement that caged animals are able to make; she paced about in a circle inspecting her situation in order thereby to transform it.

Actually, it turned out that her options were not nearly so limited as she had first feared. True, he was cruel—even dangerous—but she was clever and cunning. He was explosive, but she was patient. He was domineering and tyrannical, but she was manipulative and unforgiving. In the end, she domesticated him, and although she had not freed herself from her prison, she had at least widened the bars by enslaving him as well. And thus they spent the next thirty-eight years together in mutual slavery and mutual mastery to one another.

Often—so very often—she returned to her diary. A delicate voice, raised no higher than a whisper, speaking to itself alone. Within these parchment walls there resided corridors, rooms, cells of every dimension and coloration. Wandering now in solitude, hooded like a Cistercian monk in meditation, she pursued endless shadows of herself. With silent, catlike caution she crept up upon herself in the hope that through the shimmering distance she might view herself, catch an unguarded glimpse of herself, and discover who she really was. The slender, delicate diary knew everything about her: all of her fantasies, dreams, girlish thoughts, womanly lusts, matronly fears, and all the terrors too unspeakable to mention except in the silence of ink. Eventually, each and all of these found its own small cell within hushed cloisters wherein it dwelt forever undisturbed except by Erma's occasional furtive visits.

Meanwhile there was much to learn. Having married this late in life, she knew nothing about cleaning, cooking, tending garden and yard, or caring for a home of her own. Frankly, Erma was not at all certain that she wished to know such things or to be burdened by them. Every woman—or at least so she had been told—gravitated in an intuitive and natural way to such domestic duties. But for Erma they were only duties and

216

ones which inspired neither energy nor enthusiasm. In fact, before she met Robert she had been an accountant who loved the neat and well-ordered precision of numbers. Dust, dirt, food scraps, and grime were amorphous, disorderly materials that refused to obey any laws or rules whatsoever. Housework was a duty; it certainly was not—as Mother once had said—a privilege.

When Erma became pregnant at the age of forty-two, she was elated. It was not that she thought a woman could only thereby fulfill herself—she was much too intelligent to believe such nonsense—but rather that she now had an ally, a buffer with which to insulate herself from the cruelty of her husband. This child would be a comrade, a companion drawn of her own flesh with whom she could share her innermost thoughts much as the slender diary had previously allowed her to do. The two of them would go on walks together, share secrets, laugh together, cry together, and so entwine flesh to flesh to become the mirrored images of one another. Robert—she now understood fully and completely—had simply been the unavoidable means to this most perfect and satisfactory end. And therefore he could now be moved to the outer periphery of the circle where, at last fully domesticated, he could do no harm. And so said, it was so done.

It took Robert years to comprehend fully the weight and measure of his now radically altered role. The child looked like Erma; he talked, walked, and seemed more like her than the father. Indeed, eyes, hair, lips, and even mannerisms were all hers and not his. One day—was it out of a desperation born of certitude?—the father said to the son:

"Whom do you love the most? Your mother or me?" Instantly, he knew the answer. The mother's blue eyes looked back in a puzzled, quizzical fashion. The blond hair, the light complexion betold the truth.

"Well," Robert quietly said as if to himself, "I guess boys always love their mothers best."

Companions they were indeed; friends, comrades, and allies they became against the insensitive and highly self-interested Robert. Erma now began to write her diary through her son's eyes, and as the years unfolded so the two merged in

perspective and point of view. On February 12, 1945, Erma—
or was it her son?—wrote:

> Now it all comes out! Daddy was mad cause Mom had too good a
> time at the dance Saturday nite. I had to cough all night last night
> and Mom took me to Dr. Myron. He says I have bronchitis and he
> said to put mustard plasters on me and he gave me pills galore. He
> said the ulcers in my throat and mouth and ears were from a vita-
> min deficiency and he gave me some homicebrin which has all the
> vitamins in it. This is Mom and Daddy's 5th wedding anniversary
> and they are celebrating it by being mad at one another. He thinks
> she spends too much money. He said she was bleeding him, what-
> ever that means. Mom called the doctor for me cause I had a tem-
> perature of 103 yesterday, all night and today.

Where did mother end and son begin? Like separate roots
about a single tree, they seemed more fully to entwine even as
they grew and nourished one another.

By December 11, a Tuesday, matters had continued to de-
teriorate. Erma—or was it her son?—wrote in their diary:

> Daddy didn't come home from the 7 to 3 shift today until 9:30 in
> the evening and he sure was in trouble. He didn't get any supper.
> I am not a very good little boy these days. Mom says I am getting
> too snobbish. I won't speak to people when they talk to me.

Within the next two years, Erma had seized complete control and was now sovereign master of the household. Cruel and
unpredictable Robert had been transformed from a nightmare
to a contrite and somewhat whimpering effigy of his former
self. How had this alchemist achieved her chemical magic? It
was simple. Like a mongoose weaving in mesmerized sympathy with the deadly cobra, she had found his weak spot and
struck tenaciously with fanged teeth into the soft underbelly.
And where lay that sensitive navel within those folds of toughened hide? Precisely where one would least expect to find it:
in silence. Because for all his cruelty, for all his insensitivity,
Robert could not tolerate and could not endure silence. Angry
words, tears of beseechment, apologies, vindications, resentments, cajoling, pampering, giving-in, ego-stroking, and flir-

tations, she had tried them all and to no avail. In fact, he interpreted every kindness or compromise as weakness, and therefore his greedy anger simply fed and feasted upon all such attempts at reconciliation. But silence—simple, elemental, and elegant silence—worked every time. It was magic, a charm, and once Erma discovered its power, she never again abandoned its protection.

Erma experimented with silence in order to understand its power and complexities. For example, she discovered that partial reinforcement was far more effective than total silence. However, it was vitally important that the pauses as well as the intervals be both brief and unpredictable in their occurrences. Again, an ambiguous answer to an important question—delayed by hours or even days of its initial asking—was a major weapon in the arsenal of silence. Timing, self-discipline, patience, these were the virtues which insured success. Silence was not to be confused with either pouting or withdrawal. The latter were simply childish distractions or pranks, whereas the former was a highly sophisticated art upon which rested the very highest stakes. Gradually, as she gained greater and greater expertise, additional manipulative techniques were added such as reversal shifts, inversions, and occasionally complex circularities. It was not by plan or reason that Erma achieved such skills, but by an intuitive savvy which came to her naturally. And indeed had she been confronted, she would have denied all such accusations and believed her denial with the very greatest self-conviction. After all, a fox does not plan to run in circles or to suddenly reverse its direction in order to confuse the enemy. It does not plan; it just does. And so did Erma. And she did so very well indeed.

There seemed to be a symmetry—even a symbiosis—between the mother and the son. When one was sick, the other was also. In turn, recovery of either brought renewal of both. Each sensed when the other was in danger, and each felt the rush of relief when the danger had passed. They were mirrored reflections of one another held in union by powers darker and deeper than either could ever hope to understand. Thus secured against cruel and unpredictable Robert, they were safe insofar as they were together. And together they were for most of the time; they shopped together, gardened together, cleaned house together, and planned together against the ever present danger of cruel and unpredictable Robert. After all, he was no less than a sleeping monster. Should he wake and find one of them alone, he would be unmerciful in his rage. And that must not happen at any cost.

However, unbeknownst to either, the biological time clock that governs each of our lives was seeking out these two frightened doves huddled together for safety. It found them finally and began to separate and disconnect the delicate mesenteries that bound them together. Time is jealous of all unions that arrogantly pride themselves on being permanent. The boy one day discovered girls. Erma sensed danger in the air; she had a nose for it. The monster rolled over in his sleep, groaned once, and slept again. The boy discovered books, friends—his own friends—and Erma felt the flesh tear, the muscles recoil, the bones break. He made plans for college. She saw the black wound of separation grow larger and more grotesque in its bloody rupture. The drugged breathing of cruel and unpredictable Robert interrupted its comatose rhythm to sniff the air for blood and torn flesh.

When finally the boy left home to attend college, Erma instinctively realized that the next few weeks were crucial to her survival. The beast, the monster would sense her vulnerability—even as the predator instinctively understands the weakness of the prey—and so would strike immediately and unmercilessly. But then—in a golden moment of good fortune—she suddenly understood everything. She understood why silence worked with cruel and unpredictable Robert. She understood why he was cruel and why he was unpredictable. She understood—in a brilliant instant of clarity—the entire geometry and algebra of the last twenty years. It was so simple, so elementary and obvious. Robert, cruel and unpredictable Robert, was—underneath all the threats, intimidations, obscenities, and monstrous bullyings—quite simply a little boy. Who could believe that for all his insensitivity, coldness, and indifference, here was a fragile constitution which was deeply wounded by the slightest affront? At some deep and profound level, Erma had always suspected as much. But now all the parts fell into their respective places like the solution to a geometrical puzzle. The years of possessiveness and male dominance had simply been the cry of a child to be loved. The coarse and clumsy efforts at lovemaking had not been eroticism but materialism. She understood; she finally understood. The boy had been her ally, but more precisely he had been Robert's most feared and hated enemy. Since the son had absorbed all the maternal love available, and since Robert knew no other kind of love, he felt impoverished and orphaned. Now the orphan wished to be adopted, to take the boy's vacant place and so fulfill all of Erma's maternal instincts. He would be a good boy; there would be no more temper tantrums, no more mischievousness, no more pouting spells. He promised and she understood. She understood. And so it was!

III

Erma smoked for over sixty years. She lighted her first cigarette on her sixteenth birthday and continued to light well over 800,000 cigarettes—at the rate of two packs a day—until her death on December 6, 1979, just sixty-six days past her seventy-sixth birthday. Those nearly one million cigarettes cost her well over $30,000 to purchase and promoted countless bouts of chronic bronchitis, asthmatic attacks, pleural infections, viral and bacterial pneumonias, and finally chronic emphysema and squamous-cell carcinoma of both lungs. Why then did she do it? Why—after all that pain and suffering—did she continue to smoke?

She enjoyed it. She enjoyed having a good cigarette with a rich cup of strong black coffee. She enjoyed the quiet laughter of friends over coffee and cigarettes and Danish. She enjoyed the first full puff of the day when still weary with the lethargy of sleep she lazily reached for her Camels and inhaled the first of more than forty cigarettes that day. She enjoyed it. What more can be said? To inhale the strong rich tobacco flavor and feel its curlicues and wisps of pungent tartness is a joy, a pleasure well beyond words or description. Instantly, there is a tautness to the lungs as they come alive under the stimulation of smoke; the tongue, the lips, and even the throat seem to resonate with the slight tingle of nicotined satisfaction. There is absolutely nothing better than a cigarette after a fine meal, after a cup of rich coffee, after having made good love, just before going to bed at night. There is positively nothing that is better than a full, rich, mellow, fragrant, full-bodied, pungent, ripe, delicious, and satisfying cigarette at such times. And for these reasons—and many more as well—Erma enjoyed a good cigarette. She simply enjoyed it. What more can be said?

It is true that cigarettes were a dirty habit, as Erma would frequently admit. Her middle and index fingers had been stained a yellow ocher which resisted soap, scrubbing, or solvents. She had tried everything to remove the evidence of her addiction; nothing worked. Her teeth were stained a brown and dirty color which only worsened in the presence of plaque and refused even the cooperation of the dentist's polish and cleaning. Occasionally she would discover an ash burn here, a discoloration there upon a new sweater, a favorite skirt, or a white blouse. But such destruction and outward evidence of this dangerous practice were so rare and infrequent as to minimize their importance and meaning. The evidence of her addiction only occasionally achieved visibility. Because the habit brought her far more pleasure than pain, far more satisfaction than inconvenience, and altogether far more joy than misery, Erma could not bear to give up what had simply become part of her life.

After all, what would she do if she did not smoke? It was relaxing, and what would she do with her hands if not hold a cigarette? It was something to do, and how could she read or sew without a cigarette? It was a reassurance when she was worried or ill, and what pleasure would she have at such times without a cigarette? You see, a cigarette is more than simply a roll of tobacco which burns when lighted and smokes when inhaled. People who think of cigarettes in such terms have simply never smoked. No, a cigarette is . . . well, it is . . . a sort of . . . a kind of . . . friend. Yes, that's it exactly: a cigarette is a friend, a companion, and even an ally in times of sorrow and in times of joy.

When she had her first baby and labored in pain and sorrowful joy, her cigarettes were there to comfort her. When she fought with her husband, argued about finances, and wondered whether he was unfaithful to their marriage bed, her cigarettes were there to see her through the night. When her body ached with pain, her brow sweated with fever, and her very mortality shuddered at the prospect of death, her cigarettes were there once again. It was impossible for her to imagine the highs and lows of life unaided by her cigarettes.

Does this seem strange or perhaps excessive? If so, then you have never been in the grips of an addiction and therefore do not know its uncanny and tremendous power. Lucky you! An addiction is a silent, secret longing which craves insatiably for satisfaction and yet never once achieves it. It is a desire, a lust which devours with voracious greed the object of its longing, only to be further inflamed and eroticized by it. Accordingly, the more it gets the more it wants, the more it desires the less can satisfy it. Far more powerful than sexuality, this eroticism never even reaches a temporary orgasm of satisfaction but continues to swell with its own excesses until it destroys itself. It is a maddening and altogether bewitched vicious cycle in which, never satisfied and never exhausted, this deranged lust finally destroys itself by a power too enormous to be self-contained. There is nothing normal, sane, natural, or organic about such addictions, for they seem to be rather the disruption and deformation of natural processes whose internal logic has turned malignant and self-devouring. One is never satisfied. One is simply never, never satisfied.

Already, the first thing in the morning while still not fully awake, you can feel a gentle tug, a half-conscious reminder of an unsatisfied urge. It is just a mild discomfort, just a slight dissatisfaction, just a sense that all is not quite right, that something important is missing. But very quickly this urge becomes a craving and the craving becomes a longing and the longing becomes an obsession which grips and controls one's thoughts to the exclusion of all else: one must have a cigarette. Now the mind begins to rehearse the ritual that leads to satisfaction. From a crisp cellophaned package, you withdraw the tightly rolled cigarette by sharply snapping the package upon one clenched fist. Already the brusque smell of fresh tobacco fills the nostrils, and one can see rich brown and ocher cut leaves tightly curled within the cylinder of crisp paper. The thin stalk of packed tobacco is pulled forth with two fingertips, and you raise the lengthened stem of cigarette to your lips. There is a slight pull as dry lips meet dry dense paper, but you withdraw the blade of cigarette for just a moment to moisten the end and then place it once again upon your hungry lips. With cupped hands to protect the flame and with your head slightly turned to angle against the wind, you strike the match and carry the quivering flame to ignite the tobacco. Now for the first time you feel your body relax, the tension and pent-up energy expelled even as you inhale the fragrant rich tobacco taste. It is sheer ambrosia! It is delicious! It is satisfaction of the most absolute and focused intensity, and nothing, absolutely nothing can even begin to compare with its wanton eroticism. It is far more satisfying than any sexual orgasm, far more intense than liquor, and far more delicious than the most exotic food. The soft tissues of your mouth ooze with moist salivation, and the tartness upon your tongue only increases as you draw the heavy, lazy, bitter-rich smoke past your lips, down your throat, and into your expanded lungs. Oh, it is good. Oh, dear God, it is so good. It is everything that satisfies, that satiates, that quenches, and it is all of these in one final instantaneous release of need, craving, and thirst.

And that is why Erma smoked. And that is why she smoked for over sixty years. And that is why she smoked in spite of the many illnesses, inconveniences, and even dangers of what she herself understood to be a dirty habit. And for her it made perfect sense to do so; and for her it was well worth all the misery, pain, and sorrow it cost her; and unless you are also a smoker you will never understand the perfect logic of such illogical addictions.

There are essentially four types of bronchogenic carcinoma, distinguished by cell type: squamous cell, oat cell, large cell, and adenocarcinoma. The most common conduit of metastasis is the bloodstream; however, squamous-cell carcinoma also spreads by lymph nodes and direct invasion of the surrounding tissues. Within those airy labyrinths of honeycombed tissue, there reside the necessary ingredients for a host of different tumor types including bronchial adenoma, chondromatous hamartoma, sarcoma, and lymphoma.

Erma had squamous-cell carcinoma of both lungs, and her symptoms started innocently enough with a cough. At times, it was such a gentle cough as to be merely a tickle in the throat, while at other times it literally bent her double into paroxysms of red-faced asphyxia. But whether kind or cruel, whether a caress of the throat or a whole convulsion of the body, that cough seized her with such ferocious intensity that it remained with her until her death. She coughed day and night; she coughed when she smoked and she coughed when she didn't; she coughed herself to sleep and coughed herself awake again. She coughed herself to death.

Erma had thought about death before; she had thought about it many times, but she had not thought about it until recently. When her mother died years ago, she had marveled to touch the soft flesh turned hard as stone, to scrutinize the sculptured brow now cold as ice, and she had trembled to kiss those frozen—but so familiar—lips a last goodbye. Death was a paralytic rigidity which locked you into the small, narrow closet of your own immovable body and therein you silently screamed in claustrophobic terror throughout eternity. Yes, she had thought of death before, and now she thought of it again. She thought of death the day she had found a lump in her breast and fearfully rolling that slender yolk round and round wondered if it also were a stone of ice which sought to freeze her into rock. It was not! The lump was nothing but a cyst, but it had caused her to think of death that day, and the thought had made her tremble with sickening fear. But for some time now she had not thought of death and even came to accept all of her headaches, stomach upsets, hemorrhoids— yes, even her hiatal hernia—and a dozen other complaints as the rantings and ravings of a body which would not die or, at least, would not die soon. Actually, Erma had almost come to disbelieve in death or at least to suspect that perhaps it disbelieved in her. None of her ailments had ever been serious, and she wondered now if any of them ever would be. That is why—well, that is one of the reasons why—she didn't worry about her bronchitis.

But now she began to think about death again and even to dream about it as lovers sometimes dream of love. Always she had thought of death as dark and sinister, but in her dream he was actually beautiful, young, and strong. She dreamed herself in a foreign land where all the people were afraid of a cruel and powerful prince who ruled their lives. She found herself falling in love with these good and gentle people and decided that she would rid them of this monster who had so terrified them. One night, very near the break of dawn, she positioned herself close to the place where she knew he would be passing by. From the darkened rocks wherein she hid, she planned to leap unexpectedly and stab him with her knife. And so he came and so she leaped. And indeed, he was terrible to gaze upon, for his body was filth; his face grimaced with painful, bitter hate, and about him—upon him and everywhere within him—there was an oily, blackened slick which caused his body to shine. She recoiled in fear at first but sprang nonetheless, and as she did, his own hard eyes liquified with terror and fright in recognition of what she sought to do. Then suddenly—before she could strike—he opened his arms to embrace her and was in that instant transformed into shimmering light, strength, and lean, muscular power. He was so incredibly beautiful that it took her breath away just to look, and her heart felt faint, her knees weakened, and as she trembled with the glory of him . . . she awakened! For days thereafter, Erma could only remember the beautifully muscled youth who smiled to embrace her and forgot entirely the oily, darkened viper from whence the youth had sprang. Strange dream! Strange, indeed! And its strangeness was both glorious and awful, beautiful and ugly, frightful and so very reassuring to her. In any case, she could not forget death having once remembered him, and so, yes, she thought frequently of death these days.

She could not remember a time when she did not have bronchitis. Wheezing, tightened, suffocating, and burning bronchitis that awoke her in the night with the awful noise of her labored breathing and musically intonated her speech throughout the day. In fact, it seemed that she had always had it, and so it seemed to her friends, who could no longer distinguish the dry rustle of her words from the bronchial constrictions that informed them. Her bronchitis had been so long with her that she no longer would know herself without it. She had always had colds, and her colds had always developed into bronchitis. It was simply an old and familiar illness, and since she had also learned to treat herself, it was neither a very frightening nor a very disturbing one. Certainly, she was not afraid of it, for she knew full well, after all these years, its powers, and she knew what it could and couldn't do. It couldn't kill her, but it could make her uncomfortable. And so a vaporizer had sat upon her bedstand for years; she kept tissues, cough drops, and bronchial sprays nearby; and she bought—even with some enthusiasm—the newest medicines as they appeared upon the market shelves. Naturally, nothing really helped—she had never thought that anything would—except orange juice, a lot of rest, and staying away from chills. It was chills that had to be watched in particular, and she never went out in the winter without her heavy coat and boots. But sometimes even that was not enough, and then she had to treat herself at home. But over the years she had become quite skilled at knowing what to do to make herself feel better, and therefore she was not afraid of her bronchitis; it was not a friend but neither was it an enemy.

She did not stop smoking, nor—while battling the bronchitis—did she even lessen the amount that she smoked. When the thick, pungent smoke of her regular brand became too irritating, Erma simply switched to mentholated cigarettes. The slow rise of camphor and peppermint oils throughout her lungs always seemed medicinal and restorative to the dull, raw ache of inflammation. And yet it is the clever curse of every addiction that its pain hides behind its pleasure and so springs upon us when least expected. Erma was so anesthetized by pleasure that she therefore could not feel the dull, hard ache of pain.

IV

Early in 1978 Erma knew that she was ill; she was definitely, desperately, profoundly, and gravely ill. At first she tried to hide from herself the malevolent truth of her constant coughing, aching lungs, bone-weary exhaustion, and bloody expectorate. It was just a bad cold, but it would pass. It was bronchitis again, but it would pass as it always had. Well, perhaps this time she had a touch of pleurisy or even pneumonia, but it would pass. But Erma knew; she knew full well. And her diary—her secret friend—told the truth by showing how much she really did know:

> Got the report on my X ray. The doctor says there is still congestion and wants me to see a lung specialist. I wish I could just go to sleep tonight and not wake up in the morning. No sense in living when one doesn't amount to anything any more.

But sleep she could not, for there was the problem of Robert. Could he survive without her? In fact, had she not accepted responsibility for his well-being by accepting the role of matriarch?

For every crisis in the past she always had an answer. If her opponent was a person, then she worked her manipulative intrigue until the enemy was domesticated. If her goal was a possession to be won, a force to be resisted, or a danger to be avoided, then Erma would plot and plan until her will triumphed. But this enemy was herself! It was her very own body that now stood in open defiance and opposition to itself. Such an enemy cannot be destroyed; it must rather be tricked into healing itself instead of devouring itself, into repairing rather than destroying, into living rather than dying. And Erma was convinced that she had found the answer to this crisis: cataracts.

Yes, cataracts! She could not fight if she could not see! And she had not been able to see for some time because of these scalding, scaling, oily, and blinding cataracts which continually occluded the lenses of her eyes. Perhaps . . . just perhaps . . . there was a connection between the two! After all had not her lungs decayed in perfect and equal symmetry with her eyes! And, moreover, had not each diminished and increased, recovered and demised with the other? Of course, the whole logic of the syllogism was entirely misguided and faulty. It was the reasoning of shamans, magicians, children, soothsayers, mystics, and fools, but perhaps . . . just perhaps . . . it was also true. Who can say? In any case, it was a hope; it was some hope, a slender—infinitely thin—hope which offered itself in desperation to a very desperate person. She took that hope;

she took it in secret without telling anyone and buried it deep within her bosom. And therefore having made her plans, she now recognized her enemy, discerned his weakness, and sought to destroy him.

A cataract is a degeneration of the eye's lens in which the transparent yields to the translucent and finally becomes the opaque. The term itself comes from the Greek word *kataraktēs*, which means a rushing down or downward flow as in a waterfall's downpour. It is a beautiful word and well describes the blearing, rubberized flow of gelatinously failed vision. One sees, but one sees as if the eye were smeared with Vaseline, oil, or grease. Certainly there are many reasons for its occurrence—disease, trauma, X rays, old age—but Erma's patient records would simply note "senile degeneration." That is no doubt the true cause, but it could not have mattered less to Erma. She cared nothing for causes; she was only interested in cures, and cured of this affliction she must be if she was also to be cured of her lung cancer.

Treatment, her doctor informed her, consisted of either lens extraction or emulsification followed by irrigation and aspiration of the lens substance. During the postoperative period, he continued, there will be correction therapy which may include cataract spectacles, contact lenses, or even intraoperative implantation of an introcular prosthetic lens. Erma didn't give a damn. And she didn't care about the details; she simply wanted to see again by whatever means. For her, it was a matter of life and death. The pain in her lung grew worse each day, and she felt more exhausted after a night's sleep than before she went to bed. Something had to be done quickly.

Her operation took place on October 1, 1979; it was her seventy-sixth birthday. This was only a coincidence of scheduling, but Erma symbolized such accidents as omens and felt reassured that her decision had been well advised. It had not been a decision advised by anyone other than herself. Her doctor had advised against it, and so had her husband, her son, most of her friends, and all of her relatives down to the very last niece, nephew, and distant cousin. As usual, Erma listened to them all, ignored their advice completely, and then did things her own way. On the morning of the operation she was anxious but excited—this is often the case when one begins a new journey—and by evening she was only in mild discomfort and happy that the ordeal was over. Now the waiting would begin. As soon as the tender ocular tissue healed and the swelling subsided, she could be given her new glasses. Then she could see. And then the real fight would begin. And then she would heal herself. Erma was certain that it would happen in just this way for that is just the way in which she planned it.

By the end of October, however, the squamous-cell carcinoma—which had for months slumbered in quiet vegetation within her lung—now grew discontent and restless. Perhaps it smelled the anesthesia, discerned that repairs were being made, and became afraid. Perhaps not. Perhaps it had rested all it needed, or perhaps there was no reason at all for its arousal. In any case, it now began exploring, probing, searching, and establishing new sites, new satellites and way stations within her breasts, her bones, her brains, within the very substance and core of her. Indeed, the metastases went wild with their ranting, raving roamings, and simply conquering a new locale did not seem to satiate their inflamed and ravenous hunger for healthy tissue. Geometrically they grew—in direct proportion to their invasive powers—by mathematically squaring and resquaring conquered tissue areas until the squamous carcinoma logarithmically established a military network of battlefronts, bulwarks, ramparts, and flanks of tumorized tissue. And as the enemy forced Erma into greater and greater withdrawals, into greater and greater retreats, so also did she lose more and more territory, and in so doing she finally lost that slender thread of hope whose gentle grasp separates our lives from our deaths.

There were endless delays with the prescriptive lenses. First, the wrong prescription was sent to the laboratory and therefore the wrong lenses were returned. The prescription was found and corrected, and then it was temporarily lost again and then found again and then delayed and then finally completed. Was it inconsideration or incompetence or both that so ruled this lazy, languid opthalmologist who seemed to squander his time daily even as a silly schoolgirl postpones her chores with excuse after excuse? Did he not see? Did none of them see (doctors, family, nurses) the urgency of her situation? It was not a question of glasses but of life. Erma was in a desperate minute-by-minute fight for her existence, and the urgency of the situation was precisely that she could not live if she could not see. Those glasses were her lifeline, her salvation, and every moment mattered. But they did not understand and instead reassured her, placated and excused her anxiety with empty words, clichés, and meaningless gestures of comfort. They did not believe as she believed. And why, after all, should they, for they were living and she was dying.

Doctors, nurses, technicians, family, friends, and visitors are like tourists who pass through a country without ever becoming a part of its culture. Since they cannot speak this language of pain or eat this food of suffering or participate in these rituals of death, they therefore must always remain strangers. The surgeons and oncologists among them have watched these troubled waters many times before, but they have never had to swim in them. Husbands and wives, lovers and friends are frightened by this barren countryside of wasted tissue, open sores, dry, snoring, whiskered faces bleached white by internal metabolic furnaces, and balding, bruised bodies still smoking from fires that burn within. Neither do these tourists care to tarry along the way, for they are terrified by spectacles, visions, and happenings too shocking to recount and too terrible to recall. Rather, they wish to hurry back to their sunlit world of strong bodies, painless pleasures, and trivialities that have nothing to do with death. They are tourists, strangers, and foreigners who have been so insensitized, numbed, and anesthetized by their good health that they cannot feel the ache of death as only the diseased and dying do. And therefore as often as Erma sought to explain what it meant to die, these alien spirits of the healthy remained confused and dumbfounded by the serious urgency of death.

Erma Katherine Denbrook was no longer one of them. She was no longer a middle-class suburban housewife living among bright sunny mornings, coffee cups, bridge clubs, afternoon soap operas, evening knitting by the fireside, and good, hot, home-cooked meals. No! She was an animal—a terribly wounded and desperately ill animal—fighting for its survival.

Her world was not of theirs and no longer consisted of wicker chairs set in summer's evening dusk, of tall refreshing glasses of iced tea, of birthday presents and Christmas bells, of cool bodies seeking the hot lust of one another's loins, of shopping trips, bus tours, and country fairs, of new dresses, fresh Sunday hats perched smartly upon fashionable heads during church services, of pen pals, thank-you notes, of anniversaries, of baptisms and dinner invitations, of hot baths, clean shampooed hair, and finely talcumed bodies. No! Her world had been transformed from all of that to sweat, fever, oily brows, and aching joints; of burning lungs and thickened throats so dense with dying tissue that swallowing was impossible; of blurred vision and twisted eyes that could not straighten within their sockets; of not being able to feed yourself, relieve yourself, comb your hair, do your nails, clear your throat, or—yes, dear God—simply throw your head back and laugh effortlessly at a funny story. Transformed by her disease into an animal, she was now beyond all of that and sought only to survive. Cunning, clever, sneaky, angry, crazed, and maddened by her intense pain, she would tear, scratch, claw, and bite her way to freedom at any cost. Even as rodents devour their own limbs in exchange for freedom from leg traps, so also did Erma scorn her own flesh to bargain for such release. The tourists—doctors, nurses, technicians, friends, and family—could not possibly understand the terror of being imprisoned by a dying body. After all, they lived in a world of pleasure whereas she was in a world of pain; they were in a world of health whereas she was in a world of sickness; they were in a world of strong bodies whereas she was in the rotting prison of flesh that she had become.

Sickness—not simply mild, inconvenient illness but terrible and desperate sickness—is a suffocation unto death. Certainly it is also pain, agony, and weakness, but first and foremost one feels a claustrophobia which closes in while closing down all the essential routes of communication and openness. Before, when one was healthy, the brilliance of the world was simply too splendid and seductive to resist, and its myriad colors, melodious tones, outrageous spectacles, subtle nuances could not be ignored. Each morning upon opening one's eyes the world suddenly phosphoresced with astonishing textures and glowed incandescent with sights and sounds that could not be silenced. Immersed in the world and therefore over-whelmed by it, one was simply a natural extension of all this blazing substance whose boundaries included all that one was or saw or felt or touched or smelled or could ever be. But now all of that has changed, for those intense saturations of color have bleached to pastels, those harmonious melodies have turned to ragged noises that disturb rather than reassure, those sweet smells of summer violets and fresh breezes are now re-placed with rotting flesh, blood, pus, and antiseptics. All that is internal and inward becomes more real and substantive than the external and outward. The antennae, registers, and recep-tive curvatures of the body—formerly so delicately attuned to rhythms and vibrations not of their own pitch and meter—are now dull, unresponsive, and fallen mute. It is pain that has created this confusion, for pain has closed the circumferences and boundaries of the body, and now the inner clangs and clat-ter of disease rebound so intensely that nothing else can be heard or seen or smelled or touched save the agony of the dis-ease itself. One is reduced to an air balloon that seeks elevation and cannot find it without discarding all that is nonessential. Sandbags and people, ballasts and memories, maps, diagrams, geographic charts, and feelings, hopes, and beliefs must all be thrown overboard in order to gain sufficient elevation. Such sickness demands that we sacrifice the earth for air else we cannot distinguish ourselves from dust. So it was with Erma, and so also was it that only she could fully understand how absolute, how desperate, how final it really was with her.

By the middle of November she had lost all hope of recov-ery. Daily she was locked within the silent vault of her diseased and rapidly disintegrating body; she would lie for hours listen-ing to the transport of fluids, the erosion of tissues, arteries, vessels, veins, and cells while the ever descending veil of ex-haustion slowly closed in upon her. In dreams of wakened de-lirium, she saw herself crouched and huddled in the corner of a burning house as the violent flames furiously opened door after door in angry search of her fragile and delicate soul. Would those flames devour her with their teeth of flaming steel? Erma was not religious, but she had prayed. She had prayed to someone; she had prayed to anyone; finally, she had prayed to everyone—to saints and sinners alike—in the hope that she would be saved. She had prayed, and it had not worked. She never thought that it would work—and perhaps that was precisely why it had not—but now she was bitter. God had tricked her. She had bargained and promised, confessed and cajoled, repented and recanted, and for a time believed that she was winning. But it wasn't so, for she had been losing all along. God was unfair, unjust, unforgiving, and therefore unforgivable.

Sometimes while lying in her hospital bed, while drowning in her own fluids and listening to the systematic dismantling of her own body, she thought of springtime, of when she was a girl, of laughter and boyfriends and ice-cream sundaes. She had been lovely when she was a girl, with large almond eyes and delicate bronzed hair filled with rust and gold and chestnut. Her lips were petulant but full and succulent as rose petals. Certainly, she had never wanted for boyfriends. But each of her suitors—they were today doctors, lawyers, and manufacturers—had been dismissed as "not good enough for my little girl" by her jealous father. Only Robert—only Robert among them all—had been the one exception. She thought of ledger sheets, debit and credit columns, and the joys of being a single woman with a good job and . . . and . . . with freedom. It would be so wonderful to be free again, to be free to breathe, to no longer be suffocated by cancer, by Robert, by life! Had there ever been such a time when her lungs were not being collapsed by some force that she could not control? If so, she could not remember it. She thought of her dolls from childhood, of her diary from adolescence, and also of her son. Did he understand what she had suffered for his survival? Did he remember all of the love, care, watchfulness, and maternal jealousy with which she had guarded his young, fragile life? With silent, immobile, brooding meditation, she pondered such things.

When Thanksgiving arrived—and her cataract prescription still had not—she simply turned inward. The curtain fell, the veil descended, and Erma withdrew. She would not talk; she would not even acknowledge the presence of others. She had failed; the battle was lost; she was reconciled to death. Robert came each day with pleadings, excuses, encouragements, reassurances, and complaints. It didn't matter; it was too late. Her son was caught up in the fabric and web of his own involvements. He tried to make recompense, to apologize, to excuse himself. It didn't matter; it was too late. Her friends came with their healthy, contented lives to offer words of solace and consolation. It didn't matter; it was too late.

On December 5—it was a late Wednesday afternoon—the prescription lenses finally arrived. As if they were a precious treasure, offered in supplication and respect, so were they presented to her. Curiously, tentatively, she took the plastic omen in her hands; she thought richly of all they had promised and of the power therein contained; slowly she raised them to her scarred and muddy eyes and then flung them aside with a finalized gesture of disgust. It was too late; it was simply too late. She turned now—drawn by an internal cosmic gravity—upon the inner axis of herself and fell quite naturally, quite effortlessly forward into moonlight, dreams, and memories of fifty years ago.

Down, down—spiraling ever down into deeper and darker recesses—gentle, fragile Erma falls. Far in the distance, she hears the clanging, brittle sounds of hardened reality beckoning her return. But within these greater depths there is a soft, dense, porous cushion which seems so much more substantial than reality itself. She turns inward upon the pivot and axis of her own thoughts to dream, to float, to see more intensely than she has ever seen before. The visions here are accessible only to visionaries who can bear such intense dimensions and colorations with their saturated hues of cobalt blue, ocher yellow, reds and lavenders, emerald greens and delicate pastels that vibrate and entwine with one another in symphonic resonance. Here too are currents, flows, pressures, and eddies of immeasurable force that seem to pull and draw with gentle persuasion her aching body along their corridors. And as they flow, so also do they seem to cleanse and refresh; Erma follows the fluid avenues of light and sound with an innocent trust that all will be right. For everything here is richer, stronger, denser, and far more saturated than what she left behind. Even if she wished to return she could not, for the effort would be too exhausting, too demanding for the slender energy she commands.

Suddenly there—over there—isn't that a doorway slowly opening? She turns and hesitates . . . turns and hesitates again . . . and looks behind to see what she has left. She hears the pounding of her strained, arrhythmic heart; she feels the labored efforts of her lungs to pull clean, fresh air through the thickened green pus that surrounds her; she sees the wrinkled pale visage of herself as through a glass darkly; and she turns toward the open door. Should she walk through? It seems a benevolent, peaceful, and even tranquil entrance, and she yearns to decide, she aches to touch the doorway and to look beyond to the other side. But dare she? Should she? May she? . . . She does.

Fast approaching now the threshold—even faster than she imagined possible—it seems so easy, so natural, so right to simply walk through. But just as she is about to do so, the door is suddenly flung wide open and there appears the startling vision of a smooth muscled youth whose face is all phosphorescent with joy, exhilaration, happiness, and utter, absolute gentle benevolence. She knows him instantly, for he is the youth of her dream. And he smiles. He is the transformed vulture whose oiled wings flamed into smooth, lean muscles; whose beak whitened into straight, narrow teeth; whose blackened feathers became soft, supple skin; whose terrible, frightful terror became a gentle, gracious benediction. And he smiled. And he is smiling now as his smooth, warm body touches hers, and she feels herself ignite with the sparks of energy that are his even as they now becomes hers, and she knows that this is right. She knows now that this is how it is supposed to be. She knows that it could never have been any other way. And she knows that she is happy, truly happy for the first time, and all because he smiled. She walks through the open door and somewhere in the distance another door closes.

It is 11:23 on Thursday morning, December 6, 1979. From her bedside, all that can be seen are the eyes that turn but once in their sockets and then fall still. Her left hand—clasped round the finger by a wedding ring—clutches with a shudder the metal bars of the hospital bed; her nostrils constrict and then infinitely, eternally dilate forever. But what cannot be seen from the bedside—indeed, what is not visible from any vantage point within the room—is Erma transformed. Her gray hair darkens, her parched skin moistens, her muddy, scaled eyes clear, her youth renews itself in a single but splendid, simple but elegant rebound of energy.

When Robert learned that she had died, he was not quite sure what he felt. Was he alone, deserted, abandoned? Or was he victorious, triumphant, and finally reconciled? Slowly and with great anticipation of the moment to come, he dialed the son's phone number. The cleaning lady answered—how had he managed to afford a cleaning lady when Robert never could?—and for a moment he knew not what to do.

"No," she said, "he's not in now. Can I leave a message?"

Robert hesitated—to relish the purity of the moment—and then struck. "Yes, tell him that his mother died today."

IV

Diseases of Life

Folly and error, avarice and vice,
Employ our souls and waste our bodies' force.
As mangy beggars incubate their lice,
We nourish our innocuous remorse.

Our sins are stubborn, craven our repentance.
For our weak vows we ask excessive prices.
Trusting our tears will wash away the sentence,
We sneak off where the muddy road entices.

Cradled in evil, that Thrice-Great Magician,
The Devil, rocks our souls, that can't resist;
And the rich metal of our own volition
Is vaporized by that sage alchemist.

The Devil pulls the strings by which we're worked:
By all revolting objects lured, we slink
Hellwards; each day down one more step we're
      jerked
Feeling no horror, through the shades that stink.

Just as a lustful pauper bites and kisses
The scarred and shrivelled breast of an old whore,
We steal, along the roadside, furtive blisses,
Squeezing them like stale oranges for more.

Packed tight, like hives of maggots, thickly
  seething,
Within our brains a host of demons surges.
Deep down into our lungs at every breathing,
Death flows as, an unseen river, moaning dirges.

Charles Baudelaire
"To the Reader"

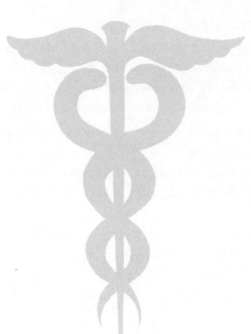

12

A Cup of Bitterness

Well, then another minute yet.
Again and again they manage to cut my rope.
Recently I was so well prepared,
and there was already a little eternity in my
        entrails.

They hold out the spoon to me,
that spoonful of life.
No, I don't want, I don't want any more,
only let me vomit.

I know life is well-done and good,
and the world is a full pot,
but with me it doesn't get into my blood,
it only mounts to my head.

Others it nourishes, me it makes sick;
you understand one spurns it.
For at least a thousand years now
I shall need to diet.

Rainer Maria Rilke
"The Song of the Suicide"

SUICIDE: Suicide is a psychological and social problem of great magnitude. It ranks tenth as a cause of death in this country, with about 20,000 taking their own lives each year. Over 200,000 people, however, make suicidal attempts, although some of these are believed to be gestures designed to elicit attention, control others, or express hostility.

Studies show that the largest number of attempts are made during the spring, and in the morning at the beginning of the week. Firearms account for about half of the deaths and hanging, sleeping pills, gas (including car exhausts), jumping, poison, drowning, and cutting arteries account for the rest, in that order. The incident is three times as high in men as in women, but women make more unsuccessful attempts. More than half the victims are over forty-five, with the rate among men increasing until old age, and among women increasing through fifty and then declining. The highest rates are among the divorced, the widowed, and the single, in that order; about 25 percent live alone. Although all occupations are represented, the highest percentages are on the professional level, especially among lawyers, dentists, and physicians.

Studies of the dynamics of suicide show that occasional cases are motivated by revenge, spite, or the desire to make others feel guilty. Sometimes these attempts are only halfhearted but succeed by accident, as when a person cuts his wrists and dies before he can be rescued. More frequently the act is motivated by a personal burden which the individual cannot bear: loss of a loved one, physical pain or disability, social or occupational failure, financial reverses, loneliness, or boredom. One of the reasons social, vocational, and financial failures precipitate suicide is that many people cannot endure loss of status and self-esteem.

In mental illness the motivation for suicide is believed to stem from unconscious levels of the personality. Two factors are most deeply implicated, and are frequently found together. First, the patient may become overwhelmed with feelings of guilt out of all relation to reality. These feelings may be a gross exaggeration of a trivial lapse, or take the form of a frank delusion. He may then try to do away with himself because he feels he is unworthy to live. Second, he may develop intense, overpowering feelings of hostility which "turn inward" and lead to self-destructiveness.

Robert M. Goldenson
The Encyclopedia of Human Behavior

I

If you had called 3471 in 1938, a thin but highly resonant voice would have answered: "Good afternoon, Schindler's Drugstore."

The voice would belong to the owner himself, and you would not easily mistake the nasal tones of that most resonant voice for any other. Had you occasion or need later on that afternoon to stop by the drugstore for a prescription and a chocolate sundae, the owner himself would service both of your purchases. For Henry Schindler was both proprietor and sales staff of that small but very well equipped country drugstore. Upon your arrival that afternoon, there would be gathered the usual clientele who frequent such places on lazy afternoons throughout the small towns of the Midwest. Near the front of the store, lined up in a regular row like bowling pins, would be the raucous high schoolers seeking delay upon delay at the soda bar in order to postpone the chores awaiting them at home. At the prescription counter would be Mrs. Henderson, Alice Marquette, or perhaps Elmer Clark, hoping to find some immediate cure of their chronic pains upon the shelves of ointments, salves, capsules, and pills. Finally, near the magazine rack would be the coarse, toughened young farm boys leisurely leafing through the girlie magazines in search of brief but intense moments of sensual eroticism.

Henry Schindler was a most unlikely centerpiece in the midst of this bizarre dinner party. Certainly, one look at him was sufficient to ascertain that he would not be in sympathy with any of his clients' reasons for visiting the drugstore that sunny afternoon. Clearly, pharmacist Schindler did not partake of chocolate sundaes; moreover, it was known that he had long been a firm believer in holistic medicine and had never so much as taken an aspirin for a headache. Finally, one cannot imagine—indeed, the very thought sends a chill up the spine—that Henry Schindler would ever drool over a girlie magazine as those young fellows to the right of the prescription counter were now doing.

No! Henry Schindler was . . . well . . . he was proper. Yes, that's the right word: he was proper and he was dignified. A dapper, thin little man, he was remarkable only for the bow ties that were his constant and singular adornment. His suits were either dark brown or plain navy, and he wore no jewelry. Neither wedding ring (though he had been married for over twenty-seven years) nor watch (although he rented the upstairs of the drugstore to a jeweler) was ever seen to adorn finger or wrist. But these ties—these remarkable, incredible bow ties— were simply astonishing. Perhaps it was a perverse kind of vanity which promoted such asceticism, or perhaps he simply preferred the bow tie center stage where the limelight could not refract off ring, watch, or clasp. For whatever reasons, all else was blackened in the theater, so to speak, in order that the bow tie might shine out with its own internal incandescence.

Except for this slight eccentricity, Henry Schindler was a most ordinary and unremarkable man. There was nothing exceptional about that patrician-shaped head or the fine and thinning hair that adorned it. There was nothing exceptional about the well-manicured hands, save they were so delicate as almost to be feminine. There was nothing exceptional either about the dapper, pencil-thin mustache that Henry daily trimmed and waxed. No, Henry Schindler was like the most regular of regular verbs, and had he been a nation rather than a person, Baedeker would have summed him up in a single line: "There is nothing here to detain the traveler."

But Henry Schindler was not a nation or a thing but a man, and a very complex one indeed. For on the inner surface of this outwardly calm exterior, there brewed storms, disasters, and hurricanes of unspeakable monstrosity. The mustache, so neatly trimmed, the well-groomed and finely chiseled head, the fragile, delicate fingertips had not the courage to proclaim what only the bow tie could silently confess.

II

Henry did not share his problems—his worries, fears, anxieties—with others, and most especially he did not share these with Beatrice, his wife of twenty-seven years. It was unmasculine, so he thought, but also he was a most private and solitary person for whom conversation and confession resolved nothing of life's troubles. As an only child, he had learned to suffer alone, in silence, and now he turned inward at the first sign of danger or disorder in the world. What had started as enforced solitude soon became a comfortable life-style, and so Henry Schindler did not complain and did not explain. Rather, he suffered until the pain was unbearable or the problem was solved.

Despite Henry's inward resolve, Beatrice knew—as only a wife can know—that grave and malevolent forces were assembling themselves for warfare within him. She suspected that Henry was in deep, even very desperate financial trouble. But she said nothing. After twenty-seven years a good wife develops a certain wisdom about these matters—about where and when to confront an issue—and Beatrice simply had not found the time to yet be ripe. Having nothing yet to say, she therefore said nothing, and her silence was so deafening that even Henry occasionally heard its piercing density. And yet she did worry. She did grieve—for, oh, how she loved this gentle man—and she did inwardly ache over his deep distractions, his unpredictable moods, and his vacant stares. The passionate side of their lives had long since turned from lust to companionship, and this was compatible and comfortable for both of them. But recently, within the past few weeks, Henry had sought to rekindle the fires of youth as if thereby he might through sexual energy resist the demons that now sought to consume him. It had been a failure, of course, and worst yet a failure which only further humiliated and degraded Henry's own critical estimation of himself. Potency and power, impotence and weakness are divisions without apparent diameters, and the decision to achieve one over the other is not a matter of will but of spirit. And Henry Schindler was surely, at this time and at this point in his life, a spiritually broken and crippled man. It was therefore this most recent failure in particular which alerted Beatrice's instincts and transformed her worry into terror, her apprehension into a chilling and frightful certainty that Henry would not survive this latest confrontation with himself. That spiritual transition from a chronic to a critical phase had been so subtle that only Beatrice, with her microscopic vision, could discern that something had died that could not be reborn. And, as usual, she was right.

III

Friday evening, October 12, the Schindlers had been invited out to play bridge with another couple. They were not close to these people—but then they were not close with anyone—and yet Henry had seemed especially interested in accepting the invitation. Frank and Thelma McAdams were about the same age as the Schindlers, in their mid-forties, and a couple who shared the same basic values. Frank was a veterinarian with a practice limited to large animals such as cattle, horses, sheep, and general farm livestock. Rarely, except as a personal favor to someone, did he treat domestic pets such as cats, dogs, or parakeets. No, Frank regarded himself as a professional veterinarian and not a sort of "jack-of-all trades" vet who tried to treat every turtle, goldfish, and frog that became the pet of some child. "Children's veterinarian" was the disrespectful way he referred to his colleagues who had chosen this easy kind of medicine. No, to be a professional veterinarian—a veterinarian like Frank McAdams was—you had to be tough. In this specialty it was not a question of simply saving animals but a matter of business, cost efficiency, and general farm economics. "Not every animal that can be saved should be saved," Frank was fond of saying. "Can the animal repay in profits its own medical bills? Does the animal's recovery belong in the debit or the credit column of the ledger sheet?"

Frank was proud that he had long ago resolved these problems for himself, and he did not respect others who had difficulty in so doing. He was not at all sure what he thought about Henry. He was a druggist, a chemist, and so he should be tough; he should have a no-nonsense attitude about him. But did he? Frank could not be sure. There seemed to be something fragile, something delicate or weak about the fellow that was disturbing to a man like Frank McAdams. "Those damned fingernails," he thought, "almost look manicured."

Beatrice, nonetheless, was having an altogether pleasant evening. She had known Thelma since high school days and liked her a great deal. She did not know quite how she felt about Frank, but that didn't matter for the moment. Also, Thelma had found the cutest scorecards down at Brenneman's; Beatrice intended to buy a few packages for herself tomorrow morning when she went shopping. Also—and this was the important thing, wasn't it?—Henry seemed relaxed and more at ease than he had for weeks. Finally, the cards were good. They were very good that evening.

Well, there was one unpleasant moment, but Beatrice had come to accept such occurrences as the natural consequence of spending an evening with the McAdamses. Naturally, it had to do with another one of Frank's unpleasant stories, and there was always—whenever the four of them got together—at least one such unpleasant story. Really, Beatrice could not imagine why Frank found it necessary to talk about such things, and she knew that he probably embarrassed Thelma no end. The stories were always coarse, frequently cruel, and sometimes just plain disgusting. Secretly, Beatrice suspected that Frank told them on purpose just in order to contrast his own masculinity with Henry's more delicate constitution. And yet, Henry always seemed fascinated by these stories and especially so this evening as Frank told his tale with the usual great relish and personal satisfaction.

The day before yesterday Frank had been called to the Nussbaum farm out on county route 214 to treat a cow with gastric torsion, or—in everyday terms—simple bloat. A large animal's stomach which hangs suspended by mesenteries, such as a cow's, sometimes will accumulate enough internal gas to float and then flip upon its axis, thereby strangulating the pyloric valve. The stomach now becomes a self-contained balloon which rapidly inflates until it produces ischemia in liver and spleen. The animal may die of shock within minutes unless the intraruminal pressure is quickly relieved. The precise treatment, of course, depends upon the animal. With dogs, such as a Great Dane, the condition is often fatal, and therefore a laparotomy may be the only effective treatment. Bloat in ruminants, like cattle, however, is more easily treated by simply counting down the rib cage to the appropriate gastric area and then inserting a catheter or hypodermic needle to release the gas. A steak knife—if nothing else is available—will also do. Frank had found a long screwdriver in his truck and simply drove the instrument in all the way up to the handle. The animal had screamed like hell, of course, but it was back to normal by that evening. "These farm animals," Frank smacked his lips in admiration, "are tough."

It seemed to Beatrice—Henry was busy inspecting his cards—that Frank had definitely winked at her as he slowly enunciated the word "tough." But Frank's next story—and actually the motivation for telling the first—was, to Beatrice's mind, definitely disturbing. In fact, it was more than disturbing; it was disturbed, cruel, and sadistic. And yet, while she found the tale to be grotesque, Henry seemed fascinated—if not strangely hypnotized—by its details.

An hour or so before Frank arrived at the Nussbaum farm that afternoon, a neighborhood dog had been found in the chicken coop where already he had killed and eaten two prize-winning hens. He was caught after a lengthy chase by the Nussbaum boys, who were big, rugged lads with deep florid faces and hair the color of burnt rust. Henry knew both of the boys quite well since they frequently invaded the quiet drugstore on Saturday afternoons to look at the girlie magazines. Henry knew as well that they routinely stole a copy or two of those issues featuring especially large-breasted women. Naturally, he had never said anything to either of the boys. It would have been far too embarrassing and also, he suspected, perhaps too dangerous.

"Well, now the Nussbaum boys"—Frank was obviously anticipating his own story with great eagerness—"grabbed this dog and tied it up with rope like a hog. Then Earl"—half turning in his chair to Henry, he said—"you know Earl, the big one that's supposed to be hung like a horse?"

"Yes," Henry softly answered with his head lowered, but with a strange luminiferous glow to his eyes as if in admiration of the cruel but erotic energy of the young farmhands.

"Well, Earl just ups and grabs an old jar of carbolic acid they had there on the shelf and poured the whole quart down the damned dog's throat."

Henry shuddered—but with a strange excitement—for as a pharmacist, he knew full well the ulcerating, greedy, devouring effects of that malevolent acid. If one was unlucky enough to get even a single drop upon the fingertip, it would burn like a white-hot coal to the very center of the finger's gentle tissues.

Dear God, carbolic acid was unmerciful; it devoured with graceless greed everything in its path, hair, flesh, bone, muscle, until exhausted and diluted by its orgy of eating, it finally came to rest in the center of the destruction it had produced.

"Well, sir, that damned dog"—Henry was awakened from his reflections by the wet smack of Frank's lips—"broke all four of its legs trying to get out of those ropes. The boys said its eyes started rolling in their sockets while that acid melted its teeth like they were peppermint drops. Hell, I guess you could see that old carbolic traveling down its throat because it tore everything out like a crowbar."

"Oh, dear God, Frank," Beatrice interrupted, "that's enough. Please stop." She had turned quite pale.

But Henry was fascinated and wanted to hear more. "Well, what happened when you got there, Frank?" he asked.

"Well, when I arrived, the dog was still alive and that was about two hours after the boys had given him the cocktail." Frank was amused by his own wit. "The mouth, lips, throat, chest were all gone. Just a big hole there. But that son-of-a-gun was still breathing. I think it was dead by the time I left, though. Isn't that a hell of a way to go?" smiled Frank.

"It sure is, it sure is," Henry whispered as to himself.

But Beatrice saw fire—definite fire—in his eyes.

Later that evening in bed, Henry was like a teenager first discovering sex. "Maybe he thinks he's one of the Nussbaum boys," she thought sarcastically. But she indulged him and suffered the humiliation of being made love "to" instead of making love "with" him. Quite simply, Beatrice adored him! And also . . . also . . . she understood. She understood that his hunger was not erotic but a frenzied fire within the caldron of his own dissatisfaction. He was a metabolic furnace devouring himself and in danger of explosion unless a relief valve was somewhere opened within him. And she sought desperately to find that valve—for, dear God, she did so love this gentle and timid man—to release whatever poisons so consumed him; and yet, she knew neither where to begin her search nor where to end it. And in the morning, at first, he did seem calmer but not thereby less tense. "Exhausted" is a better word. Henry seemed exhausted even as an epileptic is exhausted after a grand mal seizure.

IV

Henry was to meet with the bankers that afternoon at 3:30 to "finalize" the loan for his new drugstore. "Finalize," that was the word he had been using all week to describe this important meeting.

But Beatrice suspected things were not all that final; in fact, she knew the loan would not be approved. Her girlfriend Mildred, who was married to one of the bank's vice presidents, had told her last week that the president of the bank himself had refused the loan. Of course, Mildred naturally assumed— who would not?—that Henry had confided all of this information to his wife long ago. He had not. And Beatrice had remained silent. This meeting at 3:30, she realized, was simply a last-ditch effort on Henry's part to have the loan reconsidered. It would not work, Mildred had said—partly in sympathy for her friend and partly to defend her husband's bank—because Henry was already overextended on his credit line and even several months behind on his present mortgage payments. Again, Henry had said nothing to her about any of this. But Beatrice knew.

Henry knew as well. He knew that he would not get the loan, and he also knew—or at least he suspected—that Beatrice had probably figured all of this out long ago. He dreaded this day; he had loathed its coming for weeks. This morning he awoke with the icy chill of anticipation that causes one to feel almost drugged and yet to tremble as well. Each chore—shaving, eating breakfast, opening up the drugstore, filling prescriptions—was simply an obstacle in the pathway of the only destination that mattered: the 3:30 appointment with the president of the First National Bank.

Frank McAdams would not have been refused the loan. They wouldn't have dared—Henry thought in admiration— refuse old Frank anything he asked. He would go in there and explain away the whole line-of-credit business and past due mortgage payments, and by 4:00 he would walk out with that loan in his back pocket. Good old Frank. He was a corker.

Why, if they tried, if they even tried to refuse Frank McAdams, he would have hauled them into court and ended up owning the whole damn bank. That's what he would have done because Frank was tough.

But Henry Schindler was not Frank McAdams, nor would he ever be. Henry was not tough; he was weak, and weak to such a degree as only he could know. Henry would not make threats; Henry would not get tough; and Henry would not sue the bank, as he himself knew. No, Henry would take his medicine; he would drink the bitter elixir to the last drop even if it killed him to do so.

The day seemed to drag on endlessly. Mrs. Beiner came in for a refill of her prescriptions. She clung like a drowning woman to these brightly colored pills in the hope that her lung cancer would be arrested. Of course it would not, and Henry ached inwardly to aid in this self-deception while having neither the courage nor the credentials to expose it. At noon one of the Nussbaum boys came in to leaf through the girlie magazines, and Elmer Hosteteler got a refill on his digitalis. Business was the best it had been all week. But was it enough? The ledger sheets were disastrous. There were cost overruns on both major and minor purchases (two dozen gross of insulin syringes; four cartons of vaporizers; six cartons overstock on distilled water) as well as cash-flow problems (down another 22 percent on cash reserves for this month alone) and clients who did not pay their bills ($8,000 in uncollectibles with over 31 percent past due for two years or more). He had often thought about turning the past-due accounts over to a collection agency. The trade magazines listed a variety of such companies, and even at 40 cents on the dollar it was better than no collection at all. At least it would be enough to resolve his cash-flow problem temporarily with perhaps a $1,000 reserve to pay one month's back mortgage. Frank McAdams would have done so long ago; Beatrice would have as well; and yes, probably young Nussbaum would have done so also. But Henry could not. He was weak; yes, he was weak. Might as well admit to oneself what others knew so well. Henry Schindler was a weak, weak man. He admitted it; he accepted it. But what else could he do? These past-due accounts—the ones which would return

40 cents on the dollar—belonged to people like the Gerbers whose little boy, Bobby, was dying of leukemia. And they belonged to Mrs. Palmer, who was a widow on Social Security bent nearly double by rheumatoid arthritis. They belonged to Ellen and Buster Kick whose farm was about to be sold out from under them; they belonged to Bud Mason who was out of work and whose wife had terminal cancer; they belonged to Eli Snyder whose diabetes had already blinded him in one eye and was now working on the other; to the Zaugg family, the crippled Swede who spoke broken English and repaired shoes; to the barber who trimmed Henry's hair and mustache for nothing; and to Mrs. Detwilder who brought him homemade preserves once a week. These accounts did not belong to Frank McAdams, to the Nussbaum boys, or to the bankers but rather to the little, gentle, sick, and fragile people of the earth. These accounts—the uncollectibles with 40 cents return upon the dollar—belonged to people with whom Henry felt the strongest kinship because . . . well, because . . . they were weak.

It was almost 1:30; in a couple of hours he would have the answer; in a couple of hours the matter would finally be settled once and for all. Frankly, Henry had no idea what he would do if the answer was no. He would be ruined; the business would simply go—as the economists liked to put it—belly-up. He was certain that Beatrice would not understand, for she expected Henry to be the provider and protector of his family. If his father were alive—thank God he was not—he would not have understood. He would have been ashamed of his son. And even Henry did not understand; he was even ashamed of himself. He was ashamed of all that he was, of all that he might have been, of all that he had become. How the hell did it happen? What had he done wrong? Why weren't things working out? He was not stupid; he was not lazy, God knows; if anything, Henry was organized, conservative, and careful. He never took chances or made wild, irresponsible investments. Why, in fact, he was the most responsible person he knew. But wait a minute. That was it. He was responsible because he was too cowardly to be irresponsible. McAdams, the Nussbaums won by not following the rules because they were not afraid to lose. Henry, on the other hand, did not have the courage to lose and that was precisely why he never won. His weakness was his curse, and it was the complete absence of such weakness in Frank and the young Nussbaums that he most admired. Frank's stories that night had excited him—yes, they had excited him terribly—precisely because of the strange combination of cruelty and sexuality of which he knew the Nussbaums were perfectly capable, and of which he knew he was not. Henry had not the courage to be cruel—not to others and not even to himself.

v

The First National Bank of Alston was a short, squat building of red brick located in the center of town. From this vantage point, with its vaults of cash negotiables and promissory notes, it surveyed its domains. And domains they were indeed, for this bank owned directly or indirectly the entire town as well as most of the surrounding farms. The president was the recently appointed Pershing J. McAllister, who had brought to this small community the modern banking practices of the city. He was a tough, no-nonsense sort of man whose first order of business was to place a service fee wherever he could. The following day a nonrefundable $10 fee on all safety deposit boxes was charged and the yearly rental fee increased by 30 percent. There were rumors—who can say if they were true?—that McAllister had asked for only two items his first day at the bank: a list of present employees and a red pencil. In any case, by day's end four tellers, one vice president, and half the secretarial staff were unemployed. Moreover, McAllister had proclaimed the following day that he would personally review all new loan applications himself.

That was six months ago, and exactly three weeks later to the day Henry Schindler had the very great misfortune of making his loan application. After two months, he was informed in a curt and formal letter that his application had been rejected for "internal audit reasons." However, the letter went on to state, he could make reapplication in two months' time. The letter was signed by Pershing J. McAllister, President and Chief Loan Officer. Henry did reapply last month and this time asked for a personal interview, rather than a letter, to learn the results. The interview had been scheduled by the bank, without the courtesy of consulting Henry's schedule, for 3:30 this afternoon.

Henry arrived promptly at 3:30, but he was kept waiting in the outer lobby until almost 4:00. There, seated with hat in hand, he greeted—he was forced to greet—passerbys who were, at one time or the other, patrons of his drugstore. Whether it was the disadvantage of being seated when others are standing or whether everyone actually knew that he was in deep financial trouble, Henry felt transparent and without any sense of inner privacy. Altogether, it was one of the most embarrassing times of his life, and in the end he felt robbed— even raped—of his dignity.

At 4:00 he was ushered into McAllister's office. The inner sanctum—or at least Henry perceived it as such—was so dimly lit that it seemed less a room and more an enclosure of unfriendly forces. McAllister sat at his desk upon which the one available light served to illuminate the papers before him while casting all else in shades of darkness and semidarkness. It seemed to Henry to be more of a spotlight upon McAllister than a worklight intended to aid banking business. Pershing J. McAllister did not stand up; he did not even look up, but merely nodded and said: "Sit down, Schindler!" It sounded more like an order than a request, and why did he call him Schindler rather than Henry or Mr. Schindler? Perhaps, Henry thought—quickly trying to dampen the obvious insult—I just misunderstood him.

Silence . . . Silence . . . Silence . . . Then a bark of command.

"No, Schindler, it's out of the question; it's entirely out of the question. Why, good Lord, man, you can't pay your present mortgage; how in the hell do you expect to pay a larger one?"

Now, for the first time, the steel blue eyes of Pershing J. McAllister turned like machine-gun turrets in their sockets while holding Henry Schindler in target range, waiting, only waiting, for an excuse to fire.

"Well, I believe that I can handle the larger payments if I

. . . if I . . . have some operating capital," Henry tried to sound reassuring and firm.

"You believe," the guns barked, "you believe? Why, hell, man, business isn't based on belief; it's based on knowledge. How the hell have you survived this long in the clothing business?"

"Not clothing," Henry interrupted. Perhaps, he thought to himself, as soon as he realizes that I am a professional man, a druggist, this whole misunderstanding will be cleared up.

"Not clothing?" The guns were cocked to fire but looked momentarily puzzled. "What then? If not clothing, what then?"

"I'm a druggist," Henry proudly asserted, "a pharmacist."

Instantly, the guns cocked and fired another round of blue steel. "Drugs, clothing, it's all the same," McAllister triumphantly affirmed. "In banking terms you're simply a small businessman without the power to blow your own lead." McAllister smiled to himself: military terms; he liked military terms. "No! No! No! No!" McAllister fired, recocked, and fired again.

Henry felt his insides jump with every shot, and when the smoke cleared he was limp and broken. He knew the "interview" was over; he had been dismissed. Henry balanced himself as he stood to leave when suddenly, without any warning whatsoever, McAllister fired another round.

"The collection people will be in touch with you soon about the . . . uh . . . the . . . uh," riffling through what appeared to be Henry's file he found the correct figure, "yes . . . the $9,546.23 you owe in back payments on your several loans." Turning back to center-stage light, McAllister left Henry in darkness to find his own way out.

VI

Henry drove. He simply drove. Aimlessly, purposelessly, he drove through the back roads of the countryside pursuing his escape in endless circles that half completed themselves. Beatrice, dear sweet Beatrice, would be expecting him home for supper soon. Dear God, how could she be told? Dear God, how does any man tell his wife that he is a failure, a weakling, a wimp? When crushed, broken, and humiliated by life, how does one look into those eyes that have always looked to you for strength, solace, and comfort? And how—how indeed—does such a man turn lustfully to his wife in the watches of the night when he has been gelded and castrated in public?

Beatrice was both complex and simple at the same time. She was intelligent, sensitive, and certainly a better business person than Henry would ever be. Under her hand, the drugstore would have flourished. And yet she was also instinctual, primitive, and most practical in her devotions. Quite simply, she adored Henry. She knew that he was weak; she loved him all the more for it. She knew that he was not a good lover, and it didn't matter. She knew that he was afraid most of the time, and she sought to draw that fear out of him in order to absorb it herself. He was her husband, her lover, her protector—true enough—but he was also her friend, her child, and her responsibility. Can there be any doubt that she was the stronger of the two? But also can there be any question that precisely her strength consisted in disguising it as weakness? Yes, Beatrice was complex with intuitions as old and primal as time itself and as primitive as the very substance that separates men from women. She understood the darker, shadowed mysteries of this whole damned business about men and women. For all of our intelligence, sophistication, and culture, we are each of us caught up in some primal web of nature that prescribes what men can do and women cannot. She understood all of this without knowing why, and because she understood, she also realized that Henry must destroy his own demons or be destroyed by them.

By 7:30 that evening, Henry found himself thirty miles away in another town. Precisely how he arrived there was not clear, nor did it especially matter. Henry was in pursuit of his past. At first, it occurred to him to find a woman for the night; perhaps, a very large-breasted one such as seemed to appeal to the Nussbaum boys. But no! No, he discarded the idea almost as quickly as he had conceived it. Henry had never been unfaithful to Beatrice, and it broke his heart to think that he might break her heart by so doing. It also occurred to him to get drunk at one of the local bars running up and down the avenues he now silently drove through. But no! His peptic ulcer would pay him back immediately for such personal infidelity to his own body. And then instantly, intuitively, like a homing pigeon headed for its own roost, he knew where he must go and go immediately: back to the quiet solitude of the drugstore—which was still his drugstore—to plan his future.

Beatrice was definitely worried. By 8:00 that evening she had called the drugstore several times, and she had even driven there herself. But Henry was not to be found. She knew that he would be hungry, and she knew that his ulcer probably was beginning to ache. And also she wanted to take care of him. But where could he be? She suspected—yes, she knew—that he had not gotten the loan, and she grieved for this gentle, kind, and fragile man who could not share his troubles.

Henry arrived at the drugstore by 9:30 and quickly let himself in the back door. He sought the solitude and warmth of this small haven just as an animal rushes to the safety of its hiding place. For there among the pharmaceuticals, the chemistry books, the glassware he finally felt safe and secure. The substance of ideas had always been more real, more immediate and palpable for him than the thinness of things. And it was for this reason that he liked the recipes and formulas for mixing prescriptions far better than the actual pills, capsules, or ointments that were their products. Thoughtfully, affectionately, he ran his fingers in a gentle caress about the glass rim of his mortar and pestle. There, high up on the third shelf, were the graduated weights and balances that he used to equalize the apothecary scales. Here, beside his right hand, was the wooden file case in which every prescription he had ever filled was neatly filed.

"A monument," he thought, "to every ache, pain, cry in the night, and agony of health that the residents of this town have suffered for the last twenty-five years. Is there—somewhere among these oils, acids, and alkaloids—some antidote for ruin, damnation, and despair?"

Beatrice, now in utter desperation, called 3471 once more.

Henry heard the ringing as if it were a muffled voice calling from a distance. It sounded plaintive as does an urgent cry for help and yet demanding as does an order which cannot be disobeyed. But disobey Henry knew he must, for all his energy and strength had been devoured by the fear that held him huddled in this small sanctuary of Pyrex, chemicals, and gummed labels.

Beatrice hung up, redialed, and waited; she hung up, waited, and redialed again. It was a litany, a sacrificial ritual intended to sanctify by mechanical means her love and devotion. She did not, therefore, expect an answer, nor would she have known what to say had he answered.

The ringing stopped. Resumed. Stopped again. Resumed once more. It was a strangulated cry uttered in silence from slightly bruised lips, and had that damaged voice spoken clearly he would not have known how to answer it.

Perhaps he knew that she was silently calling out. Perhaps she knew that he was silently listening. Perhaps not. For Henry was, at this moment, coiled like a snake within himself while waiting, silently waiting to strike. But at what enemy in the darkness did this thin and altogether too fragile viper aim? Wherever and whenever, his first strike must be deadly accurate, for Henry had neither the strength nor the courage to strike a second time.

Turning now, slowly and rhythmically turning now upon the coiled axis of himself, Henry reaches toward the shelf above and slightly weaves with mesmerized absolution as the delicate—they are almost feminine—fingertips coil and curl about their target. Swiftly, the fangs withdraw and deposit with certain speed the bottled treasure into Henry's right coat pocket. He watched the whole unfolding of these movements as if they belonged to another and thereby constituted a sacramental ritual of which he was only an observer and not yet ordained to be both priest and celebrant.

VII

Henry's eyes smiled with contented peace as the October sky dissolved from darkness into dawn. And perfectly mirrored in duplicated miniature, the silver moon of that broken night reappeared as reflected coins phosphorescing from those unseeing eyes. Tranquil, relaxed, now finally at ease, those delicate—were they not almost feminine?—fingers entwined one another as if in loving embrace. The bow tie—just so very slightly askew—was a rich lavender with dotted highlights of emerald green. And his hair, yes, his hair was so elegant and polished in its careful curvature of comb that one almost thought it painted upon the patrician forehead of finely chiseled marble. He sat in his car, which was, of course, immaculately clean both inside and out. Henry had always been most particular about these details of life, for everything must be perfect in an otherwise imperfect world. Indeed, he had even tied with painful precision the elegant bow tie that was now the singular source of coloration to his otherwise bleached complexion of whitened stone.

Of course, Beatrice must be told! But who among us has the courage? And how should one begin? And whom should one blame? Shall we blame the coarse and rude Nussbaum boys with their fantasies of big-busted farm girls? Shall we accuse Pershing J. McAllister, who shot before he aimed his gun of financial ruin? Or shall we blame little Bobby Gerber whose white-blood-cell count now exceeds 100,000 as he lies dying of lymphoblastic leukemia, or the bending arch of Mrs. Palmer's arthritic bones, or the cavernous lungs of Mrs. Beiner slowly being hollowed out by the devouring teeth of a squamous-cell carcinoma? Who among each and all of these is responsible for the bewildered—yet strangely contented—look of eternal resignation upon the face of gentle, fragile, much-beloved-by-Beatrice Henry Schindler?

He was found by farm boys, by boys who were close to the earth and the animal smell of things. Gentle Amish lads who—sensitive to spiritual voices such as might have drawn them to this place—became the appointed messengers of disastrous news. They came upon Henry's car while searching the fields for stray calves that brilliant, blue, and brutal October morning. Suddenly, there in the grove, they saw the green Chevrolet resting like a dove upon its nest within a sanctuary of evergreens. And . . . yes . . . they saw the man inside as well. At first—so they told their parents later—they thought he was simply enjoying the splendid break of day upon the dawn. For he smiled—or he seemed to smile—at the yellow crescent of brilliant morning sun.

But then the boys looked more closely and saw not a smile

but—dear God, how their slender bodies shook with horror when they told the tale—they saw instead a sinister, oozing erosion of flesh which gaped like a grin as still it poured forth its exudate of blood, bone, and melted flesh. And oh, the mouth, the throat—oh, dear God in heaven—the entire chest had been eaten and chewed away as if devoured by some malevolent and altogether crazed animal. And still cradled in those folded hands—held as if in silent benediction by thin, almost feminine fingertips—rested the eucharistic chalice that had so consumed gentle, much-beloved-by-Beatrice Henry: a half-quart jar of carbolic acid whose rim still dripped a bloodied stew of devoured lips that dissolved even as they sought to kiss the chalice.

13

Just Looking

He watched himself see; he watched in order to see himself watch; it was his own consciousness of the tree and the house that he contemplated. He only saw things through this consciousness; they were paler, smaller and less touching as though seen through an eyeglass. They did not point to one another as a signpost points the way or a marker indicates the page; . . . on the contrary, their immediate function was to direct awareness back to the self. . . . This consciousness which was watched and scrutinized and which knew that it was being watched and scrutinized while it performed its normal functions, at once lost its naturalness like a child playing under the eyes of grown-up people. . . . Everything was faked because everything was scrutinized and because the slightest mood or the feeblest desire was observed and unravelled at the very moment it came into being. . . . He was trying to discover his own nature, that is to say, his character and his being, but all he saw was the long, monotonous procession of his states of mind. . . . Thus, the tortures which he inflicted on himself simulated possession. They tended to make flesh—his own flesh—grow beneath his fingers so that in the very throes of its

261

*suffering it would recognize that it was his
flesh. . . . Baudelaire was the man who chose to
look upon himself as though he were another person; his life is simply the story of the failure of this
attempt.*

Jean-Paul Sartre
Baudelaire

VOYEURISM: A sexual deviation in which gratification is obtained from observing the bodies or sexual activities of other people.

Voyeurs are generally young men—"peeping Toms"—who secretly watch girls or women undress, or observe couples engaged in sexual relations. An occasional voyeur is primarily interested in watching homosexual behavior or other deviant sexual activity, such as sadistic acts.

Practically all males derive sexual pleasure and stimulation from looking at female nudity. They are also curious about the mystery of sexual activity. The voyeur, however, deviates from the normal in persistently searching for opportunities to spy on others, and in deriving most or all of his sexual satisfaction from observing them. He generally achieves orgasm while looking, either spontaneously or through masturbation. Sexual response is heightened by the suspense, excitement, and danger of being caught, and it is therefore not surprising that most voyeurs do not react sexually when observation is permitted as in watching a burlesque show.

The voyeur is typically an isolated, shy individual who fears women and doubts his sexual adequacy. The peeping gives him satisfaction without risk of rejection or failure. It also reassures him of his potency. In addition, it probably serves as an outlet for aggressive, hostile drives, since peeping is a stealthy act and probably makes the voyeur feel superior to the people he is watching. Older men, sometimes married, may engage in peeping as a result of sexual frustration. In some cases, the voyeur identifies with one or the other partner in sexual relations as a result of homosexual impulses.

262

When voyeurism is the result of emotional immaturity, it can often be corrected through short-term psychotherapy; but when it is a persistent pattern and an expression of an inadequate personality, as it frequently is, treatment may be difficult or unsuccessful. Contrary to rumor, the typical peeper is not criminally inclined and seldom attacks women.

Robert M. Goldenson
The Encyclopedia of Human Behavior

I

Ernest Waltmeyer was a jeweler and had but one testicle. Neither fact, of course, was the cause of the other. It just happened that way. Still, it did bother him to be . . . well, to be . . . defective in an otherwise perfect world of full-cut carat diamonds and intricate Swiss watch movements. Probably, he would not have thought of his missing testicle had not this most delicate and fragile world which he inhabited been such a constant reminder. For a jeweler dwells within a miniature, gossamer universe in which the slightest imperfection creates chaos of cosmic proportions. And so, yes, he both remembered and forgot the missing testicle each and every day.

There was another fact of some importance about Waltmeyer: he was cross-eyed. And in order to compensate, or perhaps to reconcile, this additional deficit he constantly wore his jeweler's lens in the other eye. His intention, of course, was to achieve visual equilibrium in an otherwise disproportionate world. The effect, however, was simply terrifying! Indeed, it was difficult to discern whether Waltmeyer was looking at you or away from you, and more difficult yet to determine whether you were being magnified or miniaturized by the contradictions in his visual powers.

Each morning promptly at nine o'clock he opened his shop and each evening at exactly five o'clock he closed it. In between these times, he entertained customers and looked at the many jewels and gems that were his stock and trade. Waltmeyer loved to look at things—at beautiful things in particular—but even ugly things would do if nothing else was available. Some people in this world are especially sensitive to the touch, texture, and surface of things; unless they surround themselves with silks, furs, and satins, they do not feel whole and complete. Others can recognize the atmosphere of a place, a city, or a situation by its odor alone. Still others yet touch reality only through the timbre, pitch, and harmony of sounds. They are the musicians, the audiophiliacs of this world, and to the same degree that some are gourmets of touch, taste, and smell, they are connoisseurs of sound. Waltmeyer was none of these. No, he had tried the trumpet as a boy and hated it. He had neither an interest nor a liking for odors whether they be perfumed or foul. And Ernest Waltmeyer most definitely, most absolutely wished neither to touch nor to be touched by fabric or flesh other than his own. No, he loved instead to see things; he was quite content to peer—whether microscopically or macroscopically—at the world that surrounded him. All his delights, all the sensual and erotic pleasures of his world were inexhaustibly contained in what could be seen.

To see his world you must imagine, for a moment, darkness: utter and absolute darkness. Herein is an opaque and indistinguishable darkness of such a degree that it covers the pungency of reality like a deep, velvet death shroud. Now there to the far left appears a single, solitary sliver of light which clarifies even as it increases itself in both substance and depth. A cobalt blue, perhaps, of the deepest most intense saturation or even an ocher yellow of open and airy sunshine brightness. And as each or the other of these grows, do you also see how the thin crust of reality that surrounds them is illuminated and thereby gains both depth of substance and visibility? Now a crescent of ruby red appears, or a shell of emerald green, and each inspires and complements the other until perspective, distance, and even time seem but the ploy of various hues within and without one another. It is a trajectory of light, angle, and proportion through which reality unveils itself in blues and golds, ruby reds, greens, and elegant lavenders. This is no longer the thick, heavy world of surface, weight, texture, and tone but an altogether ephemeral ether of delicate lights and their reflec-

tions. Such extraordinary visions were for Ernest Waltmeyer
perfectly ordinary ways of seeing.

He loved to look. He loved to feel the sight of colors,
angles, perspectives, and contours. And yes . . . oh yes . . . he
also liked the sight of naked bodies. Yes, he liked such sights
very much indeed. To see the supple, satin skin of a smooth
thigh, of an ample breast, of a languid length of lazy leg was
very nice; it was very, very nice indeed to see such sights. No,
you understand, he had no desire whatsoever to touch. But he
did very much enjoy looking.

In only the most superficial and irrelevant sense does eroticism have to do with our genitals. And yet with their penchant
for theatricism and hysteria, these exaggerated organs have
drawn undue attention to themselves. The erotic, however, is
far more than the interplay of tumescence and orgasm; it is
rather a global—even a cosmic—reverberation of desire which
inundates every aspect of our composition from brain to bowel.
The Greeks understood this and saw that "eros" is a desire
seeking possession of itself, a fragmentation yearning for unity,
a polarization of opposing forces seeking harmony, and not
merely a glandular confusion. Ernest Waltmeyer also understood these things and therefore regarded his desire to peek,
to peer, to watch as more than crude pornography but rather
artistry of the highest form. Not everyone would agree, and
many would fail entirely to understand these subtle distinctions. Accordingly, Waltmeyer always conducted himself with
the greatest propriety and dignity, not for his sake alone but
for the sake of others as well. He did not—no, he absolutely
did not ever—look at anyone who did not desire to be seen.
Moreover, when he did look, it was with aesthetic vision and
not mere sexual gawking. The difference—for those sensitive
and sophisticated enough to perceive it—was enormous.

These were "matters of the heart"—as he chose to regard
them—and far too private, too personal to be shared with anyone. Rather, they were his own secret and most intimate concerns. Certainly his customers would never understand!
Certainly his wife Emily would not understand the very precious and divine nature of these nocturnal peerings, peekings,

and viewings. It was, therefore, with the greatest precision that Waltmeyer guarded his inner life from all unauthorized invasions.

II

Connie Daniels turned, and then half turned again, pirouetting as she postured in front of the tall bedroom mirror. She was completely naked save for the soft blue Chinese slippers that she wore upon her slender feet. The carved mirror of walnut and cherry woods was an heirloom dating back to over three generations of great-grandmothers, grandmothers, and mothers, and it seemed to watch her intently even as she watched it. Cupping her delicate breasts from beneath with full hands, she raised their weight and carefully watched the teased, puckered response of her reflected nipples. They were not the pink, delicate nipples of a girl but the long, brown, slender nozzles of a woman who has suckled her young. For Connie Daniels was not a young girl, nor did she have such a fragile blush to her body. Rather, there was a taunt, ripe, and altogether experienced texture about her which suggested a beauty about to fade instead of one about to bloom. And yet even now the slightest breeze, the lightest touch upon her breasts was enough to arouse her. Perhaps it was the publicity of these private caresses, the eyes of this reflecting mirror, or even the whole ancestry of its communal belonging that made her feel all the more naughty and wicked.

At thirty-eight Connie Daniels was still a very fine looking woman. Oh, yes, she was a very fine looking woman indeed. The poetic Keats would have seen within her "silver moons, that, as she breathed, / Dissolv'd, or brighter shone, or inter-wreathed / Their lustres with the gloomier tapestries." Her rich, thick auburn hair sparkled with highlights of strawberry, blonde, and red and showed not a trace of gray while still being as soft, luxurious, and moist as it had been twenty years before. The lines about her eyes, such as they were, seemed so delicate as to be complementary, and neither furrow nor crease interrupted that vast smoothness of cheek, brow, and chin. Oh yes, she was a very fine looking woman indeed! But it was especially her eyes that could not be forgotten; those eyes that haunted her former lovers far into the loneliness of their nights when no longer were they permitted to touch her. Those eyes, dear Lord, those eyes of emerald green whose amber yolks and flecks of chestnut brown only served to intensify the rich, luxurious weight of her ambergris hair. Yes, she was a fine looking woman, indeed, with full pouted lips of ruby red and soft shallows to her dimpled cheeks. Her body was the full, sensuous, and enriched body of an experienced woman rather than the thin, frail impoverishment of innocence. Her hips flared out from a slender waist in perfect proportion to the soft and delicate curvature of her breasts. A thick and luxurious tuft of pubic hair descended from the soft arch of her belly to the swell of her thighs. Whether in contrast or in competition it cannot be said, but the pale transparency of her skin seemed to illuminate and focus every other feature of this remarkable body. Truth to tell, Connie Daniels was sensual; so absolutely erotic that even she had fallen quite in love with herself and sought at times—at times like these before the mirror—to seduce herself.

She knew, of course, that Ernest Waltmeyer often watched her undressing. She was disgusted. She was also—strange to say—very aroused to be so watched. Physically, erotically, and in every other way she found Waltmeyer repulsive, and the very thought of entwining her body within his anemic and weakened thighs was nauseating. His penis—or so she imagined—would be a slender flaccid affair weakly erupting its discharge and so leaving her and him quite unsatisfied. No, dear God, no, she would never consider sex with a man such as Ernest Waltmeyer. But it was very exciting to know that he sometimes watched her and that it excited him to do so.

Why? Well, she was bored. Leo, her husband for the past twelve years, had never been a passionate lover and recently seemed to have lost entirely what little passion he once had. Even when he did summon the energy forward, so to speak, it was an insipid and uninspired effort. And when finished, he would immediately turn over, yawn, and fall asleep. She yearned, she dreamed of a man with a golden body of tanned, rippled muscles who would take her in his arms. The two great powerful hands—shaped more like the claws of some degenerate animal—would grasp with fury the cup of each rounded buttock and slowly knead the moist and pliant flesh. His penis would be thick, massive, and his entrance into her delicate body would be forceful and even savage to a brutal degree. And yet he would neither apologize nor even seem to notice the pain he caused her as the thick muscled loins pounded like jackhammers into the depths of her body. Then in a twisting contortion of quivering bodies, they would climax together. The fantasy humiliated and aroused her at the same time, for within this degradation there gathered the storm of her power to excite, to draw savagely the lust of such men to her body. It made her feel a woman in the fullest sense to be so humbled by a sexual power she could arouse but then could not control. Leo was certainly not such a man, nor was Ernest Waltmeyer, and such fantasies were drawn from the wellspring of her boredom with life. She had every desire to cheat on her husband, but she simply did not have the courage. Therefore, Connie Daniels contented herself with seducing but never satisfying the very safe, very timid Ernest Waltmeyer who simply liked to look.

And even now she knew that he was there outside her window and even now she could feel the cold stare of his confused eyes upon her body. And always it was the same with her and with him, for they seemed to form a union within diversity as the one watched and the other felt herself being watched. As if by silent, subtle prior agreement, he would creep cautiously on cat's feet through the bushes to the vaulted edge of the windowsill to stare in raptured adoration. And silently she, in turn, would acknowledge his arrival by first removing her shoes, then slowly unrolling her stockings by lazy turns down the length of her long, languid legs, and finally removing a slender laced garter belt with great decorum. All of this took a long time—a very long time, for Connie never hurried herself— and she always acted with the greatest modesty. She next undid her dress, button by button, until it slowly slid down the length of her body and into a heap upon the floor. Then standing in only bra and panties, she turned full face as if to confront Ernest Waltmeyer. He, of course, rapidly ducked below the window ledge. Slowly then he reappeared, and slowly she re-

moved one strap and then the other until the cups of her bras-
siere freed the fleshly, quivering mounds of soft jellied breast.
Why did it give her so much pleasure to taunt and tease this
gentle, weak, and impotent man? Did she hate him? Did she
hate all men? Next she removed her panties by slowly sliding
the satin from off her rounded hips until she was completely
naked. Was that a gasp heard from the window? Never mind,
for the show is over; she is bored, and Ernest Waltmeyer is
dismissed. She closes the blinds, shuts off the lights, and goes
to bed.

III

Upon occasion—after such an evening's performance—she
might visit the jewelry store the following afternoon. He was
always most courteous, dignified, and very, very discreet.

"Good afternoon, Mrs. Daniels."

"And a very good afternoon to you, Mr. Waltmeyer."

"May I show you something?"

"On the contrary, Mr. Waltmeyer."

"I beg your pardon."

It was a game, of course, a vast and very elaborate game in
which each contestant understood the rules very well. To what
profit or to what advantage each participated in this game can
be neither ascertained nor foretold. She no doubt was tanta-
lized; he no doubt was eroticized. She no doubt was bored; he
no doubt was desperate. Their mutual needs seemed to stand
in stark contradiction to one another, and yet they both needed
and attracted one another. It was a strange union, a symbiosis
born of the need to see and of the need to be seen.

Life-styles such as these—held corseted and bound within
carefully controlled limits—often appear normal and even
commonplace. It takes an eruption—an incident of volcanic
proportions—to disconnect the union of the two and thereby
reveal each for what it really is in isolation from the other. Exactly such an incident occurred one day in the person of Johnny
Martin, who dissolved the umbilical tie uniting Mrs. Daniels
and Mr. Waltmeyer with a single glance of pure, unadulterated
lust.

IV

Johnny Martin was sixteen years old and certainly a young man with much growing left to be done. However, it was rumored that one area in particular had definitely reached full growth even at this tender age. And it was, in fact, this one area in particular that absolutely interested the matronly Mrs. Connie Daniels.

She set out to seduce him. Why? Oh, dear God, why indeed? Why do we do these stupid, dangerous, and ill-advised things? Because we are compelled—quite beyond reason and even good common sense—to satisfy some primal and primitive drive within us. Yes, she was as if possessed, and it was just the thought of all that abundant—and no doubt unexercised—meaty manhood that drove the poor woman nearly mad. So despite all good counsel, quite in violation of all that is right or wrong, with no regard to what is appropriate or inappropriate, sensible or sane, mad or demented, she proceeded forthwith to make her plans.

"Perhaps," she inquired of him one day, "a young man such as yourself might wish to earn some money gardening."

"But I know nothing about gardening," was his quick reply.

"I myself will teach you," so she assured him, "absolutely everything you need to know."

So said, so done! He arrived the following afternoon for his first lesson. Young men, of course, must often be led to where they wish to go. An older, more mature fellow needs only the invitation of a sleek thigh or supple breast to point the way; but young boys are innocent, clumsy, awkward, and so they need to follow rather than lead. Follow he did: through the living room, past the dining room, but not to the garden.

Connie Daniels's bedroom was in many ways a theater, even an amphitheater, planned for the singular purpose of visual delights. Perhaps she had been influenced in these decisions by her long "association" with Waltmeyer. The colors were all muted and intensely feminine in order to promote both tranquillity and eroticism, for it was intoxication that she sought to paint upon the walls, within the drapes, and everywhere that she could be seen. Peach, lavender, and a dash of ocher punctuated the eiderdown quilt, the lace and the frill of everything. And discreetly placed at an angle to her bed—so as not to be too obvious—was her dressing table with full-length mirror and a smaller mirror to the right in white porcelain frame. "Vision," the great photographer Ansel Adams used to observe, "is nothing but light and angle."

How true this prophecy was within the very photographic life of Mrs. Connie Daniels. Everything that happened within this peach and lavender room must be focused and illuminated to high visibility lest it escape the ever watchful eye of Waltmeyer. She had made her preparations well, for while he delighted in looking, she, in turn, was most delighted to be seen. And so they were—the two of them—but mirrored reflections of one another.

By this time, young Johnny was nervous beyond belief. In his most innocent mind, he had already deduced the general sense of what was happening as Connie proceeded to fill in the particulars.

"Would you like to remove your shirt before you start to garden? It's such a warm day, don't you think?"

"Well," creaked the cracking voice desperately trying to locate its masculine tone, "I was afraid it might get dirty."

"Yes," she reassured him, "it'll be clean as a whistle when you finish planting your beautiful garden."

She removed his shirt; she removed her own. Quick as a flash, she removed her undergarments and quick as a flash his own were removed as well. She removed her jewelry, and then naked they stood before one another. The reports of young Johnny's growth were not in the least exaggerated. In fact, it would have been almost a laughing matter to see this boy's head on a man's body were not the occasion such a solemn one. For his part, young Johnny was simply astonished. He had never realized that there were so many . . . well, so very many "things" to a woman's body. The soft inviting thighs, the ample billowing breasts with taut nipples were facts of which he had already some premonition. But he was not at all prepared for her long sleek and slender neck with its delicious perfumed fragrance. Nor was he at all prepared for the wild ringlets of cascading hair, the red pouted lips, her half-closed eyes, or her labored, heavy breathing, all of which simply drained the energy from him. At first, he reached out to touch her—most tentatively and with the greatest hesitation—but suddenly she enveloped him in her golden arms, tight hips, soft belly, buttock, and breast. He felt absorbed, and as he entered her so it seemed that she entered him as well. They turned and twisted like a double helix on a single axis. And as they expanded and contracted, so they also reabsorbed one another. Dissolving, as separate mixtures into one another's composition, they reassembled the integrity of themselves when it was finished. It was . . . well . . . it was . . . it was quite simply delightful.

Of course, Waltmeyer saw it all. And he was disgusted! This was pornography; it was not art. Nonetheless, he stayed to the end, but not without considerable discomfort. Nor did it go unnoticed—by this most keen observer of human nature—that young Johnny Martin possessed two very large, two very powerful testicles.

v

It was several weeks before Waltmeyer could summon the courage once again to return to his customary perch beneath Mrs. Daniels's bedroom window. In the meantime, he was haunted almost daily by visions of her supple breasts, her smooth belly, arched thigh, and slender neck. And, yes, he was haunted also by young Johnny's most perfectly formed testicles. In certain ways, breasts and balls are one. Each is an encapsulated gland which distinguishes the feminine from the masculine, and each has the power to inspire and to excite. "Yes, yes," Waltmeyer admitted, but only to himself, that he was excited—very, very excited—by Martin's strong young testicles. They were the essence of masculinity and yet so fragile and smooth as to be almost feminine. Finally—and this was the most important point—they were two rather than one. Why had Johnny been blessed with two fine testicles rather than cursed with only one?

Breasts are so strange in their power to attract. After all, they are nothing more than milk ducts intended to nourish the young. And yet, the long, slender slope of a ripened breast capped by a delicate nozzle of pink flesh can be devastating in its eroticism. Oh yes, to lift the heavy weight of that tender teat, to so loosen it from brassiered confines, is absolutely arousing. And is it not a liquor of intoxicating power to trace with lazy finger that long channel of fragrant cleavage in a ripe, well-developed woman in her thirties? And such a woman was Connie Daniels.

A woman in her full maturity—not a girl or a child, but a woman—is the most perfect of God's creatures. The full growth and development of every muscle, fiber, sinew, and aspect of such a woman has now been achieved. In her teens or even early twenties, she is still imperfect, unripened, and immature. But at thirty, her hips have widened to their full, sensuous arch. The slight curvature of womb forms now a soft dome of belly above the inviting loins. Finally, her breasts have just the right proportion of bounce and stretch to give them fullness and weight. Moreover, she is no longer a novice but rather an experienced and educated connoisseur of pleasure who is not intimidated by lust but feels perfectly comfortable in its presence. To enter such a woman is—dear God—it is to feel the very earth tremble. And to know that herein is the full, rich fertility of a woman within whose loins rests the promise of birth, life, and renewal is an almost sacred experience. Connie Daniels was such a woman. Oh, my, yes, she was such a woman.

And now for the first time, Ernest Waltmeyer yearned for her; he yearned and he ached with jealous passion for the moisture of her flesh. And he hated as well. He hated with envy and bitter scorn those two most powerful testicles of young Johnny Martin. A transformation had occurred within him from the passive act of seeing to the active desire of doing. Why had he been so aroused from his dogmatic slumbers? And why must he now long, desire, wish for what he could not possess? Before it had been so very easy since all he wanted to do was look. But now—how he wished it were otherwise—he wanted more. Yes, he wanted much more, and the aching pain of these confused longings drove him near mad with their endless taunting.

VI

"Mrs. Daniels, it's a pleasure to see you again."

"Thank you, Mr. Waltmeyer, I assure you the pleasure is all mine."

"May I show you something? In fact, may I insist upon showing you something?"

"Thank you, yes, I should like to see something that might please a young man."

"His age? May I inquire?"

"Oh yes, perhaps sixteen or seventeen."

"No doubt a relative, Mrs. Daniels?"

"No doubt, Mr. Waltmeyer."

"Well, then, may I recommend a Christian emblem, Mrs. Daniels? Good, moral young men of today are not embarrassed to show where their sentiments lie."

"His sentiments, however, do not quite lie in that direction, Mr. Waltmeyer."

"I see," was all that could properly be replied.

"I rather thought," she absentmindedly rearranged the delicate lace of her bodice as she spoke, "that an engraved bracelet might be nice."

"But do you think perhaps that such a gift might be seen as too . . . well, too . . . ," he struggled for the right word.

"Perhaps too personal," he finally succeeded in stating his sentiments perfectly.

"No!" she quickly affirmed without being quite certain whether the jeweler's lens or the crossed eye had her in focus.

"No, given the circumstances, I think that is not a possibility, Mr. Waltmeyer."

"Dear me," was all that he could reply.

VII

Johnny Martin had always been frightened of Waltmeyer. It was his eyes and especially his habit of looking through you rather than at you that disturbed him. Still, his was the only jewelry store in town, and Johnny badly needed to find a gift for Connie's birthday, which was tomorrow. Thus, on Tuesday afternoon—after school, of course—he entered the small shop at 132 West Prospect Avenue. A faint bell announced his arrival upon first opening the door. The store was empty of customers and very tranquil that quiet afternoon with only the peaceful ticking of a clock in the background.

"Good afternoon, Johnny." Waltmeyer seemed to immediately appear from nowhere in particular.

"Hi, Mr. Waltmeyer, how are you?"

"I am very good, son, and you?"

"O.K. I need a gift for a friend."

"A lady friend, I presume."

Young Johnny blushed to admit that it was so. "Yes, a lady friend."

"Young or old, may I inquire?"

"Well, actually somewhere in between."

"I see. Well, in that case, it must be a relative and not a girlfriend, wouldn't you say?" Waltmeyer did so enjoy taunting this innocent, naive, young lad with the child's face and the man's testicles.

"Yeah, I suppose so."

"May I recommend a Christian article of jewelry. So many of the more mature ladies these days wish to identify themselves as persons of Christian character and morality by means of the jewelry they wear."

"Well, I don't think so," Johnny responded.

"You don't think she's a Christian, Johnny?" Waltmeyer quickly countered.

"No, I don't think that's what I am looking for," Johnny just as quickly explained.

"I see," Waltmeyer lowered his voice even as he lowered his eyes.

While young Johnny made his selection from the velvet tray, and Waltmeyer observed him, it was virtually impossible not to peer with jeweler's lens beneath the clothed body to the hidden nakedness. Indeed, it was difficult—and hardly worth the effort—not to recall the twisted tangle of nude hips and loins vigorously pumping intense pleasure from one another. Neither was it easy, even though Waltmeyer was not an auditory person, not to recall the hushed mews and small squeals of pleasure that issued from Connie's parted ruby lips. It was difficult not to hear again the labored, hurried breathing of Johnny Martin as he buried that tousled head in those moist, fertile, alabaster loins of Mrs. Daniels's. So lost in thought, he barely heard Johnny triumphantly announce:

"I'll take this one, Mr. Waltmeyer."

"Good choice, Johnny, a very good choice."

VIII

What was to be done? What was to be done? Monsters, de-mons, and devils of all degree had been released within the gentle soul of Ernest Waltmeyer, and without his permission. Why had he been so unfortunate that fateful night to view a scene of such unadulterated lust that he could not now forget? How simple it had been just to look, to passively and longingly gaze at what could never be his. But now he wanted more; he desired and lusted for more than he ever thought possible, and the desire would not extinguish itself but only further inflamed and renewed itself. Something must be done.

Came Thursday evening around ten o'clock, and once again Ernest Waltmeyer found himself outside of Connie Daniels's bedroom window. She was not alone! There, twisted in a sexual pretzel of inventive lust, was the supple young body of Johnny Martin entwined about the experienced loins of his mature mistress. Moreover, within and without this tangle of twisting flesh, there glittered the unmistakable gold of Waltmeyer's jewelry, which had been purchased and exchanged by each of the bodies now before him.

His hand searched himself for the missing testicle but in vain, for instead he merely found a hollow emptiness. Mean-while the strong, powerful testicles of young Martin seemed almost to vibrate with swollen seeds. Ernest Waltmeyer was near the breaking point; he could stand no more! He could tolerate no more pain, no more self-loathing, and no more emptiness within. In an instant he knew what must be done. And . . . so . . . he did it!

Waiting anxiously for the bodies to announce by their trem-bling a crisis beyond recall, he threw the window open and announced: "I see you; I see you both."

Instantly, of course, the once withering bodies separated with a resounding wet pop as they both stared in horrified amazement at Waltmeyer. And then, as if to plunge the mur-derous, self-destructive dagger in even further, he added: "And you disgust me."

He had forced the moment to its crisis and given the secret affair public visibility. It isn't done! It simply isn't done! Poor Connie was left with no alternative. She called the police and pressed charges at once.

Mrs. Daniels explained to the officers that while she was instructing young Johnny Martin in his piano lessons, Waltmeyer had appeared at the window and exposed his genitals. She could not be certain—after all, it was very dark—but she said that something was definitely missing that ought to be there. Waltmeyer did not deny either charge, and in truth, his silence was as much an indictment as was the accuracy of Connie Daniels's identification.

The jewelry store, of course, was closed. Waltmeyer was not jailed, but he was placed in the state mental hospital for observation and subsequently therein committed. Connie Daniels grew eventually bored with young Johnny, and he—as young men often do—grew disrespectful of her. Each separated from the other to pursue sensual delights of a more exotic sort. There is no evidence that either of them were transformed by virtue of having known one another. Rather, it seems that their lives merely touched—like the arcs of a continuous circle—without ever unifying or integrating themselves.

V

Acute and Chronic Diseases

That learning, thine ambassador,
From thine allegiance we never tempt,
That beauty, paradise's flower
For physic made, from poison be exempt
That wit, born apt high good to do,
By dwelling lazily
On Nature's nothing, be not nothing too,
That our affections kill us not, nor die,
Hear us, weak echoes, O thou ear, and cry.

John Donne
"A Litany: The Doctors"

14

Faces Frozen in Time

*Parkinsonian disorders, of one sort or another,
were perhaps the commonest of these disorders, although their appearance was often delayed until
many years after the actue epidemic. Post-
encephalitic Parkinsonism, as opposed to ordinary
or idiopathic Parkinsonism, tended to show less in
the way of tremor and rigidity—indeed, these were
sometimes completely absent—but much severer
states of "explosive" and "obstructive" disorders, of
akinesia and akathisia, push and resistance,
hurry and impediment, etc., and also much severer
states of the complaint—perseverative type of akinesia which Gowers had compared to catalepsy.
Many patients, indeed, were swallowed up in
states of Parkinsonian akinesia so profound as to
turn them into living statues—totally motionless
for hours, days, weeks, or years on end. The very
much greater severity of these encephalitic and
post-encephalitic states revealed that all aspects of
being and behavior—perceptions, thoughts, appe-
tites, and feelings, no less than movements—could
also be brought to a virtual standstill by an active,
constraining Parkinsonian process.*

Oliver Sacks
Awakenings

281

THE PARKINSONIAN SYNDROME: In Parkinsonism the facial muscles exhibit an unnatural immobility. The eyes have a somewhat staring appearance, and spontaneous ocular movements are infrequent. The attitude of the limbs and trunk is one of moderate flexion. The limbs are moderately flexed and adducted, but the wrist is usually slightly extended. The fingers are flexed at the metacarpophalangeal and extended or only slightly flexed at the interphalangeal joints, and adducted. The thumb is usually adducted, and extended at the metacarpophalangeal and interphalangeal joints.

Voluntary movements exhibit some impairment of power, but more striking is the slowness with which it is performed. In general the movements which are carried out by small muscles suffer most. Hence the patient shows weakness of the ocular movements which are characteristically jerky, of the facial movements, characteristically associated with tremor of the eyelids on closure of the eyes, and of movements concerned in matication, deglutition, and articulation. The speech in severe cases is slurred and monotonous, owing to defective pronunciation of consonants and lack of variation in pitch. Movements of the small muscles of the hands are also markedly affected with resulting clumsiness and inability to perform fine movements. The patient has increasing difficulty in writing, and the handwriting tends to be smaller—micrographia. Certain associated and synergic movements suffer conspicuously. Swinging of the arms in walking is early diminished and later lost. Emotional movements of the face are reduced in amplitude, slow in developing, and unduly protracted.

There is no sensory loss in Parkinsonism, but many patients in the later stages complain of pains in the limbs and spine, and extreme restlessness is a common symptom. Flushing of the skin and excessive sweating are occasionally seen, and excessive greasiness of the face, and salivation occur in encephalitic Parkinsonism. This is also the cause of oculogyral spasm, now rarely observed. This symptom consists of spasmodic deviation of the eyes, usually upwards, which the patient is unable to overcome, which occurs paroxysmally and may last for minutes or even hours. Parkinsonism is not necessarily associated with any mental disturbances, though such may of course be an independent effect of the disorder causing Parkinsonism.

Roger Bannister
Brain's Clinical Neurology

I

Friedrich Schwarz walked with a slow, purposeful shuffle across the carpeted tile of the sunporch and back into the cool, darkened living room. It was nearly 85° outside on that July afternoon, and the heat almost suffocated him. He was an old man—almost seventy-six—but looked older and was often mistaken for a man in his eighties. Indeed, Friedrich Schwarz often felt like such a man in his eighties, and lately he questioned the purpose, reason, and sense of his continued existence. He had not always done so. There were times when he thought life so rich and marvelous that it astonished him to realize how much he possessed, and only when he began to lose it, did he also realize how truly impoverished a man can actually become.

What had he lost? Well, not material things to be sure. In fact, his business was doing better under his sons than it had ever done under his own management. Neither had he lost his prestige, position, and place in the community. Indeed, he had finally achieved in his seventies what he had desired all his life: the respect of others. Friedrich Schwarz was a respected man, and people now spoke about him with a certain awe and reverence in their voice. Moreover, they wanted to be his friend, and no one had ever wanted to be his friend before. Nor had he lost the love of his good and dignified wife Bess, who seemed more maternal and more concerned about him than at any other time in their fifty years of marriage.

What then had he lost? He had lost his health; over the past ten years he had watched himself become feeble, infirm, and elderly. As the days became weeks and the weeks became months and the months finally became years, Friedrich Mueller Schwarz became an old, decrepit man. Now when he walked, it was with the slow, rigid movements of an ancient, elephantine creature whose brittle, clumsy legs threatened to break under the monster that they supported. His skin felt like hide and was waxed slick with a greasy, oily sweat which reappeared as quickly as it was wiped clean. Moreover, tremors continually shook his enormous body as if there festered within him both small and large quakes rumbling deep inside in order to erupt several centuries later upon the wasted, barren, forgotten surface. At first, it had only been his left arm that shook and then his left side. But gradually—like seascapes and oceanic waves that eventually must meet the shoreline—these local disturbances became global events which rose precipitously to greet the terrible disintegrations that descended. That was years ago, and as time passed the right side of his body became affected as well, and now both sides shook in discordant harmony like a symphonic orchestra led by two different conductors. He was rent asunder as the two halves of his body obeyed different measures set by different metronomes that could not be coordinated.

Friedrich Schwarz had been diagnosed with Parkinson's disease ten years before and despite treatments and medications had grown steadily worse every year thereafter. Before that he had not been sick a day in his life except, of course, for that terrible illness when he was sixteen. It was 1929; Friedrich had just finished his junior year of high school and was about to start a summer job. But one afternoon he came home in a sweat with a terrible headache and dizziness. For the next week or so his whole pattern of sleep was turned upside down, and often he was unable to sleep at all during the restless night but then would fall into an exhausted sleep throughout the day. There had also been something the matter with his eyes—he could no longer remember exactly what it was—and the doctor came nearly every day to see him. Later his mother had said that it was brain fever and that lots of other people were sick with the same thing. Since that time, however, he had been fine and had not even missed a day's work until the Parkinson's started.

It was a shame—he thought, and others did as well—that such a terrible disease should strike such a good man. They felt sorry for him—and he did as well—because Friedrich Schwarz was a self-made man who deserved a better life than this one. He came from a family of artisans and master craftsmen who made their living through carving and woodworking. In 1854 his father, Heinrich Guttermensch, had met and married the very lovely Rebecca Mueller and soon thereafter the couple left the rich and dense beauty of the Schwarzwald in Germany to make their fortune in America. This they had done by frugality, hard work, and simple, sheer German stubbornness. As time went on, Heinrich established himself as a craftsman and cabinetmaker in this country, dropped the awkward sounding Guttermensch—adopting instead the name Schwarz from the German Black Forest—and invested his money in a nearly bankrupt organ factory. By the turn of the century, the Schwarz Organ Factory was one of the leading suppliers of handmade wooden pipe organs in the United States, and by the 1920s it was beginning to compete with some of the great European organ companies. Then, of course, the stock market crash came, and the family lost nearly everything except the organ factory. But that was enough, because they were survivors, and by the 1940s they had gained back everything that had been lost. Father Heinrich eventually retired, and his only son, Friedrich, continued the family trade.

Friedrich and Elizabeth Schwarz had three children, and each received an education appropriate to their role in the family business. Eitel was always the mathematician, and therefore his father decided that he should become an engineer in order to apply these natural skills to designing organs. Johann—or John as the family called him—was the musician, and he was sent to Oberlin College for a degree in music with special attention to the organ. Virginia would, of course, marry, for that is what a woman did. But she would marry a businessman, her father had made that understood, who could make a contribution for her to the family business.

Friedrich Schwarz was a strong man, and he had succeeded in life by maintaining perfect control over every aspect of his life. Even upon his retirement from the business, he had conceived an arrangement to control the various factions in the family and thus keep each in check and balance with the other. To Eitel, the eldest, he gave a noncontrolling percentage of stock and made him the president of the company. To John he gave an equal share of stock and put him in charge of all production operations as well as installation and tuning of the organs. Virginia was given the largest share of stock—more than both of the boys' stock combined—and in fact held enough to have controlling interest. However, it was firmly understood that she would have no voice whatsoever in the day-to-day op-

erations or management of the firm. After all, she had her responsibilities to her husband. Having insured that the children
would continue in harmony with one another—because they
had to—their father felt content and confident to retire. And
then the Parkinson's hit him.

The Parkinson's was the one thing that he could not control,
although he certainly tried for the first few years; instead it
gained control over him. He hated the tremors, and he hated
the rigid way in which he walked, and he hated all the other
outward and inward signs and symptoms of the disease. But
more than these, he hated most the degradation and humiliation that the illness cost him. Friedrich Schwarz had always
been a proud and dignified man with a majestic bearing, dignity, and grace to all his movements. Extraordinarily handsome
with coal-black hair, dark intense eyes, and the robust complexion of a German peasant, he had always been self-assured
about his good looks. Indeed, they had served him well
throughout the years and probably made it possible for him to
court and marry Bess, to do well socially, and even to influence
important business associates to his way of thinking. His strong
and powerful features—of which he was justifiably vain—were
like a royal stamp which imprinted itself upon all of his children. The same strong, determined jaw and the same intense
dark eyes were stamped upon each of their faces in such a way
that no one could doubt to whom they belonged. He was proud
of this ownership and proud of his features, but the Parkinson's
had even taken some of these away along with everything else
that it had stolen.

Today, the square-cut jaw sagged and trembled while the
intensity of his eyes had long since emptied out to a sad, insipid
stare. His face, once so flushed with vibrant life and energy,
was now pale and pasty with a greasy waxen shine to it. Those
powerful arms and massive hands which once had carved such
beautiful wood now trembled like falling leaves upon dying
branches, and when he walked it was with a stooped and
discordant gait which brought pity and sympathy rather
than pride and recognition. The Parkinson's—that damnable,
blasted viper—had robbed him of so much that what remained

no longer seemed to matter. Friedrich Mueller Schwarz no longer gave a damn whether he lived or died.

II

From 1916 until 1927 the disease encephalitis lethargica killed millions of people around the world; it spared no country including the United States, England, France, Germany, and Austria. It first appeared in Europe in the city of Vienna during the winter of 1916 and rapidly spread within three years to the rest of the world. There were different names given to the ailment, and it disguised itself by different symptoms which were often hard to diagnose. In England, for example, it was called sleepy sickness, in America brain fever, and in Germany *Schlafkrankheit*. Wherever it appeared, it did so with an amazing mimicry of other illness and was often misdiagnosed as multiple sclerosis, polio, or even rabies. The agility of the disease to assume and change masks so rapidly made identification by clinical symptoms alone nearly impossible. The viral agent responsible for the disease was finally isolated by the Austrian neurologist Constantin von Economo, who lived from 1876 to 1931. Using specimens taken from autopsied brain tissue as well as comparative studies with monkeys, Economo was successful in demonstrating both the presence of the virus in brain tissue as well as its infectious nature.

Actually, this was not the first appearance in history of encephalitis lethargica, but it was the first outbreak on such a global and worldwide scale. Outbreaks of a disease with similar symptoms had appeared in 1672, 1673, and 1674 in and around London. In 1675 Dr. Thomas Sydenham described his standard treatment for such an illness, which he called "febris comatosa."

> Even when bad treatment has brought on a brain fever, and the brain fever has become so obstinate that it cannot be got rid of at once (it being unsafe to attempt to cure it by bleeding beyond the limits described, and by purges), it will at its own good time go away under the aforesaid regimen. To promote this there is nothing like shaving the head. This I always order; neither do I lay on a

plaster. I only recommend a little cap to make up for the hair that has been shaved off, and just to keep off the external cold. By these means the brain is much refreshed and restored, so that by slow degrees it overcomes those hot impressions that excite frenzies. ["Schedula Monitoria," p. 197]

Throughout the 1700 and 1800s there continued to be episodic outbreaks in Germany (1712), Italy (1889), and elsewhere of a neurological disease whose clinical profile seems to suggest encephalitis lethargica. But from 1916 until 1927 the disease became pandemic, and nearly five million died before the siege was finally over.

Of those infected with the virus, nearly 40 percent died of the disease itself. In those who recovered, however, there was a flatness, a sense of intellectual exhaustion which often remained with them for the rest of their lives. Still others, however, showed no aftereffects of the illness for nearly fifty years until they reached the age of sixty or seventy and then were diagnosed with Parkinson's disease. Such a person was Friedrich Schwarz.

The curious and misunderstood connection between a virus in one's youth and the shaking palsy in one's old age was suspected but not established until quite recently. For example, Sir William Osler in *The Principles and Practice of Medicine* suggested such a connection in 1892. "In some instances the disease has followed directly upon severe mental shock or trauma. Cases have been described after the specific fevers. Malaria is believed by some to be an important factor, but of this there is no satisfactory evidence" (p. 926).

Today, the relationship between encephalitis lethargica and Parkinsonian syndromes is well established, and the following text from *Brain's Clinical Neurology* (1973) is typical of this acceptance.

During the epidemic of encephalitis lethargica (1916–1926), Parkinsonism sometimes developed acutely, or within a year or two of the acute illness. Since the greatest incidence of that disease was in early adult life, for many years after the epidemic most patients with encephalitic Parkinsonism were under the age of 40. This, however, is no longer true, but it is probable that most cases occur-

ring before the age of 40 are examples of encephalitic Parkinsonism. [Bannister, p. 249]

Oliver Sacks, in one of the most authoritative and perhaps
elegant books written on Parkinson's disease in this century,
devotes an entire section to sleeping sickness and its relationship to the Parkinsonian symptoms that might appear ten,
twenty, thirty, forty, or even fifty years later.

> Nearly half the survivors became liable to extraordinary crises, in
> which they might experience, for example, the simultaneous and
> virtually instantaneous onset of Parkinsonism, catatonia, tics, ob-
> sessions, hallucinations, "block," increased suggestibility or nega-
> tivism, and thirty or forty other problems; such crises would last a
> few minutes or hours, and then disappear as suddenly as they had
> come. . . . Not infrequently a single, sensational moment-of-being
> is "caught" by a crisis, and preserved thereafter. Thus Jelliffe
> (1932) alludes to a man whose first oculogyric crisis came on dur-
> ing a game of cricket, when he had suddenly to fling one hand up
> to catch a high ball (he had to be carried off the field still entranced,
> with his right arm still outstretched and clutching the ball). [*Awak-
> enings*, pp. 18–19]

Economo once compared the Parkinson patient to an "ex-
tinct volcano," and it certainly makes sense to do so. Resting in
silent slumber for years on end, the malevolent virus works like
a thief in the night to do its damage. One is reminded of those
termites which burrow into the darkest, deepest recesses of
wood to devour and decay the pulpy substance while leaving a
thin, imaginary covering of solidity and health on the surface.
One day, however, the system strains, the support bends, and
the wood breaks in the center to reveal a rotted hull of damage
beyond repair. It takes time—indeed, it takes years—for such
a catastrophe to happen, but when it does, the damage is absolute.

III

Deep within the protective insulation of the brain, there rests
a small structure no larger than a thin strip called the substantia nigra. It is what it appears to be, and that is essentially a

small, black body or substance. The pigmentation of the cells comes from their heavy concentration of melanin—a polymer of indole 5, 6-quinone, and 2-carboxylic acid that darkens in the skin when exposed to sunlight—which is missing in the substantia nigra of the Parkinson patient. But the size of the structure is astonishingly outranked by its importance, for within the slender anatomy and physiology of this black body rest the secrets of calm, integrated movements, of steady hands and perfect poise, of dignity and grace, of balance, equilibrium and symmetry, of easy flexible smiles and warm unfrozen faces.

To disturb or destroy the delicate aspects of the substantia nigra is to risk holocaust and disaster on a scale that the body is ill equipped to handle. All the tremors, palsies, shakes, gyrations, frozen movements, and awkward shuffles of Parkinsonism will erupt like a volcano should this sleeping structure be disturbed. Weighing less than an ounce, it has the power to rock and shake hundreds of pounds for dozens of years and ceases its endless vibrations only when the body dies, at last insensitive to the bizarre and mismanaged commands.

James Parkinson, an English physician who lived from 1755 to 1824, first described the syndrome and symptomatology of the disease named after him in the early 1800s. But it was nearly another hundred years, in 1917, before Economo drew a connection between patients with a history of encephalitis lethargica who later developed Parkinsonism and damage to the substantia nigra. A number of other researchers—including J. G. Greenfield, an English neuropathologist who lived from 1884 to 1958—confirmed this finding within the next several years through autopsy and tissue samples. The final piece of evidence was supplied in the 1920s when it was realized that the substantia nigra played a role in maintaining chemical syntheses by means of its anatomical structure. Accordingly, structural damage to this black body caused corresponding functional imbalances in brain chemistry.

Anatomically, the substantia nigra lies within the midbrain, or mesencephalon. This whole area is sometimes called the isthmus cerebri because it acts as a connecting link between the pons Varolii and the cerebral hemispheres. If one were to cut or cross section the mesencephalon, the substantia nigra would come into view as a dark, pigmented layer of cells which divides the upper and lower portions of the midbrain into two unequal sections. The larger, rear section is called the tegmentum, while the small forward portion is the crusta, or pes. The lamina of the substantia nigra is curved with the concave portion pointed upward, and it runs from the external lateral groove to the internal oculomotor sulcus (fig. 14.1).

The role of the substantia nigra in human behavior still remains a mystery in many of its more elegant and esoteric functions. Since it lies within the region of the reticular formation, it perhaps contributes to certain important duties of that system such as motor and autonomic functions. Moreover, it is also known that the reticular activating system plays an important role in consciousness, sleep, wakefulness, and general awareness. In animal studies, stimulation of this general area

Fig. 14.1 Transverse section of the midbrain. Adapted from Frank H. Netter, *The Nervous System,* vol. 1 of *The CIBA Collection of Medical Illustrations* (Summit, N.J.: CIBA Pharmaceutical Co., 1962), p. 69.

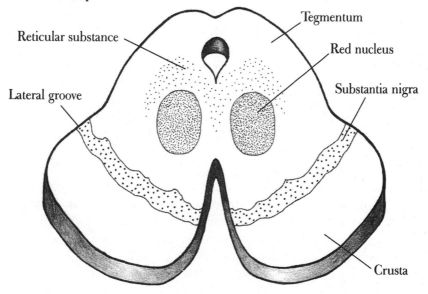

will lead to arousal reactions, and it is known that cells within the reticular formation's nuclei are especially sensitive to anesthetics. The Soviet neuropsychologist A. R. Luria explains some of these activities in *The Working Brain*.

> It was shown that besides the activating portions of the reticular formation, it also has inhibiting portions. Accordingly, whereas stimulation of certain nuclei of the reticular formation invariably led to activation of the animal, stimulation of its other nuclei led to changes characteristic of sleep in the electrical activity of the cortex, and to the development of sleep itself. This fact, as observations showed, applies equally to the brain of animals and man; that is why, when the Soviet surgeon Burdenko stimulated the wall of the third ventricle during neurosurgical operations, a state of sleep was induced artificially in the patient on the operating table. [p. 52]

The Italian neurophysiologist Giuseppe Moruzzi was the first researcher to show that stimulation of the midbrain's reticular activating system in the sleeping cat could control the sleep and arousal patterns of the animal. In collaboration with Horace Magoun, he published his results in a classic paper titled "Brainstem Reticular Formation and Activation of the EEG" in the first volume of the journal *Electroencephalography and Clinical Neurophysiology*. In their study, the EEG pattern was the same whether the cat was awakened by electrode stimulation or in a normal way by a loud sound. Mark and Ervin report a wide range of responses from active rage to utter passivity in the cat by stimulating various regions of this midbrain area. Stimulation, for example, "in a wide area in the limbic brain of an awake and freely moving cat with implanted electrodes turns the animal into a Halloween cat—its back arches, it growls and spits, its hair bristles, and its pupils widen. . . . Cats so stimulated have attacked rats, other cats, large dogs, teddy bears, and experimenters" (*Violence and the Brain*, p. 30). Whatever role the substantia nigra plays in human behavior, it would appear to involve complex and sophisticated mechanisms that have important emotional and intellectual overtones. Indeed, the cognitive and affective deficits in Parkinson's disease are highly suggestive of midbrain disorders. Oliver Sacks—who dedicated *Awakenings* to A. R. Luria—describes such patients. "They would be conscious and aware— yet not fully awake; they would sit motionless and speechless all day in their chairs, totally lacking energy, impetus, initiative, motive, appetite, affect or desire; they registered what went on about them without active attention, and with profound indifference" (p. 14). But what role physiologically and neurochemically does the substantia nigra play in brain function? The answer to that question took over sixty years to answer, from Sherrington's hypothesis of the synapse in 1906 to Cotzias's therapeutic administration of L-dopa in 1967.

The English neurophysiologist Sir Charles Sherrington (1857–1952) was nearly ninety-five when he died. At the time of his death, he was acknowledged to be the most important figure in neurology during the past century and perhaps in the history of the field. He shared the Nobel Prize in 1932 with Edgar Adrian for their work on the function of neurons; he was teacher and friend to all of the great figures in neurology including Harvey Cushing and Wilder Penfield; and there was not an area of neurology to which he did not make a major contribution. In 1906 he published a remarkable book titled *The Integrative Action of the Nervous System.* In this work he argued against the accepted neuron theory and in favor of his claim that the nervous system actually consists of discontinuous cells that communicate with one another across a gap, or what he called a synapse. It had been argued by such greats as Golgi and Bielschowsky that neurons were much like blood vessels in that there were long, continuous lengths in which cells were connected together like the wires of a cable. Indeed, empirical and anatomical evidence on large nerves such as the vagus nerve seemed to make the point obvious and a matter of common sense. Sherrington's formulation, however, went entirely against such claims by arguing that nerve cells do not connect with one another and indeed do not even meet. Rather, they communicate across the synapic gap or bridge by means of certain chemical transmitters called neurotransmitters. To make matters even more incredible, Sherrington did not make his claim on the basis of microscopic or observational evidence but rather simply by comparing data from neurophysiological studies on nerve trunks with neurobehavioral data from reflex actions. He was absolutely right, and since that time we have discovered dozens of different types and kinds of neurotransmitters including acetylcholine, epinephrine, and a number of biogenic amines. These neurotransmitters are released by small buds or vesicles at the end of nerve axons and flow across the neural synapse, thereby continuing the nerve's transmission on the other side (fig. 14.2).

But what if the transmitter or transmitters are destroyed, or their chemical structure is damaged? Should that be the case, the message may be either not relayed at all or transmitted in a garbled and distorted form. Given the delicate nature

Fig. 14.2 Typical synapses. Adapted from Ernest Gardner, *Fundamentals of Neurology* (Philadelphia: W. B. Saunders CO., 1968), p. 69.

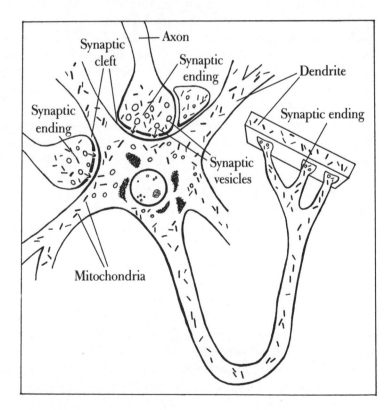

of the midbrain's anatomy, such physiological and chemical possibilities might well spell disaster, and that was exactly what Cotzias in 1967 hypothesized happened in Parkinson's disease. There had been claims as early as 1960 by researchers like Horykiewicz that damage to the substantia nigra created metabolic problems in the production and transport of the neurotransmitter dopamine, but it was Cotzias who actually discovered a method of administering L-dopa so that it could pass the otherwise impenetrable blood-brain barrier.

L-dopa is manufactured under a variety of names including Bendopa, Larodopa, and Dopar. These drugs are not dopamine itself but synthetic variations of levodopa (laevodihydroxyphenylalanine), which is the natural precursor of dopamine. Its effect is merely to give symptomatic relief; it does not correct or reverse any of the structural damage already done to the substantia nigra. Moreover, it is effective in only about half of the patients who use it and, as Oliver Sacks documents so well in *Awakenings*, often produces unexpected and unpredictable results in different patients. Its advantages are that it can relieve some of the tremors, instability in walking, rigidity, and bradykinesia. But its drawbacks and side effects run the gamut from nausea through duodenal ulcer to cardiac irregularities and even an exaggeration of Parkinsonian symptoms. Rose R. is a remarkable example of the drug's ironic qualities. She was a charming woman—indeed, when Harold Pinter wrote the play *A Kind of Alaska* based upon Sacks's *Awakenings*, he was charmed enough by Rose to make her one of the principal characters—who was placed on several L-dopa regimens from 1969 to 1972. At first, the drug had astonishing results, but then she began to run into crisis after crisis, and Sacks finally concluded that "she is a Sleeping Beauty whose awakening was unbearable to her, and who will never be woken again" (p. 79). There is no cure for Parkinson's disease, and at best the medications available are palliative measures that relieve the appearance but not the fact of the disease.

IV

Friedrich Schwarz experienced the thick, tight, tense claustrophobia of his own body as a suffocating force which threatened to drown him with its inertia. Imagine being locked into a dark, damp closet so small that you cannot even move your arms sufficiently to break the seals of sweat that weld together armpits, groin, legs, toes, and fingertips. One feels as if a thick, gelatinous glue were clinging to every ribbing of flesh, sticking the skin together into sweating pockets. You try to stretch here or there and you hope to break this seal or that, but nothing works. Finally, you go so nearly mad with the damned, greasy, wet suck and sweat of the whole matter that even death would be better than this rigid claustrophobia. And yet death is not an escape that you can readily manage with this frozen, rigid torso which moves like a rusted suit of armor.

He hated what he had become. He hated himself and his degradation, but especially he hated the look of pity in the eyes of his wife. A man—any man, but especially a proud man— needs to be able to do certain things. He needs to be able to hold his wife and love her; he needs to have strength to defend her; and he needs to open doors for her, lift things too heavy for her, carry things she should not carry, and be the foundation of their relationship. Friedrich could do none of these things. He had once been able to do so. But he could not anymore. He had become a burden, an invalid and he was no longer a husband but an aging, sick, disgusting child.

It had happened so gradually and subtly that one day it seemed he was well and the next gravely ill; one day he was young with a strong, supple body and the next he was an old, old man with rusted, rigid limbs; one day he could feel the power of being a man and the next he was a wasted crater of disaster and disease who walked with the dying crunch of a mortally wounded animal. What in the hell had happened? He wanted to know. He needed to know. Damn it, he at least had the right to know what the hell had happened.

What happened? Dear Friedrich, do you really wish to know? Can you stand to know the truth?

Then so be it!

For what happened within your sleeping body while it rested, while it pleasured itself in lovemaking with Bess, while you worked, and while you laughed is not for the tame of heart to hear or for the sorrowful to learn. It is bitter truth drawn from the bowels of an indifferent universe, and it may crush your illusions of what is right and wrong about the way you lived your life. For this is a story of defeat, of decay and degradation, of slow death and disintegration. But you have asked, and therefore you shall be answered.

As soon as the outward symptoms of your sleeping sickness disappeared some fifty years ago, the virus that caused them bore deep within your fevered brain, and there it slumbered and fasted, awoke with famished tongue to feed itself, and slumbered and fasted once again. Safe within the dense coils of pinkish-gray brain tissue, it hibernated in this unusually warm and fragrant jungle of neuroglia for years on end. Consuming the fruits that abounded on that dark island of brain substance called the substantia nigra, it lived like a recluse in shy retirement. But while it slept, it also lived and bore its young, devoured tender morsels of your brain, nursed its generations upon your flesh, and so exhausted the food that sanctified it. Meanwhile, Friedrich, you died a little each hour and each day that it lived within you, but you did so in the quietest of ways. There was no pain, bleeding, headache, or swollen tissues to betray the terrible destruction being done. A tremor here or a rippling of muscle there might have warned you had you been aware, but you were not. These are subtle matters which become apparent only when it is too late and the damage is beyond recall.

The first outward signs of your disease began to appear nearly fifteen years ago. By this time, the production of dopamine in your brain had been slowly diminishing for years until now there was such a scant supply that its effects were becoming noticeable. Your right hand started to twitch and tremble when it was at rest, but the slow palsied motions may have been so minute that even the slightest movement disturbed and masked their visibility. Therefore, they chose the night to make their fateful appearance when you and Bess were sleeping. Nor did she notice your smile grow strained and stationary while all the muscles of your face froze their tension into a flat, smooth mask which stared without expression. Slowly the blinking rate per second of your eyes was cut in half and then in quarters until finally you did not look but rather vacantly gazed instead. Meanwhile, the tensile strength of your lips weakened and that firm, masculine jaw line began to sink and sag while the parting lips fell open in a drooling expression of dumbfounded confusion. Neither did you notice your leg begin to drag behind you and your walk become a shuffling gait instead. Meanwhile, the forefinger and thumb of your right hand flexed inward and started an endless rolling shake as if you held therein a pill which you continually rolled upon its circumference. All of these movements were slow and methodical—as is the disease itself—unless you became excited or embarrassed, and then the tremors accelerated, the palsy increased, the pill rolled faster, and what had been subtle was now exhibitionistic in the most undistinguished and flagrant sense.

When you walked it was as a lead pipe rolls with stiff, unbending motions that refuse grace, measure, and poise. There was a mechanical catch and jump to your upper body which resembled a cogwheel drive as it ratchets from one metal space to the next and moves with an interrupted spacing which is neither smooth nor even in execution. Soon it was difficult to walk at all, and each beginning step was hesitant, prolonged, and tentative until sheer momentum supplied what your willpower lacked. You bent more gradually to the ground as do birds when they peck or animals when they paw. So equipped with this body of stony immobility, you shuffled and scuffed across the floor and not infrequently became stuck between destinations like a windup toy that has simply run down.

Your speech also slowed to a hesitant slurring which lost pitch and cadence to become a monotonous, soft rumbling which occasionally jumbled words and intonations into a mismanaged word salad. Others could barely hear you, and they concentrated less on what you said and more on your desperate attempts to say it. As time went on, the effort simply grew out of proportion to the reward, and it was easier to remain silent. And so you did.

Locked more and more deeply into yourself, you fell through that center axis which connects us to others, and so resting deep within yourself you floated in a somnolent and solipsistic universe of your own. Here there are no lights and open places but rather stony margins, plateaus, and rigid cliffs that hem you in and confine your movements on all sides. In this hardened world, all motion is frozen by time, and the simplest tasks unfold in slow-motion mimicry of a more normal, elastic, and fluid reality to which you are now refused access. Your world is a frosty, frozen place of diminished movements that continue to slow day by day.

And yet for all the terrible anguish and claustrophobia of this place, it could be worse. At least, your world is gelatinous and jellified rather than being one of bizarre tics, festinations, and propulsions, wild choreiform movements and crazed jerks, jacks, interruptions, and swinging torticollic spasms. You have chosen, Friedrich, a world slowed down rather than one sped up, and your life will end as a slow, moving tortoise finally arriving at its destination rather than as a quick-paced lemming which hurls itself suicidally over a cliff through frenzy and frustration.

15

The Marble Palace

My spirit is too weak; mortality
    Weighs heavily on me like unwilling sleep,
    And each imagined pinnacle and steep
Of godlike hardship tells me I must die
Like a sick eagle looking at the sky.
    Yet 'tis a gentle luxury to weep,
    That I have not the cloudy winds to keep
Fresh for the opening of the morning's eye.
Such dim-conceived glories of the brain
    Bring round the heart an indescribable feud;
So do these wonders a most dizzy pain,
    That mingles Grecian grandeur with the rude
Wasting of old Time—with a billowy main,
    A sun, a shadow of a magnitude.

John Keats
"On Seeing the Elgin Marbles"

HODGKIN'S DISEASE: Hodgkin's disease is a primary neoplasm of lymphoid tissue. The characteristic pathologic findings of Hodgkin's disease distinguish it from the other primary lymphoid tumors, usually called the non-Hodgkin's lymphomas. The disease was first recognized by Thomas Hodgkin in 1832, when he de-

300

scribed seven cases based on their peculiar clinical and gross pathologic findings. Subsequently, only three of Hodgkin's original cases were shown to contain the Reed-Sternberg giant cells now considered necessary to establish the diagnosis. The disease has been of great interest because of its infectious-disease-like symptoms and findings, its epidemiologic characteristics, its associated immunologic abnormalities, and its responsiveness to therapy. A uniformly fatal disorder when first recognized and if untreated, the majority of patients with Hodgkin's disease can now be cured of their neoplasms.

The presenting and subsequent clinical manifestations of patients with Hodgkin's disease can be extremely varied and considerably influenced by the effects of therapy. A common typical presentation is the observation, usually by the patient, of a painless, enlarging mass, most commonly in the neck, but occasionally in the axilla or inguinalfemoral region. Upon examination, this is found to be a discrete, rubbery, painless lymphadenopathy, very often with enlarged lymph nodes in close proximity. In other patients, a chest roentgenogram, taken for unrelated purposes, reveals a moderate or even massive mediastinal enlargement with associated lower cervical lymphadenopathy which was not apparent to the patient. Though these typical presentations may occur at any age for any histopathologic type, these patients are usually between 15 and 35 years of age and have the histologic subtype of nodular sclerosis.

Almost all patients with Hodgkin's disease develop increasingly severe systemic symptoms as their disease progresses beyond control. High continuous fever, severe night sweats, malaise, fatigue, anorexia, and weight loss are all characteristics of the terminal picture of patients with Hodgkin's disease. Generalized pruritus is seen in a proportion of patients during their course.

Calabresi, Schein, and Rosenberg
Medical Oncology

I

San Pietro Patti is a small town on the northern coast of Sicily near the volcanic Mount Etna. It has no industry, houses no government offices, and boasts no wealthy or famous citizens. So small, barren, and poor is this place that it has significance only for the residents and for one man in particular who lives in the northern region of Tuscany. He is Antonino Gentile, who lives near Florence and makes his living as a marble merchant. This most gentle man comes often to San Pietro Patti, making the twelve-hour trip by car or sixteen hours by Rapido express train to sit for hours beside the Carrara marble tomb that he built for his daughter Angelina, and perhaps eventually for himself as well.

Cold to the touch but smooth and slick as glass, this white marble from Carrara is the finest in all the world. It was to Massa-Carrara that Michelangelo came to quarry his stone, as did all the great sculptors of the Florentine Renaissance including Desiderio da Settignano, Benedetto da Maiano, Mino da Fiesole, and Benedetto da Rovezzano. Combing the mountain ranges of the Apuan Alps around Carrara, they searched for gleaming blocks of pure white marble free from veins and cracks. The chunk of stone eventually to become Michelangelo's magnificent David was originally a block of Carrara marble over eighteen feet tall which was loaded onto a barge and floated down the waterways to Florence. Nearly four hundred marble quarries operate out of the Colonnate, Fantiscritti, and Torano valleys, employing most of Carrara's 70,000 residents and Massa's 63,000 citizens. Within these sheer, staggering walls of towering stone there still reside the building blocks of countless churches, government buildings, municipal courts, and whatever else can be made of marble. In one of the hundreds of small cutting and polishing shops that sell marble to consumers around the world, Antonino Gentile has established a business which allows him a new car every two years, a comfortable home, and funds sufficient to support his remaining daughter and her husband and two children. And yet after all these years, he still recalls his sweet Angelina, who now lies brittle and smooth as stone in a marble tomb outside of San Pietro Patti on the northern coast of Sicily.

II

Within the next year, more than eight thousand new cases of Hodgkin's disease will be diagnosed in the United States alone. That figure has been steadily rising over the past few years until now Hodgkin's disease is one of the most prevalent types of cancer in young people, along with the leukemias. It is a disease which prefers males to females, the young to the old, the urban dweller over the rural, the single child to one with many siblings, the more highly educated to the less educated, and has a particularly high incident in young men living in underdeveloped countries. If there are other children in the family, they have a fivefold greater risk of developing the disease, and this figure rises to ninefold if the siblings are of the same sex. The cause of Hodgkin's disease is unknown, but an early history of infectious mononucleosis, appendectomy, or tonsillectomy seems to correlate significantly with later diagnosis of the disease. Whether there is actually an infectious agent present is not certain, but during studies completed in 1981 Gutensohn and Cole found some interesting epidemiological parallels that suggested an infectious pattern similar to paralytic poliomyelitis.

The English physician Thomas Hodgkin—"well known morbid anatomist of Guy's Hospital," as Sir William Osler described him—earned a place in medical history by first presenting seven cases of this lymphoma in 1832. He was greatly aided in formalizing the parameters of the disease by several other prestigious researchers including Wilks, Virchow, Billroth, and Cohnheim. Three of these cases described by Hodgkin demonstrated the presence of the Reed-Sternberg cells that are now considered crucial for a definitive diagnosis (see fig. 15.1). Osler, writing in 1892 in *The Principles and Practice of Medicine*, considered the disease to be always fatal and offered little advice in the manner of treatment except for the palliative administration of arsenic, "which should be stopped where unpleasant effects are manifested," or the use of Fowler's solution three times a day and sometimes phosphorus, "which should be used if the arsenic is not well borne" (p. 750). Today, the grim prophesies of Osler have changed somewhat, but only when the disease is arrested in its early stages.

There is perhaps no truer aphorism applied to medicine than the ancient claim that "qui bene dignoscit, bene curat." Diagnosis is an art, and differential diagnosis is truly genius under stress. Hodgkin's disease may present itself with classical and unequivocal symptomatology, but more frequently it is a malevolent Trojan horse which masquerades in a variety of disguises that often appear trivial, benign, and perfectly innocent.

Instead of pain, discomfort, or other alarming symptoms, there may be nothing more than a simple, localized itching—pruritus—which gradually becomes more severe and more generalized. At first, it seems innocent and insignificant because there are no skin eruptions, lesions, or other irritations, and in young women especially pruritus may be the only systemic symptom present. Perhaps it is only a slight fever which disappears in a few days and does not reappear again for weeks or even months. Or one may awaken in the middle of the night drenched in sweat but feel perfectly fit the following morning. Perhaps it is no more than a slight weight loss—is it the success of a new diet or instead the beginning signs of an ominous disease?—or nothing more than a general listlessness which seems no worse than an early case of spring fever. It is nothing in particular but everything in general, and one is confused about these diffuse symptoms which seem meaningless taken one by one but collectively are the signature of an illness faintly written.

One patient was driving to a local beauty contest when she noticed in the rearview mirror a small lump on her neck. It was so small that only in reflected light was the rounded nodule visible. Another young woman felt a swollen gland at work one day and thought no more about it until the rubbery painless mass continued to enlarge and she consulted her family doctor. Biopsy showed a discrete lymphadenopathy although she had no other presenting symptoms. Then there was the teenager who noticed a "couple of rocks" in his neck one day while driving his truck to school and was brought to a surgeon by his alarmed parents. Actually, he had known about the "rocks" for nearly a month but didn't think they were very important.

Hodgkin's disease is subtle, secretive, and even shy about disclosing itself. But once it decides to come out of the closet, it does so with fury and vengeance. A Notre Dame football player felt fine until he went to visit his girlfriend one weekend and doubled over in pain so severe that the frightened girl's family had him admitted to a local hospital; X rays revealed a massive mediastinal enlargement. A variety of complex diagnostic devices including bone marrow and liver biopsies, lymphography, and even exploratory surgery such as laparotomy may be necessary in order to arrive at a diagnosis. There have even been some cases of Hodgkin's disease that successfully eluded identification until autopsy. It is not merely that the symptoms are multiple, subtle, and episodic; the delicate balance of remissions and acute attacks orchestrates to produce a medical puzzle which only a sleuth or logician can finally penetrate with the arm of reason.

III

She wanted to be a doctor. When her parents moved back to Italy from the United States, she seized the opportunity and enrolled at once in medical school at the Università di Roma. Did she perhaps already sense the stirrings of some disaster within her and hope to learn enough to cure herself? Who can say? She said that she wanted to help the sick and dying but perhaps did not realize at the time that she was one of them.

With a quick intelligence and a strong memory for details and facts, Angelina easily consumed the endless pages of the anatomy and physiology texts. By the end of the first semester, she had received almost perfect marks in every subject and was known as a special student by her professors. The second semester was nearly completed when she traveled to Massa to spend the Easter vacation with her parents. She knew that she was tired, and she looked it, but everyone is exhausted by the end of the first year of medical school, and she thought no more about it. By the end of the year, however, she was so utterly exhausted that for nearly a week it was impossible to do much more than sleep and recuperate.

Earlier in the month she had come down with her third cold since January, and perhaps the fever, swollen glands, and general listlessness only contributed to her exhausted condition. It is impossible to say which caused which and whether she was sick because she was exhausted or exhausted because she was sick. She presented such an alarming picture to her parents upon arriving in Massa that summer that they both insisted she see Dr. Scollini at once. She did. He was not alarmed, for he remembered his own first year in medical school at Università di Messina; he prescribed plenty of bed rest, sunshine, some broad-based antibiotics, and, of course, a distraction from medical textbooks.

By week's end most of the symptoms were gone and she felt much better. The low-grade fever still persisted and the still tender swollen glands ached at night enough to awaken her sometimes, but she decided to just forget the whole matter, put it out of her mind, and see how she felt in a month's time.

Sometimes she would wake in the middle of the night, and drenched in sweat while aching at her neck and groin, she would get out of bed to walk about the moonlit grounds. Around the villa her father had built a high fence which provided seclusion as well as protection, and within she would stroll in bare feet to feel the soft grass upon her toes. She was a romantic, this Angelina, and she dreamed of grand and glorious things such as finding a man who was as gentle and kind as her father but as brilliant and successful as she hoped to be. With the exasperated impatience of youth, she wanted everything and she wanted it at once. Within the hour, she would be back in bed, exhausted by her dreams and exertions to fall to sleep once again in restless fits.

She was not getting better, and by June she knew that she was ill, perhaps even desperately so. The sweating, sleepless nights continued, but to this disturbance were added other symptoms. For instance, she began to itch at night and even sometimes during the day. But it was an odd, discontinuous itching which seemed diffuse, with no localized point or place to scratch relief. And then there was the fever that she thought had gone nearly a week ago but now was back again. It was not high and it was not even apparent unless she took her temperature, but now she was alarmed enough to check her temperature every day. And every day there the fever was again. She had tried to forget the whole affair, thinking it was just her hypochondriacal nature, and so two nights before she had agreed to go out with a boy who asked her to a dance. They stopped for some wine on the way home, and after just one glass she became violently ill with pain such as she had never known before. But most important—and this her mother had noticed with alarm—was her weight loss. At first it was a few pounds and then a few pounds more, but with a frame that looked right at 123 pounds, she had already dropped to 112 in a matter of weeks.

When her chest began to ache and she had some trouble speaking, Angelina knew that the symptoms could no longer be ignored. Her parents were alarmed enough to agree immediately when she suggested a complete physical at one of the surrounding hospitals. The nearest and the best was the Hospital of Santa Maria della Scala at Siena, seventy kilometers south and still within the Tuscany province. And so there it was that her parents took her one mercilessly warm day in July.

Hospitals in Italy are a strange confusion of bureaucracy and compassion born out of socialized medicine and the Italian's natural desire to help anyone in distress. The patient is often delivered over to a system of benevolent inefficiency in which it truly can be said that "obscurum per obscurius" prevails. Scheduled appointments, tests, diagnostic routines, and even operations all occur accordingly to approximate timetables that are followed only in an approximate way. One may complain, become angry, irritable, and outraged, but such behavior is fruitless and merely elicits a helpless shrug of powerless commiseration on the part of the offending official. So it was with Angelina Gentile.

A room was supposed to be waiting for her, but it was not ready until three days later. When she was finally ready for her tests to begin, she was told that Dr. Trupallino had already left that afternoon for an extended weekend and nothing could be done until Tuesday. They protested; it did no good. Nothing could be done until Tuesday. Tuesday, he decided to stay another day and would not be back in the hospital until Wednesday, when the Gentiles were assured that the tests would begin. They did. It was worth the wait, for Antonino Trupallino, M.D., was an eminently qualified hematologist who had studied at Rome, Harvard, and the Sloan-Kettering Institute under the immunologist Bob Good before returning to his hometown of Siena. He spoke the perfect, flawless, and elegant Italian that only Florentines can speak, and his English was nearly as good. Moreover, he was kind, generous, and expansive in his gracious manners as only the cultured Italian can be. The Gentiles felt fortunate in finding such a doctor and—being Italian themselves—could quickly forgive inconveniences if asked to do so in a courteous and courtly manner.

Trupallino already had a hunch about the diagnosis as soon as he read the records sent from Massa by Dr. Scollini. It was not the swollen glands or the night sweats that bothered him, but three factors that stood out in contrast to all the other symptoms. First, the Pel-Epstein pattern of fever with several days of high fever and then an unexplained period of normal temperature before the fever returned once again. He had seen this pattern in countless other cases at Sloan-Kettering, and it had proved to be one important diagnostic that he saw recurrent in Hodgkin's disease. Second, the curious incident with the wine, which brought Angelina such pain that she recalled the matter weeks later to her doctor. Finally, there was the generalized itching—the pruritus—that had originally awakened her in the middle of the night and had grown worse over the last few weeks. Taken individually, none of these symptoms was definitive of anything and especially not of Hodgkin's disease, which is difficult enough to diagnose even in its classic forms. But taken collectively and in constellation with her swollen glands, her mediastinal pain, her voice difficulties—which suggested some involvement of the recurrent laryngeal nerve—and her history of infections, they pointed to a pattern that spelled out Hodgkin's disease like a magnet arranging discordant iron filings into polar divisions.

The definitive factor would be the presence of the giant Reed-Sternberg cells in a blood sample. The pale cytoplasm of these cells contains one or two large nuclei with chromatin clumping and deep, acidophilic nucleoli (fig. 15.1). So important is the presence of this finding that a truly definitive diagnosis of Hodgkin's disease is lacking without it. The cells appear against a background of other mixed cell types but stand out in contrast due to the transparent zone around the huge nucleolus and the spherical nucleolus whose margins are smooth with homogeneous eosinophilic staining behavior.

Oddly, it is only when lymphocytic depletion occurs that

the Reed-Sternberg cells appear to be numerous. Otherwise, their appearance is rare and uncommon in lymphocytic proliferation. Moreover, these cells—or ones at least that are visually indistinguishable from them—occur in other conditions as well such as infectious mononucleosis. But this did not appear to be mononucleosis, and even without the blood workups, Trupallino was certain what the findings would be.

By Friday afternoon they had enough information available to confirm Hodgkin's disease advanced to at least stage II and possibly stage III. By stage III, the disease has affected both sides of the diaphragm and usually affected the spleen as well. Stage II is limited to lymph nodes on one side of the diaphragm alone, but the distinction was really academic in Angelina's case, for if she was not in stage III at present she would be within the next week. In short, Angelina Gentile was desperately ill with cancer of the lymphatic system and in a very advanced stage of the illness.

IV

There are no conservative approaches to a disease such as Hodgkin's. An aggressive combination of chemotherapy and radiotherapy must be instituted as soon as possible. Depending upon the stage of the disease, the remission rate may be as high as 95 percent or lower than 50 percent, and in stage III the

Fig. 15.1 Reed-Sternberg giant cells

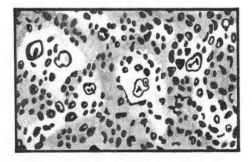

figure is somewhere in the 60 percent range. Angelina was in stage III, and her chances of recovery were about 60 to 40 depending upon a host of different factors.

She was given radiotherapy of 4,000 rads for three weeks' time as well as combination chemotherapy. This course of treatments followed the MOPP program developed at the National Cancer Institute by DeVita and co-workers in 1970. The program makes use of mechlorethamine (nitrogen mustard), Oncovin (vincristine), procarbazine, and prednisone administered in combination of two-week courses for six cycles. Between each cycle of treatment, there intervenes a two-week rest period. The recommended treatment cycle is shown in figure 15.2. In 1980 DeVita published fifteen-year follow-up studies of his MOPP program that showed remission rates of

Fig. 15.2 MOPP chemotherapy for Hodgkin's disease The original combination chemotherapy for patients with advanced Hodgkin's disease, MOMP, consisted of drug combinations of mechlorethamine, Oncovin, methotrexate, and prednisone administered for two-and-a-half months. This program was modified in 1964; the regimen period was extended from two-and-a-half months to six months; and procarbazine replaced methotrexate. Adapted from Vincent T. Devita, Jr., and Stephen Rosenberg, *Cancer: Principles and Practice of Oncology* (Philadelphia: Lippincott, 1985).

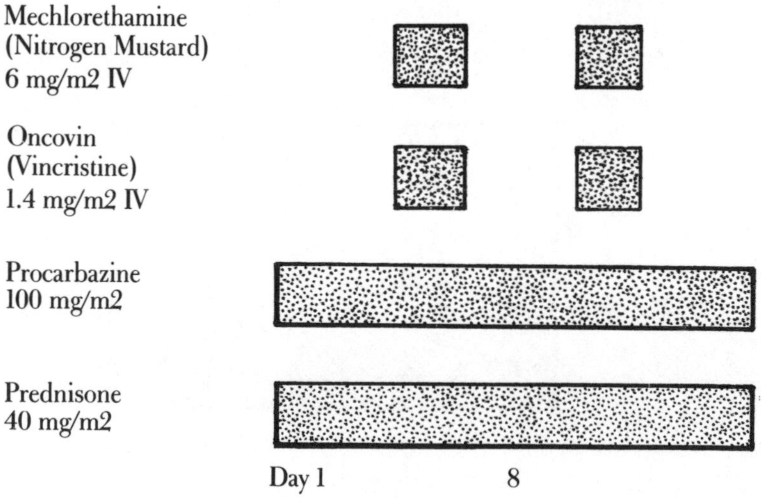

Mechlorethamine
(Nitrogen Mustard)
6 mg/m2 IV

Oncovin
(Vincristine)
1.4 mg/m2 IV

Procarbazine
100 mg/m2

Prednisone
40 mg/m2

Day 1   8

80 percent for patients in stage III and stage IV of the disease. Of these, 68 percent remained in remission for the next ten years. Relapse for the first year after treatment is high, with declining incidences over the next four years; and remission at the five-year level is considered a "cure" of the disease.

The chemotherapeutic program was not pleasant for Angelina, and she began to show signs of toxicity within the first few days. She immediately became nauseated and for nearly three days could hold nothing down. Then, at just about the time that she adjusted to the continual bouts of vomiting, she discovered that her hair was beginning to fall out. She had been told to expect this, but in a young woman gifted with abundant, luxurious hair it was still not easy to accept. Actually, it seemed to be one thing after the other. By the end of the month, she knew that she had missed her period, but she also knew that she was not pregnant. The doctor confirmed that this was probably another side effect of the medication, but he had not mentioned it since not all patients have the problem. In the end, however, it all seemed to be too much since her glands were still swollen, she was still losing weight and having night sweats with fever, and the chemotherapy was simply exhausting her. In short, she now had all the symptoms of Hodgkin's disease as well as these new symptoms of chemical toxicity.

Some treatments are worse than the disease they are intended to cure, and cancer therapy seems to be a remarkable case in point. One of the things people fear the most about cancer is the manner in which it degrades and deforms the grace, beauty, and appearance of the person. But hair loss, nausea, weakness, and various necrotic skin processes are less symptoms of cancer and more signs of chemical and radiation toxicity. Perhaps the day will come when cancer can be treated in some manner besides cutting, burning, poisoning, and radiating the person who suffers from it. There remains so much that is medieval, superstitious, and absolutely ineffective about these treatments that every cancer patient must seriously weigh the benefits of death to those of disease. Table 15.1 shows some of the side effects of prednisone, mechlorethamine, vincristine, and procarbazine. No wonder she felt sick. Moreover, consider the fact that Angelina was not taking just

Table 15.1. Side effects of chemotherapy

Prednisone	*Vincristine*
Congestive heart failure	Nausea
Hypertension	Weakness
Loss of muscle mass	Convulsions
Ulcerative esophagitis	Numbness
Pancreatitis	Vomiting
Pathological fractures	Depression
Thin fragile skin	Neuritis
Osteoporosis	Pharyngitis
Convulsions	Pain
Facial erythema	Headaches
Impaired wound healing	Enterocolitis
Hemorrhage	Loss of reflexes
Petechiae	Anorexia
Increased sweating	Hair loss
Abdominal distension	Sensory loss
Headaches	Paresthesia
Menstrual irregularities	Slapping gait
Glaucoma	Muscle wasting
Psuedo-tumor cerebri	Leukopenia
Latent diabetes	
Peptic ulcer	

Mechlorethamine	*Procarbazine*
Vomiting	Leukopenia
Herpes zoster (Shingles)	Anemia
Amenorrhea	Petechiae
Petechiae	Insomnia
Hemorrhage	Nightmares
Deafness	Delirium
Tinnitus	Coma
Secondary malignancies	Fever
Oral ulcerations	Pruritus
Hemorrhagic cystitis	Infertility
Pulmonary fibrosis	Hair loss
Jaundice	Tremors
Clot formations	Footdrop
Darkening of skin	Psychosis
Bone marrow depression	
Anemia	

one of these drugs but all four and also undergoing radiation treatment. She was not getting well. In fact, she was getting much worse.

By the end of the summer, some of her symptoms were in control, but others were not. For example, her high fevers continued, she lost more weight, and she rarely slept through the night without waking in a cold, drenching sweat. But now there was a new problem in addition to these unresolved ones. She began to have neurological symptoms that were being caused by an epidural mass compressing the spinal cord. On August 17 it was decided that an operation was necessary in order to prevent further neurological damage and possibly paralysis. The operation was performed on August 24, and the pressure on the cord was temporarily relieved. The question, however, was whether there would be a recurrence of the lesions and also whether the tissue would properly heal given her general condition and the number of chemotherapeutic agents she was receiving.

By the end of September, there was evidence of new spinal compression from additional spinal masses, and the incision from the first surgical intervention had still failed to heal. Meanwhile, she had already had significant muscle and sensory loss in her lower extremities and could no longer maintain control of her sphincter. The epidural space that had been opened by surgery was now exposed to infection, and with her lowered resistance a number of small spinal epidural abscesses began to form in and about the area.

Angelina—beautiful, bright, and happy Angelina—was dying, and there was nothing that could save her. She accepted this fact long before her parents did and even before Dr. Trupallino could bring himself to realize that he had failed his patient. But one knows when one is dying, and despite the best defenses that we provide, it is impossible to hide the truth from ourselves. Actually she had sensed the revolt and resignation of her body weeks before but wanted to protect her parents from a fact that she accepted but knew they could not. She had never been afraid of death; she was simply afraid of abandoning her parents. But now the pretense could no longer be maintained, and it was insane to believe that the inevitable could be prevented by more of Trupallino's hideous medications or her mother's fantasied and reassured hopes that each day she looked better when, in fact, each day she looked worse.

It was therefore with relieved resignation and accepting despair that the Gentile family bundled their daughter up one day in early October and brought her home to the stone and stucco villa outside the city limits of Massa. The ambulance made the trip from Siena in less than two hours, and the two handsome young men—nearly her own age and possible suitors in any other situation—carefully brought the stretcher down the ramp and across the yard to enter the back door of the house. It was the first time in months that she had been out of the hospital, and it was a beautiful, sunlight day such as only Italy in early October can truly experience.

Her hair was thinned to bare ribbons and strands hung upon the anemic white flesh; she was thin and wasted and pale as a ship beached upon the shore, and she shivered with cold on that hot and humid day. The grass was as verdant green as springtime in England, with that rich saturation of color which never leaves the Italian countryside even in winter months. She wanted to be lowered down to the ground and allowed to lie there on the grass for just a moment, perhaps one of the last moments that she would ever have to do so. Such a request— in one so desperately ill—would have been refused in anyone with even a chance of recovery. To Angelina, however, it was instantly granted, for no one had any illusions that she could be wounded more mortally than she already had been.

For a few blessed moments she lay there in the splendor of the grass pretending that she was alone or with a lover and then smashed the fantasy with the resigned wave of an exasperated hand and was taken inside to darkness and to death. The next few weeks were the worst of the entire illness, and she paid more mercilessly for those few moments of blissful splendor in the grass. Chills and torrential tremors of pain, anguish, and fever raked her body back and forth over the dying embers of her disease until finally there was nothing left for her to feel and no pain terrible enough to pierce the tough hide of dying flesh that surrounded her. She was nearly paralyzed from the chest down, and by the end of the week she was practically blind as well. By the end of the next week, she took nourishment and eliminated through a series of plastic tubes mounted upon her bed. Daily her family would come to visit, and sometimes she would recognize them and sometimes she would not.

From the bedroom door she hardly looked human to her older sister Maria. And Maria—who worked for years as a nurse—had seen enough of disease and death not to be easily shocked. But now before her she saw a sack of whitened skin and bones seemingly tied together with tubes and living only as do sea creatures that anchor their spineless bodies to heavy rocks for support and then suck nourishment from the water around them, all the while passively weaving back and forth with each new oceanic wave and current. A blind, unthinking, unfeeling, dumb creature she had become, now reduced to merely the place of congregation for the misshapen tumors that crowded about her body. She endured a pain which she could no longer understand and had not even the strength left to protest the outrage of such an ungenerous, ungrateful, and undeserved fate.

When she finally died on October 27, it was as flowers do. The blossoms simply fell from their petals and wasted away. It was nearly an event of celebration while also being the most awesome disaster the family had ever suffered. The pain was unbearable; her loss was incomprehensible, and they refused it at the very same moment that they were most grateful for it. It had been nearly seven months since that Easter vacation when she first came home exhausted, but Angelina had died weeks before these wasted remains finally agreed to stop breathing. For Angelina, for her mother, and for her sister as well, it was finally finished. But for her father, for Antonino Gentile, it was just beginning. Indeed, for him, it had not even started!

v

The women prepared and cleaned the body, dressed her in a white satin gown, and placed small silk slippers upon her feet. It was a ritual as ancient and old as the Italians themselves; it

315

was women's work to moan and cry while cleansing away the last dry visage of sickness. Meanwhile, her father was engaged in a higher, more sacred and exalted task as he roamed the rich Carrara countryside in search of marble. From a distance he looked like a crazed and demented Michelangelo desperately seeking the stone that would become his David.

To understand Antonino Gentile's fervor, it must be realized with what rapture he worshiped the stone. Those clean, straight-lined surfaces of the white, virginal rock were nearly mystical in symbolic significance for him. Should heaven and hell betray us, should disease and death destroy us, then at least the stone shall still console us. For it has the power to withstand time, erosion, and all the destructive forces of nature. In our hour of greatest suffering—when we have been abandoned by gods and men—the stone will suffice. Its hard, clean lines can neither rot nor decay; its cool chill will never be consumed by fever; and when death challenges the stone, it will be mastered by a substance which cannot die. And so while the women found solace in their tears, Antonino Gentile was comforted by the stone.

The place, time, setting, and arrival of the stone must all be perfect. He would personally attend to this planning as precisely as a priest arranges the instruments of the Eucharist. For days on end, he combed and searched the Fantiscritti valley looking for just the right angle and natural cut of virgin marble. Finally in despair and desperation, he began moving east while ever widening his search in larger and more elaborate concentric circles. Even to his undirected wanderings, there had to be a partial method else his madness would consume him.

One day, quite by accident, he came to the end of his quest in the quarries of Piastre nearly four miles east of the beginning of his search. At first, he could not be sure that he had found it, but then he was as sure and certain as one is when the heart's desire is finally satisfied. He had found it. It was a triangular block of shining white marble with no veins or interruptions to disturb the sanctity of its surface. It would be difficult to unlodge and recover—given the terrible height and angle of its placing—but well worth every effort and expense. And indeed it was expensive. Four workmen labored nearly a week to extract the reluctant marble, which dug its ivory teeth even more deeply into the massive vein of rock as it was coaxed, beguiled, bullied, cursed, hammered, pulled, and gutted from the safety of its hiding place. Finally, it relented and with absurd passivity slipped into the arms of the steel and leather harness that lifted it loose and free. Loaded onto transport rigs, the stone was taken to Pietrasanta Marina near the port city of Viareggio on the southwest coast of the Tyrrhenian Sea. Traveling now by water, the sacred marble began its pilgrimage down the coastline past Porto San Stefano, Rome, and the Lido di Ostia as well as the three major ports of Naples, weaving in and out the land's curvature to Cetrano and Amantea, and through the straits at Messina where the Tyrrhenian meets the Ionian Sea. Now swinging up to the north, it passed Spadafora, Barcellona, and Pozzo di Gotto to complete its journey at San Pietro Patti on the northern coast of Sicily. Angelina—cold as the stone she will become—had already arrived with her wailing sisters, mother, aunts, and cousins. For the first time—for the very first time since this whole damned despair began—Antonino Gentile is beginning to feel that the universe has ceased its chaotic trembling and started to orbit symmetrically once again.

They worked day and night in shifts of four hours on and four hours off. It was the best they could do. The recumbent marble still carried within it all the lethargy and inertia of its fight and so passively resisted every effort to mold, form, and transform its brittle hardness into the liquid flow of a mausoleum chamber. Throughout Angelina's sickness, her father had sat by helplessly watching the women comfort her and felt impotent at his powerlessness over the universe, death, and the treachery of the illness that consumed her. The Sicilians are a proud and noble race of men who have been conquered and abused so frequently by fate that they have learned to wait for revenge until the appropriate moment. But that moment always comes. It must come, for that is the way of the universe to make compensation for its deficiencies, to right its wrongs, to revenge its injustices. And make no mistake about it: death is unjust and greedy and unmerciful. Even death must be revenged. He would humble its power, destroy its pride by cre-

317

ating a mausoleum for his Angelina that was as magnificent as that of Mausolus, king of Caira, erected by his queen Artemisia in the fourth century B.C. With Donne, he sought to humble death, for "mighty and dreadful . . . thou art not so," and certainly not in battle with the stone.

When the marble palace was finally completed, Angelina was gently, lovingly placed inside by her father. She wore the white satin dress and silk shoes her mother had dressed her in, but this ceremony between Angelina and the stone was witnessed only by her father. Here within these cool marble walls, he was in charge, and it was altogether fitting that he should be afforded the privacy of his domain. He carried her light and fragile body as one would lift a doll and laid her on a center platform of marble carved to resemble a lounging chaise. Carefully, he parted and arranged her hair to fall precisely over the white marble and turned to kiss farewell the white, stark face that already had become as statuesque and alabaster as the stone itself. Then closing the mausoleum doors and locking them against the knockings of death, he withdrew to witness what he had created.

It was a perfectly detailed stone palace in miniature with turrets, rolling arches, block stone walls, and walkways with guard towers attached. But the most amazing thing of all—and that which the residents of San Pietro Patti would never grow tired of talking about—was the hugh stone angel that had draped its submissive and weeping form across the palace as if in mortal bereavement of the contents that lay within. Its enormous alabaster wings seemed to nearly vibrate in stony silence with misery, and one could almost see the arched back heave and fall in exasperated despair. Gazing upon its face with a tearful eye arched to the sun, no one could be mistaken about the most perfect resemblance of that angel's face to Angelina Gentile.

16

The Vegetative Heart

*I am afraid of cities. But you mustn't leave them.
If you go too far you come up against the vegetation
belt. Vegetation has crawled for miles toward the
cities. It is waiting. Once the city is dead, the vegetation will cover it, will climb over the stones, grip
them, search them, make them burst with its long
black pincers; it will blind the holes and let its
green paws hang over everything. You must stay in
the cities as long as they are alive, you must never
penetrate alone this great mass of hair waiting at
the gates; you must let it undulate and crack all by
itself. In the cities, if you know how to take care of
yourself, and choose the times when all the beasts
are sleeping in their holes and digesting, behind
the heaps of organic debris, you rarely come across
anything more than minerals, the least frightening
of all existants.*

Jean-Paul Sartre
Nausea

INFECTIVE ENDOCARDITIS: Subacute "bacterial" endocarditis
(SBE) is a smoldering bacterial infection of the endocardium usu-

ally superimposed on pre-existing rheumatic or calcific valvular or congenital heart disease. Bacteremia following a respiratory infection, dental work or cystoscopy is often the initiating event, but in many instances the source of the infection is not known. Streptococci, especially "Streptococcus viridans" and "S. faecalis" are the usual etiologic agents; straphylococci are occasionally responsible, but virtually any microorganism, including fungi, can cause endocarditis.

Bacteria lodge on the endocardium of valves (usually aortic and mitral) and multiply. Fibrin and platelet thrombi are deposited, forming irregular friable vegetations which break off to give emboli to the brain, peripheral arteries, or viscera. Embolic nephritis or true glomerulonephritis sometimes produces renal failure. Shedding of bacteria into the blood stream from the involved valves may produce mycotic aneurysms which, however, rarely rupture. Active rheumatic carditis may be present, SBE produces mild to moderate systemic symptoms: cerebral, renal, splenic, or mesenteric emboli; heart failure; or any combination of these. The onset usually follows bacteremia from one of the sources cited above within days or weeks.

Acute bacterial endocarditis (ABE) is a rapidly progressive infection of normal or abnormal valves usually developing in the course of heavy bacteremia from acute infections such as staphylococcal sepsis, postabortal pelvic infection, or intravenous injection of narcotics. It may also occur as a complication of cardiac surgery, transurethral prostatectomy, or surgery on infected tissue. Hemolytic staphylococci and candida are prominent causes of endocarditis.

Acute endocarditis produces large, friable vegetations, severe embolic episodes with metastatic abscess formation, and rapid perforation, tearing, or destruction of the affected valves or rupture of chordae tendineae.

Krupp and Chatton
Current Medical Diagnosis and Treatment

I

When Alexander Fleming returned to his laboratory on September 3, 1928, he began the day by disinfecting a stack of culture plates. Around ten o'clock, D. M. Pryce stopped by to chat and found Fleming in somewhat of a foul mood. He complained about the amount of work there was to be done as well as the general mess of his laboratory, and then, as if to emphasize his complaint, Fleming showed Pryce one of the culture plates before transferring it to the Lysol bath. Suddenly, Fleming stopped in midair, Pryce recalled, looked at the plate again, and muttered to himself, "That's odd." In the center of the plate was a spot of mold, about the size of a nickel, which had inhibited the growth of staphylococcal colonies around it. Alexander Fleming was forty-seven years old, and he had just discovered penicillin.

At just the same hour in Cambridge, a child lay critically ill with rheumatic fever in Addinbrooks Hospital. Across the Atlantic Ocean in America there were more children dying of rheumatic fever as well as endocarditis and various types of bacteremia, septicemia, and a host of other such bacterial infections. Fleming's discovery came too late for them as well as thousands of others who would die miserable deaths from staphylococcus and streptococcus infections.

By 1939 the structure of penicillin was still a mystery, and supplies of the organically produced mold were in short supply; they would so continue until 1957 when John Sheehan finally discovered the secret of synthesizing the antibiotic. For nearly thirty years—from 1928 until 1957—a series of scientific and political battles were fought over this drug, with angry disputes about its discovery, its properties, and its resistance to being synthesized. In one of these encounters of the violent kind, the fiery Ernst Chain and the rigid Sir Robert Robinson became so furious at one another that "Robinson rose from behind his desk, seized a bottle of ink, and hurled it at the rapidly retreating figure of Chain," shouting "I don't want to see that wretched little man again" (Sheehan, *The Enchanted Ring*, p. 29).

Throughout these controversial years, patients continued to die of bacterial infections that could have been cured by the availability of penicillin. One of these children was Christopher Campbell, who was diagnosed in the spring of 1950 with subacute bacterial endocarditis. The first treatment of any patient with penicillin had occurred only nine years before in 1941, and it was another eight years before the secret of the beta-lactam ring was fully understood, thus enabling Sheehan to synthesize the molecule. Christopher Campbell's illness in May 1950, therefore, marked a certain middle ground in the quest that involved international powers, children's lives, the reputation of several prominent scientists, and the age of anti-biotics.

II

Christopher Campbell was going to celebrate his eighth birth-day at the end of May, and he did not want to be sick. But for the past three weeks, it seemed to be one thing after the other. First his back tooth began aching so much that he couldn't get to sleep at night, and the dentist decided that the tooth would have to be pulled. However, since he was just getting over a bad cold, his parents decided to wait for a while. Then about a week ago, he woke up with a sore throat, and despite the fact that he was always trying to avoid school, his mother decided that this time there was good reason for keeping him home in bed. The next day he was a little worse with a fever in the morning, but that went away by suppertime. On Wednesday the fever was back along with a rash of small purple and red hemorrhagic spots across his chest and even inside his mouth. That was when Christopher's mother called the doctor.

In 1949 doctors still made housecalls and still carried their small black bags filled with medicines and instruments. It was near the end of the day when Dr. Bates finally arrived at the Campbells' house, and he carried himself up the three flights of stairs with a weariness that only a small-town doctor in 1949 could truly appreciate. His day had started at 5:30 that morning, and now nearly twelve hours later he still had three more housecalls to make. In that space of time, he had told a young woman of eighteen that she had leukemia and there was nothing that he could do to help her; he had visited two elderly sisters and advised them to sell their house and enter a nursing home; he had delivered two babies and told a third mother that there were serious complications with her pregnancy; and he had treated five cases of influenza, hospitalized a man with third-degree burns over 65 percent of his body, and spent nearly an hour reassuring a neurasthenic, hypochondriacal widow that there was nothing organically the matter with her. Frankly, Bates had had just about enough.

Charles Wilson Bates, M.D., was fifty-one years old, and in three years he would be dead of massive coronary thrombosis. Had he known this prognosis and eventuality, it would not have changed the way in which he lived the remainder of his life. He was committed—he was even obsessively driven—to rescuing patients in distress. Despite the fact that he lost many more than he saved and that even those successfully rescued were not always grateful, he was driven nonetheless, for they were rescued not for their sake but for his.

He was a bear of a man standing well over six feet tall and weighing past the three hundred mark on the scales. Such proportions in a person of lesser energy would have suggested slovenly fatness, but in Bates there was a symmetry and grace which made him seem big, impressive, and powerful. With amazing grace and speed, he moved like a bear stalking its prey, and so he moved today with great, solid footfalls that fell with a dull, loud thud as he climbed the three flights of stairs to Christopher's room. As he entered the small back bedroom, he brought with him all the smells and scents of early May, which gave a wet, earthy texture to the dry sickness of the place. Bates seemed to collapse rather than sit in the bedside wicker chair and with a violent wheeze of exertion threw his head back to mutter "What a hell of a day." It took him a moment to collect himself, and during that time he said nothing, nor did anyone speak to him. Then, as if suddenly becoming aware for the first time of Christopher, he turned to examine him.

One big hairy paw unbuttoned the boy's pajama top while Bates used the other to adjust the stethoscope to his ears and then quickly switched hands to run the silver disk over the boy's chest. He muttered all the while with quiet instructions such as "Now breathe deep . . . that's it . . . there, now, sit up and breathe in deep . . . now hold it . . . that's it . . . now breathe again," and all the while he cocked his head like a parrot to listen intently while staring at the ceiling. But for all of Bates's intensity, energy, and sheer animal power, there was also a gentleness about him that seemed to contradict his brutish size. As he sat in the wicker chair, which creaked and groaned with each motion of the stethoscope, his softer features came into focus. From this perspective, one saw an entirely different person, whose warm doelike eyes, luxurious curls of chestnut hair tipped with gray, and soft full cheeks were nearly the features of a child or perhaps a violent cupid.

Bates was certain of his diagnosis as soon as he saw the petechiae—from the Italian meaning "fleabite"—that covered the boy's chest. He dismissed leukemia and thrombocytopenia purpura with hardly a second glance, but there still remained the question of whether this was acute rheumatic fever or acute bacterial endocarditis. Within a few minutes he had also dismissed both of these possibilities and needed only to confirm his hunch that this was a classic case of subacute bacterial endocarditis. There was a clear mitral valve insufficiency which was apparent in all positions but especially when the boy was bent over. Bates pressurized one or two fingernail beds and saw the characteristic splinter hemorrhages appear. Now he was certain that this was subacute bacterial endocarditis, but he was less certain that anything could be done for the boy. The year was 1949, and supplies of penicillin were still in short supply. In addition, if Christopher showed an allergic reaction to the penicillin then he would surely die, for endocarditis was almost uniformly fatal without antibiotic therapy.

III

Fleming's fermentation process for producing penicillin was expensive and time-consuming and yielded small, impure samples. As a consequence, after nearly ten years the available supplies of penicillin were insufficient for either treatment or research. World War II, however, created an emergency need for the drug, and on June 28, 1941, President Roosevelt instituted Executive Order 8807 establishing the Office of Scientific Research and Development, one of whose top priorities was to discover a means for synthesizing penicillin. By 1942—the year in which Christopher Campbell was born—penicillin research in the United States and England was classified Top Secret.

To whom the honor should be given for the discovery of penicillin has always been a subject of debate. It is agreed that Alexander Fleming first made the discovery of *Penicillium notatum* mold, but it is argued that he never really understood the medical significance of his own discovery and that the honor rightfully belongs to H. W. Florey and Ernst Chain. The committee that awarded the Nobel Prize for the discovery in 1945 waffled on the issue and made the award to Fleming, Florey, and Chain "for the discovery of penicillin and its curative effect in various infectious diseases."

In truth, none of these three was actually the first to use *Penicillium* mold in the treatment of infections. That honor properly belongs to the great Lister, who had first successfully treated a patient at King's College Hospital in 1882 with mold probably from the species *Penicillium chrysogenum*. Actually, Joseph Lister's interest in the subject was already evident nine years earlier in his presentation to the Royal Society of Edinburgh on April 7, 1873, when he discussed *Penicillium glaucum*.

On May 25, 1940, Florey began his first experimental work on the antibiotic properties of penicillin. Using laboratory mice, he exposed the population to *Streptococcus pyogenes* and then inoculated half of the group with penicillin. Within twenty-four hours, the untreated population were all dead while the medicated ones were perfectly healthy. Florey was not a physician and therefore could not himself treat human subjects, but he did have a medically qualified colleague at Oxford's Radcliffe Infirmary, Dr. Charles M. Fletcher, who had a patient dying of breast cancer. There was no thought in anyone's mind, of course, that the poor woman would benefit from the treatment, but the real question was whether or not she would be harmed by it. Guinea pigs, for example, are extremely reactive to penicillin and die quickly of allergic response. Would the same also be the case with human subjects? It was; within an hour's time she showed unmistakable symptoms of toxic reaction. There were two conclusions to be drawn from this dramatic failure. The first was that penicillin was itself toxic to human subjects, and the second was that only the impurities in the fermentation broth were toxic. Florey decided to assume the latter and sought to produce a purer sample of penicillin for the next patient. On February 12, 1941, Dr. Fletcher introduced another hopelessly ill patient to Florey. He was a policeman who had widespread bacteremia from a cut which had become infected with streptococcus. In addition to open sores all over his body, the man also had septicemia throughout his lungs, bones, eyes, and other vital organs. He had hours to live without treatment and agreed to any extreme measure including the possibly toxic penicillin. Florey's treatment continued for five days, and during this time he conserved his meager supply of penicillin by extracting trace amounts from the patient's urine that were then purified and reused again. Throughout the course of the five days, the patient improved markedly and would no doubt have recovered had the supply of fermented penicillin been sufficient. However, the patient needed the antibiotic more quickly than it could be supplied, and he finally died. The third patient was a boy of four who had massive staphylococcal infections on his face and who responded very well to the initial treatment. Florey had hoped that his short supplies would be adequate for a child, if not for an adult, and this proved to be the case. But once again the patient suddenly died. There then followed several successful treatments in a row including two boys of fourteen and fifteen, a baby with a bladder infection, a patient with a carbuncle, and five with eye infections. By the time that Florey's results were published in *Lancet* in 1941, the news media already had the story, and penicillin was being called a wonder drug.

IV

Christopher Campbell spent his eighth birthday in the hospital. With him in the same room were two other boys with subacute bacterial endocarditis, and of the three only one would be alive by summer's end. Dr. Bates lost no time in having the boy admitted, and as soon as a positive diagnosis of endocarditis had been confirmed by blood culture studies, he was started on penicillin G by IM (intramuscular injection usually into the gluteal muscle). In 1950 a few thousand units of penicillin three times a day were regarded as an adequate therapeutic dosage;

just thirty years later that recommendation has increased to six million units a day.

These elevated figures reflect the increased resistance of certain streptococcus and staphylococcus strains through their ability to produce the enzyme penicillinase, which destroys the antibiotic properties of penicillin. For example, enterococcal endocarditis is so resistant to penicillin G that either very high dosages must be given (20 to 50 million units) or a combination therapy of streptomycin and ampicillin used instead. The range of synthetic drugs today makes it possible to provide substitutions that were not available in 1950. Staphylococci resistant to penicillin G are often sensitive to methicillin or nafcillin. Dynapen, veracillin, azapen, staphcillin, and unipen are all synthetic compounds unaffected by penicillinase. There are presently hundreds of different synthetic antibiotics (including the penicillins, tetracyclines, erythromycins, and cephalosporins) that can disrupt the metabolism of gram-positive pathogens such as streptococcus and staphylococcus.

Streptococcus viridans is an a-hemolytic streptococcus and is the most frequent cause of subacute bacterial endocarditis resulting from infected teeth or dental surgery. Bacterial seeds from the infected site are released into the circulatory system and begin to swim like semen seeking an ovum to fertilize. They rendezvous with the genius of lovers, seeking one another within the gentle waving cusps and valves of the heart. Of the several valves that compose the heart, the aortic and mitral valves are most often infected by endocarditis. The mitral valve is shaped like a bishop's miter, rests between the left atrium and the left ventricle, and consists of two large opposing cusps with smaller cusps at each end. The primary purpose of this valve is to regulate blood flow between the two chambers while also preventing the filling of the aorta during distension of the ventricle. It also becomes a favorite site for rheumatic heart disease, which is found in the majority of patients who later develop subacute bacterial endocarditis.

Rheumatic fever is an acute inflammation caused by a Grade A streptococcal infection. There are five sites where the disease can manifest itself—joints, brain, heart, subcutaneous tissue, and skin—and consequently the symptomatic profile can vary greatly. Moreover, the symptoms may be so subtle as to produce a subclinical illness that is often not recognized and not treated until sometime later. It has been estimated that as many as 2 percent of elementary school children in the United States have had a mild to a severe case of rheumatic fever, and most of these are asymptomatic. Scarring of the mitral valve—or occasionally the aortic or tricuspid valve—is the most common effect of the disease. Valvulitis will thicken and often distort the mitral valve, causing distortion and fusion of the valve's cusps and leaflets. Either mitral stenosis or aortic regurgitation is usually the long-range effect, in which the valve is so constricted in its diameter as not to operate sufficiently (i.e., mitral insufficiency, or stenosis) or so sloppy and dilated as not to close properly, thus permitting backflow or regurgitation. The symptoms of the disease—fever, aching joints, skin rash, and arthritic inflammations—usually will subside within three weeks. Damage to the heart valves remains, however, and is heard as a murmur or sometimes a soft blowing sound accompanying the heartbeat. Aortic regurgitation is usually heard below the sternal border and resembles a whoozing or gentle blowing on the diastolic stroke, whereas mitral stenosis is heard above the apex as a presystolic murmur.

Subacute endocarditis seizes the opportunity to vegetate these damaged valves. Irregularities in the valve's surface and structure permit pockets of inflammation and infection to form. As the creeping vegetation seeks out other defects in the cardiac wall, it will also establish fulminating colonies along the valve's leaflets as well as within the fissures, fractures, and swollen contours of the valve's rim. Eventually the inner surface of the pericardium will be inflamed with vegetative growth, and it is from this inflammation of the heart's interior lining that the disease gets its name. "Endocarditis" is an infection of the heart's inner pericardial lining.

Microscopic examination of the vegetative lesions shows a meshwork of fibrin masses that have trapped—like a spider with its web—a collection of red and white blood cells along with the streptococcus bacteria themselves. The vegetation is granular with a greenish-gray or greenish-yellow appearance, and it is sometimes also crusted with lime salts. One can but be reminded of the strange fungus that encrusts trees and rocks at particularly humid times of the year. As the vegetation continues to germinate and flower, it sends blossoms, seeds, and pollen throughout the body. Plaques of the original lesion break loose to become emboli that manifest themselves in several different ways. Small hemorrhages may appear on the palms of the hands and soles of the feet; they are called Janeway lesions after the American physician Edward Janeway (1841–1911), who first described them. Osler's nodes show up on the fingertips and pads of the feet as small discolorations with a slightly raised edge usually about three millimeters in diameter. Careful examination of the eye may serve the initial diagnosis through the appearance of small hemorrhages in the ocular fundi called Roth's spots.

As the emboli continue to break loose from the parent site, they colonize areas in the brain, kidneys, spleen, and elsewhere. Some of these will cause tissue damage simply by infecting specialized and vital areas, but other emboli will create local abscesses that further infect large areas and then become secondary centers for spreading the disease elsewhere. Death will come—and the disease is always fatal without antibiotic treatment—from pulmonary or cerebral embolism or from cardiac or renal failure. Sir William Osler described the effects of the disease from autopsy in *The Principles and Practice of Medicine*.

> The substance of the valve may lose its translucency, and the only change noticeable is a grayish opacity and a slight loss of its delicate tenuity. In the auriculo-ventricular valves these early changes are seen just within the margin and here it is not uncommon to find swellings of a grayish-red, somewhat infiltrated appearance, almost identical with the similar structures on the intima of the aorta in arterio-sclerosis. Even early there may be seen yellow or opaque-white subintimal fatty areas. As the sclerotic changes increase the fibrous tissue contracts and produces thickening and deformity of the segment, the edges of which become round, curled and incapable of that delicate apposition necessary for perfect closure. [p. 600]

It is remarkable that for all the internal damage being done, there is really very little external and visible distress. The patient is being torn apart but feels little pain and shows only minor symptoms or none at all. One is reminded of a sleeping volcano in which the internal pressures and heat gradually reach an explosive point and then erupt with an absolute violence unpredictable from its cool and calm exterior. A low-grade fever may be the only initial symptom—it rarely peaks above 102° F—and it may be irregular or absent for several days before returning again. Occasional aches and pains in and about the joints, some chills, and a feeling of weakness may be experienced, but usually these are without any cardiac symptoms. The heart does not usually race, beat arrhythmically, or cause pain, and all of the hemorrhages, petechiae, splenomegaly, emboli, and heart murmurs are often later symptoms that appear only once the disease is well established. There are other disorders—such as the lymphomas, leukemias, lupus, tuberculosis—that present similar initial symptoms but whose course and treatment demand radically different measures. A history of rheumatic fever or severe infection from streptococcus is often helpful, but definitive diagnosis is incomplete without blood cultures. The incubation of blood samples taken from the patient usually will culture the specific bacteria type within a week's time. And yet occasionally this diagnostic measure is also not foolproof because 10 to 15 percent of patients with endocarditis may still have negative blood culture results.

V

While Christopher Campbell continued to fight the creeping vegetation of endocarditis, John Sheehan continued to fight the pessimism of a scientific community which had given up any hope of synthetizing penicillin and its various derivatives. The problem was the mysterious beta-lactam ring. Nearly twenty-five years elapsed before this incredibly complex but also incredibly simple problem was finally solved by John Sheehan and fellow researchers. On March 1, 1957, Sheehan applied for U.S. Patent no. 643,260 describing the synthesis "of penicillins from synthetic 6-APA and the preparation of the synthetic penicillin V by attaching the side chain prior to closure of the beta-lactam ring."

The beta-lactam ring is the most important ingredient in

the synthetic production of penicillin molecules. When the ring is closed and intact, the molecule retains its antibiotic properties. However, when the ring is open or otherwise disturbed, the compound is rendered useless. It was this problem which frustrated scientists for twenty-five years and caused them to despair of ever finding a solution. Sheehan himself compared the problem to "that of attempting to repair the mainspring of a fine watch with a blacksmith's anvil, hammer, and tongs" (*The Enchanted Ring*, p. 7). In short, the technology for solving the mechanical means of closing the beta-lactam ring simply was not available.

It was on a Sunday afternoon while catching up on his journals that Sheehan stumbled upon a solution to the mysterious beta-lactam ring. He had been leafing through past issues of several scholarly journals in chemistry when he came upon a discussion about the preparation of carbodiimides. Carbodiimides had long been used as drying agents in certain reactions, but Sheehan now thought that these compounds might lend themselves as coupling agents to facilitate the closure of the beta-lactam ring in the synthesis of penicillin. The whole chemical problem with which he had been struggling reduced to a question of bonding together a carbon atom with a nitrogen atom. When this bonding takes place, the beta-lactam ring closes, and penicillin achieves its antibiotic properties. Working with his postdoctoral student George Hess, he began to explore his hunch and "all in all, it appeared that in carbodiimide I had found the ideal reagent for closing the beta-lactam and, eventually, for completing that last troublesome step in the synthesis of penicillin" (ibid., p. 142).

Sheehan and Hess published the results of their preliminary research using the carbodiimide compounds, but almost immediately there were problems. To begin with, other researchers complained that the published results could not be duplicated, and Hess even found his own results to be unpredictable from one experiment to the next. Sheehan lamented that "no one, not even our own group, could reproduce our sythesis of peptides with DCC reliably" (ibid., p. 144). But fortunately, the solution to the problem once again proved to be resolved simply by rewriting the formula to increase the quantity of acid-bearing molecules. The original formula included equal molar equivalents of carbodiimide, the carboxyl-bearing molecule, and an amine-bearing molecule. In practice, however, the weights and measures necessary for determining precisely equal amounts were not precise enough and thus every combination became unpredictable. Sheehan made "sure that the instructions called for a slight excess of the acid-bearing molecule in the reaction. With this slight alteration in the experimental instructions, most of the problems disappeared" (ibid., p. 145).

Sheehan's plan called for a total synthesis of penicillin by chemical means, without the use of any organic fermentation processes. He wanted to close the beta-lactam ring by use of the carbodiimide dicyclohexylcarbodiimide which was powerful enough to effect closure but in a reaction sufficiently mild so as not to damage or deform other aspects of the molecule. Using penicillin V—produced by natural fermentation process—Sheehan first opened the beta-lactam ring by alkaline hydrolysis and then closed it back up again with DCC. In effect, he first destroyed the antibiotic effects of penicillin by opening the beta-lactam ring and then reconstituted those same properties by closing it up again. The secret to synthesizing penicillin rested entirely with this ability to open and close the beta-lactam ring, and Sheehan had finally discovered a method of doing so.

VI

Christopher's parents kept careful records of his temperature and pulse throughout July and August 1950; those for July 1–23 are shown in table 16.1. And so it went, day by day and week by week until the end of August. There were days when his temperature would be normal but his pulse rate was alarmingly high, and other days when his pulse was regular and slow but his temperature high. There seemed to be no rhyme or reason to these unpredictable fluctuations, and about the time that he appeared to be getting better, the ominous charts would foretell the opposite. He came to hate these daily charts nearly as much as the double shot of penicillin that he got three times a day. Every reminder of this awful disease brought forth a new vision of the deep, yellowish-green vegetation that slowly grew within him. It suffocated and engulfed—like a dense, desperate moss—his rapid, feverish heart.

Sometimes he would awake in the middle of the night and actually feel the clotted vegetation burrowing through already thickened chambers of his heart. At these times, a heavy suffocation would spread over him as if the greasy, glossy green of the bacterial plant had rooted itself into his very soul and was now sending long shoots of tangled ivy twine throughout the rest of his body. He felt, or seemed to feel, the vicious plant creep and crawl within his chest and wrap its spider arms about lungs, liver, abdomen, and even the tender sensitive parts of his sex. Everywhere he was being invaded by a vegetation which grew and thrived upon the very destruction that it created. Like a saw-toothed plow which furrows up black, loamy soil, so did the devouring teeth of this disease masticate his

Table 16.1. Temperature and pulse for A.M. and P.M.

July 1950	8 A.M.		12 Noon		4 P.M.		8 P.M.	
	T	P	T	P	T	P	T	P
1 Fri.	98.6	98	99.4	89	99.2	81	99.0	79
2 Sat.	98.0	84	99.2	84	98.8	74	99.0	80
3 Sun.	98.4	78	99.0	86	98.6	88	99.2	84
4 Mon.	98.2	85	99.3	79	99.6	81	98.8	72
5 Tues.	98.2	83	99.6	83	100.0	94	99.6	71
6 Wed.	99.0	90	99.8	93	98.2	72	99.2	76
7 Thurs.	98.6	92	99.2	84	99.2	90	99.6	83
8 Fri.	98.2	75	99.0	82	99.4	76	98.8	82
9 Sat.	98.8	87	99.2	83	99.4	76	99.0	86
10 Sun.	98.2	83	98.0	82	99.4	82	99.0	80
11 Mon.	Back in the hospital for tests							
12 Tues.	Back in the hospital							
13 Wed.	Back in the hospital							
14 Thurs.	98.0	74	98.6	87	99.2	72	98.2	76
15 Fri.	98.4	83	98.8	95	98.4	84	98.2	85
16 Sat.	98.2	88	99.4	89	98.4	84	98.2	85
17 Sun.	98.6	92	99.0	74	99.0	88	98.0	90
18 Mon.	98.0	75	98.0	89	98.8	73	99.0	76
19 Tues.	98.0	73	99.2	70	99.4	93	99.0	74
20 Wed.	98.6	84	98.6	74	98.8	78	98.6	74
21 Thurs.	98.6	71	99.0	74	98.8	72	98.6	82
22 Fri.	98.0	72	99.0	90	98.8	80	99.0	90
23 Sat.	98.2	70	98.6	74	98.8	85	99.4	86

flesh in order to devour it; and as the tendrils ate, so did they also grow until his flesh became its actual food. Meanwhile, he was being suffocated, slowly suffocated by the greedy, malevolent growth. He could neither flee nor escape, for he was imprisoned within this greasy green prison of rotting flesh that continued to liquify into a yellow syrup of suppuration and seeping sores. Chest, legs, arms, fingertips as well as face, ears, nose, and mouth were frightful avalanches of bubbling sores that erupted from within and then spread out everywhere upon the glossy surface. The vegetative volcano that roared and stormed within him created internal storms of raging fever and racing pulse that appeared upon the calm exterior only after the interior had been thoroughly cooked and baked in fire to extinction. He was dying from the inside out as this hungry, greedy plant blossomed forth to replace the child wherein it fed. The very thought of the monster filled him with a nauseous claustrophobia, and yet he had no choice but to submit passively to its will and therein to suffer.

Bates was his salvation. To the boy he appeared to be a kind of god, a magician, a wizard of muscle and bulk who drew forth sorcery from his black bag with the elegant ease of a showman. Wherein resided all this power, strength, and energy of a healer who could stand between him and the terrible dark vegetation that sought to destroy him? Every day the burly, massive man who moved with the quiet grace of a dignified dying elephant would disturb the quiet of his upstairs bedroom with his entrance. First, there would be the loud thud of heavy footfalls echoing down the hallway and then a sputtered cough as he entered the room and slowly eased his wheezing frame into the nearest chair.

"How're you doing, pal? How's my boy today?" Meanwhile, Bates would already be filling a glass syringe with the white, creamy fluid of penicillin. Cocking his head like a parrot and staring through the glass barrel to the light, he would measure out the correct ccs and then plunge out the air pocket before looking back to the boy.

"Guess you're used to this by now, son. Let's try the right hip today." There would be a quick, sharp stab of pain and then that congested, bursting sensation as the thick, milky fluid forced its way into the heavy meatus of the hip muscle.

Afterwards, he might ease back into the comfort of the wicker chair, withdraw and light a cigarette in a single movement, and relax for a moment before his next housecall.

"Hell of a day, hell of a day," he would mutter to himself while the blue cigarette smoke curled up and around the violent cupid's face. "Don't ever be a doctor, son. No, don't ever be one. It's a hell of a life. No time to yourself. Never see your family, always on the go, son. No, be a lawyer or buy your own business, but don't be a doctor. Not worth the price of your family and your health."

Lost in reflection, muttering to himself as if alone, Bates cocked his parrot head toward the ceiling and watched the lazy blue smoke rise from his nostrils. Already his own heart was a twisted wreckage of broken tissue and bleeding muscle from dozens of small cardiac infarctions and two major heart attacks that had nearly killed him. The next one would come in less than three years, and its violence would literally blow the valves out of his heart while the wheezing, still beating stump bled itself to death. Perhaps Bates had some premonition of his own borrowed life and times and therein sought to save a fragment of himself by rescuing Christopher from the clinging vegetation of endocarditis.

Suddenly, the mighty bulk gave a great shudder and shook itself loose from the chair. "Gotta go, pal, see you tomorrow. You're doing good."

And then he was gone. Long after Bates died, the boy could still recall the warm, fragrant smells that he always brought with him and the powerful earthy strength of the man. He could not help wonder if Bates, by some metaphysical magic known only to himself, might possibly have traded his own life for the boy's.

VII

May 29, 1953, marked the twenty-fifth anniversary of Sir Alexander Fleming's first scholarly paper on penicillin. Years before, on the morning of May 10, 1929, he had posted to the editors (one of whom was Howard Florey) of the *British Journal of Experimental Pathology* a paper "On the Antibacterial Actions of Cultures of a Penicillium with Special Reference to Their Use in the Isolation of B Influenza E." The paper was accepted for publication and appeared a month later in issue 3, volume 10 of the journal. In the meantime, he had received innumerable honors including the Nobel Prize and the Gold Medal of the Royal College of Surgeons, which had only been awarded twenty times before in 144 years; and he had also been knighted by the queen of England and was now known as Sir Alexander.

The next day, May 30, 1953, Christopher Campbell would celebrate his eleventh birthday. He was completely recovered from endocarditis—with only a slight mitral stenosis—and back in school again. Charles Wilson Bates, M.D., had been found dead on Thursday morning the week before by his wife when she could not wake him from a peaceful night's sleep. He had died quietly and quickly in his sleep without a trace of the great anguish and misery that had pervaded his life for the past five years. Autopsy showed that death had occurred from a rupture of the papillary muscle so severe as to destroy the mitral valve completely. Death was nearly instantaneous.

March 11, 1955, was a bright Friday morning and Sir Alexander was to receive yet another award at a dinner to be attended by Eleanor Roosevelt and Douglas Fairbanks, Jr. He would be seventy-four years old on August 6 and had told friends just the night before at the Chelsea Arts Club that "I've never felt better in my life." His son Robert had come round with his fiancée, and they spent part of the evening viewing pictures through a new stereoscopic projector which had just arrived that day from America. While in the bathroom the next morning, however, Sir Alec suddenly felt weak and very nauseous. His wife ordered him to bed, against great protests, and called their family physician. Dr. Hunt had wanted to come immediately, but Fleming was feeling better and told him to attend to his other patients first. He was certain that it was not his heart but "rather something going down the oesophagus to the stomach," he told his wife Amalia. With that, his head fell forward and he died instantly. Sir Alexander Fleming had died of a coronary thrombosis (MacFarlane, *Alexander Fleming*, p. 242).

The great diagnostician Sir William Osler had often wondered whether physicians die of the very diseases they treat and hoped that his own body would be autopsied. Harvey Cushing, the neurosurgeon, had studied under Osler and requested the same be done to him upon his own death. Accordingly, when Cushing died on October 7, 1939, of congestive heart failure, Dr. Milton Winternitz, assisted by Harry Zimmerman, performed an autopsy the following day and discovered a colloid cyst about a centimeter in circumference in the third ventricle of Cushing's brain.

On March 18, 1955, at exactly noon, Fleming's ashes were placed within a crypt in St. Paul's Cathedral. The eulogy was delivered by C. A. Pannett, who concluded with the observation that "we can almost see the finger of God pointed to the direction his career should take at every turn" (ibid., p. 243). Surely it is curious that these three lives—Fleming's, Bates's, and Christopher Campbell's—should interweave in such extraordinary ways and yet do so in the most ordinary and natural of ways.

References

References

Abrams, Albert. *Diagnostic Therapeutics*. New York: Rebman Co., 1910.

Ackerknecht, Erwin. *A Short History of Medicine*. Baltimore: Johns Hopkins University Press, 1982.

Adrian, Lord. *The Physical Background of Perception*. Oxford: Oxford University Press, 1967.

Aizzolaztti, G., M. Matelli, and G. Pavesi. "Deficits in Attention and Movement Following the Removal of Postarcuate (Area 6) and Prearcuate (Area 8) Cortex in Macaque Monkeys." *Brain* 106(1983):655–73.

Alpers, Bernard J., and Elliott L. Mancall. *Essentials of the Neurological Examination*. Philadelphia: F. A. Davis Co., 1971.

Ansley, David. "Werewolves Might Be Real." Akron *Beacon Journal*, May 31, 1985.

Bannister, Roger, ed. *Brain's Clinical Neurology*. London: Oxford University Press, 1973.

Baudelaire, Charles. *Flowers of Evil*. Trans. Roy Campbell, ed. Marthiel and Jackson Mathews. New York: New Directions Press, 1955.

Berkow, Robert, ed. *The Merck Manual*. 14th edition. Rahway, N.J.: Merck & Co., 1982.

Bernstein, Lionel. *Renal Function and Renal Failure*. Baltimore: Williams & Wilkins Co., 1965.

Braunwald, Eugene, et al., eds. *Harrison's Principles of Internal Medicine*. 11th edition. New York: McGraw-Hill, 1987.

Brecher, Ruth and Edward, eds. *An Analysis of Human Sexual Response*. London: Andre Deutsch, 1967.

Brown, P., et al. "Diagnosis of Creutzfeldt-Jakob Disease by Western Blot Identification of Marker Protein in Human Brain Tissue." *New England Journal of Medicine*, 314, no. 9(1986):547–51.

Browne, Thomas. *Religio Medici*. Birmingham: The Classics of Medicine Library, 1981.

Byron, Lord. *Selected Poetry and Letters*. Ed. Edward E. Bostetter. New York: Holt, Rinehart and Winston, 1961.

Calabresi, Paul, Philip Schein, and Saul Rosenberg. *Medical Oncology: Basic Principles and Clinical Management of Cancer*. New York: Macmillan, 1985.

Campbell, R., T. Landis, and M. Regard. "Face Recognition and Lipreading." *Brain* 109(1986):509–21.

Castiglioni, Arturo. *A History of Medicine.* New York: Alfred Knopf, 1941.

Cousins, Norman. *Anatomy of an Illness.* New York: W. W. Norton Co., 1979.

Crosby, Elizabeth, Tryphena Humphrey, and Edward Lauer. *Correlative Anatomy of the Nervous System.* New York: Macmillan Co., 1962.

Cushing, Harvey. *Consecratio Medici.* Boston: Little, Brown & Co., 1928.

———. *The Medical Career.* Boston: Little, Brown & Co., 1940.

———. *Selected Papers on Neurosurgery.* New Haven: Yale University Press, 1969.

• ———. *Tumors of the Nervus Acusticus and the Syndrome of the Cerebellopontine Angle.* Philadelphia: W. B. Saunders Co., 1917.

DeVita, Vincent T., Jr., and Stephen Rosenberg. *Cancer: Principles and Practice of Oncology.* Philadelphia: Lippincott Publishing Co., 1985.

Al-Din, A., M. Anderson, and E. Bickerstaff. "Brainstem Encephalitis and the Syndrome of Miller Fisher." *Brain* 105(1982):481–95.

Donald, David Herbert. *Look Homeward: A Life of Thomas Wolfe.* Boston: Little, Brown & Co., 1987.

Donne, John. *The Complete English Poems.* New York: Penguin Books, 1977.

Eichenbaum, H., et al. "Selective Olfactory Deficits in Case H.M." *Brain* 106(1983):459–72.

Eliot, T. S. *The Complete Poems and Plays.* New York: Harcourt, Brace & World, 1962.

Eliott, Frank A. *Clinical Neurology.* Philadelphia: W. B. Saunders Co., 1971.

Fenichel, Otto. *The Psychoanalytic Theory of Neurosis.* New York: W. W. Norton & Co., 1945.

Fox, William Lloyd. *Dandy of Johns Hopkins.* Baltimore: Williams & Wilkins, 1984.

Fulton, John F. *Harvey Cushing: A Biography.* Springfield, Ill.: Charles C. Thomas, 1946.

Gabr, M., et al. "Progeria, A Pathological Study." *Journal of Pediatrics* 57, no. 70(1960):70–77.

Gardner, Ernest. *Fundamentals of Neurology.* Philadelphia: W. B. Saunders Co., 1968.

Gatz, Arthur, ed. *Manter's Essentials of Clinical Neuroanatomy and Neurophysiology.* Philadelphia: F. A. Davis Co., 1973.

Gellhorn, Ernst. *Biological Foundations of Emotion.* Glenview, Ill.: Scott, Foresman and Co., 1968.

Geschwind, Norman. *Selected Papers on Language and the Brain.* Boston: D. Reidel Publishing Co., 1974.

Goethe, Johann Wolfgang. *Goethe: Selected Verse.* Ed. and trans. David Luke. Baltimore: Penguin Books, 1964.

Goldenson, Robert. *The Encyclopedia of Human Behavior.* New York: Doubleday & Co., 1971.

Gunther, John. *Death Be Not Proud.* New York: Perennial Library, 1965.

Guyton, Arthur. *Structure and Function of the Nervous System.* Philadelphia: W. B. Saunders Co., 1972.

Haskell, Charles, ed. *Cancer Treatment.* Philadelphia: W. B. Saunders Co., 1984.

Ho, D., et al. "Isolation of HTLV-III from Cerebospinal Fluid and Neural Tissues of Patients with Neurologic Syndromes Related to the Acquired Immunodeficiency Syndrome." *New England Journal of Medicine* 313, no. 24(1985):1493–97.

Hopkins, Gerard Manley. *Poems and Prose of Gerard Manley Hopkins.* Baltimore: Penguin Books, 1961.

Hughes, A. F. W. *Aspects of Neural Ontogeny.* New York: Academic Press, 1968.

Hurst, Willis J., ed. *The Heart.* 6th edition. New York: McGraw-Hill, 1986.

Jamal, G., et al. "Myotonic Dystrophy." *Brain* 109(1986):1279–96.

Judd, T., H. Gardner, and N. Geschwind. "Alexia without Agraphia in a Composer." *Brain* 106(1983):435–57.

Juncos, J., and F. Beal. "Idiopathic Cranial Polyneuropathy." *Brain* 110(1987):197–211.

Kahn, E., et al. *Correlative Neurosurgery.* Springfield, Ill.: Charles C. Thomas, 1955.

Keats, John. *Selected Poems and Letters.* Boston: Houghton Mifflin Co., 1959.

Kennedy, G., G. Clements, and M. Brown. "Differential Susceptibility of Human Neural Cell Types in Culture to Infection with Herpes Simplex Virus." *Brain* 106(1983):101–19.

Kennedy, Richard. *The Window of Memory: The Literary Career of Thomas Wolfe.* Chapel Hill: University of North Carolina Press, 1962.

King, Lester. *Medical Thinking.* Princeton, N.J.: Princeton University Press, 1982.

Krupp, Marcus A., and Milton J. Chatton. *Current Medical Diagnosis and Treatment.* Los Altos, Calif.: Lange Medical Publications, 1975.

Kulics, Albert. "Sensory Discriminability Comparisons in Human and Monkey with Implications for the Study of Central Nervous Correlates." *Annals of the New York Academy of Sciences* 299(1977):244–54.

Lewis, Jefferson. *Something Hidden: A Biography of Wilder Penfield.* Toronto: Doubleday & Co., 1981.

Logigian, E., et al. "Myoclonus Epilepsy in Two Brothers." *Brain* 109(1986):411–29.

Lorenz, Konrad. *On Aggression.* New York: Harcourt, Brace & World, 1963.

Lund, R. D. *Development and Plasticity of the Brain.* New York: Oxford University Press, 1978.

Luria, A. R. *Higher Cortical Functions in Man.* New York: Basic Books, 1973.

——. *The Man with the Shattered World.* Cambridge: Harvard University Press, 1987.

——. *The Mind of a Mnemonist.* Cambridge: Harvard University Press, 1987.

——. *The Working Brain.* New York: Basic Books, 1973.

McCleary, Robert, and Robert Moore. *Subcortical Mechanisms of Behavior.* New York: Basic Books, 1965.

MacFarlane, Gwyn. *Alexander Fleming.* Cambridge: Harvard University Press, 1984.

Mark, Vernon, and Frank Ervin. *Violence and the Brain.* New York: Harper & Row, 1970.

Mayo Clinic. *Clinical Examinations in Neurology.* Philadelphia: W. B. Saunders Co., 1971.

Merritt, H. Houston. *Textbook of Neurology.* 7th edition, ed. Lewis Rowland. Philadelphia: Lea & Febiger, 1984.

Moruzzi, Giuseppe, and Horace W. Magoun. "Brainstem Reticular Formation and Activation of the EEG." *Electroencephalography and Clinical Neurophysiology,* 1(1949):455–73.

Netter, Frank. *The CIBA Collection of Medical Illustrations: The Nervous System.* Summit, N.J.: CIBA Pharmaceutical Co., 1962.

Nelson, Waldo. *Textbook of Pediatrics.* Ed. C. Vaughan, J. McKay, and R. Behrman. Philadelphia: W. B. Saunders & Co., 1979.

Nowell, Elizabeth. *Thomas Wolfe: A Biography.* New York: Doubleday & Co., 1960.

344

O'Connor, Flannery. *The Complete Stories*. New York: Farrar, Straus & Giroux, 1975.

———. *The Habit of Being*. New York: Farrar, Straus & Giroux, 1979.

———. *Mystery and Manners*. New York: Farrar, Straus & Giroux, 1969.

———. *3 by Flannery O'Connor*. New York: New American Library, 1962.

Oppenheim, H. *Diseases of the Nervous System*. Philadelphia: J. B. Lippincott Co., 1904.

Osler, William. *The Principles and Practice of Medicine*. New York: D. Appleton & Co., 1912.

Passingham, R., V. Perry, and F. Wilkinson. "The Long-Term Effects of Removal of Sensorimotor Cortex in Infant and Adult Monkeys." *Brain* 106(1983):675–705.

Paulus, W. M., A. Straube, and T. Brandt. "Visual Stabilization of Posture." *Brain* 107(1984):1143–63.

Penfield, Wilder. *The Excitable Cortex in Conscious Man*. Liverpool, Eng.: Liverpool University Press, 1973.

———. *The Mystery of the Mind*. Princeton, N.J.: Princeton University Press, 1975.

———. *No Man Alone*. Boston: Little, Brown & Co., 1977.

———. *Speech and Brain Mechanisms*. Princeton, N.J.: Princeton University Press, 1959.

———, and T. Rasmussen. *The Cerebral Cortex of Man*. New York: Hafner Publishing Co., 1968.

Perkins, Maxwell. *Editor to Author: The Letters of Maxwell E. Perkins*. Ed. John Hall Wheelock. New York: Universal Library, 1950.

Physician's Desk Reference. Oradell, N.J.: Medical Economics Co., 1987.

Pope, Alexander. *The Poems of Alexander Pope*. Ed. John Butt. London: Methuen & Co., 1963.

Pribram, Karl. *Languages of the Brain*. Englewood Cliffs, N.J.: Prentice Hall, 1971.

Reed, Charles, Irving Alexander, and Silvan Tomkins. *Psychopathology*. New York: John Wiley & Sons, 1964.

Resbick, L., et al. "Intra-Blood-Brain Barrier Synthesis of HTLV-III-Specific I_gG in Patients with Neurologic Symptoms Associated with AIDS or AIDS-Related Complex." *New England Journal of Medicine* 313, no. 24(1985):1498–1503.

Rilke, Rainer Maria. *Translations from the Poetry of Rainer Maria Rilke*. Trans. M. D. Herter Norton. New York: W. W. Norton & Co., 1962.

Robertson, D., et al. "Isolated Failure of Autonomic Noradrenergic Neurotransmission." *New England Journal of Medicine* 314, no. 23(1986):1494–97.

Rossetti, Christina. *Goblin Market and Other Poems*. Oxford: Oxford University Press, 1951.

Rushmer, Robert. *Structure and Function of the Cardiovascular System*. Philadelphia: W. B. Saunders Co., 1972.

Sacks, Oliver. *Awakenings*. New York: E. P. Dutton, 1983.

——. *A Leg to Stand On*. New York: Summit Books, 1984.

——. *The Man Who Mistook His Wife for a Hat*. New York: Summit Books, 1985.

——. *Migraine*. Los Angeles: University of California Press, 1970.

Sartre, Jean-Paul. *Baudelaire*. Trans. Martin Turnell. New York: New Directions, 1967.

——. *Nausea*. Trans. Lloyd Alexander. New York: New Directions, 1964.

Scully, R., E. Mark, and B. McNeely, eds. "Case Records of the Massachusetts General Hospital." Case 6–1983. *New England Journal of Medicine* 308, no. 6(1983):326–32.

——. "Case Records of the Massachusetts General Hospital." Case 24–1985. *New England Journal of Medicine* 312, no. 24(1985):1560–67.

——. "Case Records of the Massachusetts General Hospital." Case 38–1985. *New England Journal of Medicine* 313, no. 12(1985):739–47.

——. "Case Records of the Massachusetts General Hospital." Case 22–1986. *New England Journal of Medicine* 314, no. 23(1986):1498–1507.

——. "Case Records of the Massachusetts General Hospital." Case 39–1986. *New England Journal of Medicine* 315, no. 14(1986):874–85.

Selzer, Richard. *Confessions of a Knife*. New York: Simon & Schuster, 1979.

——. *Letters to a Young Doctor*. New York: Simon & Schuster, 1982.

——. *Mortal Lessons*. New York: Simon & Schuster, 1974.

——. *Rituals of Surgery*. New York: Simon & Schuster, 1974.

——. *Taking the World in for Repairs*. New York: William Morrow & Co., 1986.

Severo, Richard. *Lisa H*. New York: Harper & Row, 1985.

Sheehan, John. *The Enchanted Ring*. Cambridge: MIT Press, 1984.

Sherrington, Sir Charles. *The Integrative Action of the Nervous System*. New Haven: Yale University Press, 1947.

Shorter, Edward. *Bedside Manners*. New York: Simon & Schuster, 1985.

Shryock, Richard. *The Development of Modern Medicine*. Madison: University of Wisconsin Press, 1974.

Siegel, Bernie. *Love, Medicine, and Miracles*. New York: Harper & Row, 1986.

Sloper, J., P. Brodal, and T. Powell. "An Anatomical Study of the Effects of Unilateral Removal of Sensorimotor Cortex in Infant Monkeys on the Subcortical Projections of the Contralateral Sensorimotor Cortex." *Brain* 106(1983):707–16.

Smith, C. U. M. *The Brain*. New York: Capricorn Books, 1970.

Spaans, F., et al. "Myotonic Dystrophy Associated with Hereditary Motor and Sensory Neuropathy." *Brain* 109(1986):1149–68.

Swinburne, Algernon Charles. *The Works of Algernon Charles Swinburne*. Philadelphia: David McKay Co., n.d.

Sydenham, Thomas. *The Works of Thomas Sydenham, M.D*. Birmingham, Ala.: The Classics of Medicine Library, 1985.

Szentagothai, J., and M. Arbib. *Conceptual Models of Neural Organization*. Cambridge: MIT Press, 1975.

Thomas, P., et al. "Chronic Demyelinating Peripheral Neuropathy Associated with Multifocal Central Nervous System Demyelination." *Brain* 110(1987):53–76.

Thorowald, Jurgen. *The Century of the Surgeon*. New York: Pantheon, 1957.

Turnbull, Andrew. *Thomas Wolfe*. New York: Scribner & Sons, 1967.

Valenstein, Eliot. *Great and Desperate Cures*. New York: Basic Books, 1986.

Wagensteen, Owen and Sarah. *The Rise of Surgery*. Minneapolis: University of Minnesota Press, 1978.

Wall, Patrick, and Ronald Melzack. *Textbook of Pain*. London: Churchill Livingstone, 1984.

Walser, Richard. *Thomas Wolfe, Undergraduate*. Durham: Duke University Press, 1977.

Weatherall, D., J. Ledingham, and D. Warrell, eds. *Oxford Textbook of Medicine*. Oxford: Oxford University Press, 1984.

Williams, Tennessee. *In the Winter of Cities*. New York: New Directions Press, 1964.

Wolfe, Thomas. *The Autobiography of an American Novelist*. Cambridge: Harvard University Press, 1983.

——. *The Complete Short Stories of Thomas Wolfe*. Ed. Francis Skipp. New York: Charles Scribner & Sons, 1987.

——. *From Death to Morning*. New York: Charles Scribner & Sons, 1935.

——. *The Hills Beyond*. New York: Harper & Row, 1941.

——. *Look Homeward, Angel*. New York: Charles Scribner & Sons, 1929.

———. *The Notebooks of Thomas Wolfe*. Ed. Richard Kennedy and Paschal Reeves. Chapel Hill: University of North Carolina Press, 1970.

———. *Of Time and the River*. New York: Charles Scribner & Sons, 1935.

———. *The Story of a Novel*. New York: Charles Scribner & Sons, 1936.

———. *The Web and the Rock*. New York: Sun Dial Press, 1940.

———. *A Western Journal*. Pittsburgh: University of Pittsburgh Press, 1967.

———. *You Can't Go Home Again*. New York: Harper & Row, 1940.

Wyngaarden, James, and Lloyd Smith, eds. *Cecil's Textbook of Medicine*. 17th edition. Philadelphia: W. B. Saunders Co., 1985.

Young, J. Z. *The Memory System of the Brain*. Oxford: Oxford University Press, 1966.

Zilboorg, Gregory. *A History of Medical Psychology*. New York: W. W. Norton & Co., 1941.